Neuroimaging in Epilepsy: Principles and Practice

Neuroimaging in Epilepsy: Principles and Practice

Edited by

Gregory D. Cascino, M.D.
Chair, Division of Epilepsy, Mayo Clinic and Mayo
Foundation; Professor of Neurology, Mayo Medical School,
Rochester, Minnesota

Clifford R. Jack, Jr., M.D.
Department of Diagnostic Radiology, Mayo Clinic
and Mayo Foundation; Professor of Radiology,
Mayo Medical School, Rochester, Minnesota

With 30 Contributors

Foreword by

Jerome Engel, Jr., M.D., Ph.D.
Professor of Neurology and Anatamoy and Cell Biology,
UCLA School of Medicine, Los Angeles

Butterworth-Heinemann
Boston • Oxford • Johannesburg • Melbourne • New Delhi • Singapore

Butterworth-Heinemann

 A member of the Reed Elsevier group

Every effort has been made to ensure that the drug dosage schedules within this text are accurate and conform to standards accepted at time of publication. However, as treatment recommendations vary in the light of continuing research and clinical experience, the reader is advised to verify drug dosage schedules herein with information found on product information sheets. This is especially true in cases of new or infrequently used drugs.

Recognizing the importance of preserving what has been written, Butterworth-Heinemann prints its books on acid-free paper whenever possible.

Library of Congress Cataloging-in-Publication Data
Neuroimaging in epilepsy : principles and practice / edited by Gregory
     D. Cascino, Clifford R. Jack, Jr. ; with 30 contributors ; foreword
     by Jerome Engel, Jr.
          p.   cm.
     Includes bibliographical references and index.
     ISBN 0-7506-9716-4 (alk. paper)
     1. Epilepsy--Imaging.   2. Magnetoencephalography.   3. Epilepsy-
-Magnetic resonance imaging.   I. Cascino, Gregory.   II. Jack,
Clifford R.
     [DNLM: 1. Epilepsy--diagnosis.   2. Magnetic Resonance Imaging.
3. Tomography, X-Ray Computed.   4. Tomography, Emission-Computed.
5. Epilepsy--surgery.   WL 385 N49338 1996]
RC373.N48   1996
616.8'530754--dc20
DNLM/DLC
for Library of Congress   96-32628
                                                                 CIP

British Library Cataloguing-in-Publication Data
A catalogue record for this book is available from the British Library.

The publisher offers discounts on bulk orders of this book.
For information, please write:

Manager of Special Sales
Butterworth-Heinemann
313 Washington Street
Newton, MA 02158-1626
Tel: 617-928-2500
Fax: 617-928-2620

For information on all B-H medical publications available, contact our World Wide Web home page at http:/www.bh.com/med/

10 9 8 7 6 5 4 3 2 1

Printed in the United States of America

*To Frank W. Sharbrough III, M.D., Professor of Neurology at the Mayo Medical School,
and to our families, Teresa, Matthew, Gregory Joseph, and Mary Cascino,
and Barbara, Madeline, and Alex Jack*

GDC and CRJ, Jr.

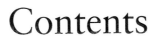

Contents

Contributing Authors

Nayef Al-Rodhan, M.D.
Division of Neurosurgery, Yale University School of Medicine, New Haven, Connecticut

Samuel F. Berkovic, M.D., F.R.A.C.P.
Department of Nuclear Medicine, Austin Hospital, Melbourne, Australia

Richard A. Bronen, M.D.
Associate Professor of Diagnostic Radiology and Surgery (Neurosurgery), Department of Diagnostic Imaging, Yale University School of Medicine, New Haven, Connecticut

Gregory D. Cascino, M.D.
Chair, Division of Epilepsy, Mayo Clinic and Mayo Foundation; Professor of Neurology, Mayo Medical School, Rochester, Minnesota

Sylvester Chuang, M.D.
Department of Pediatrics, Hospital for Sick Children, Toronto, Canada

Alan Connelly, Ph.D.
Institute of Child Health and Great Ormond Street Hospital for Children, London, UK

Jerome Engel, Jr., M.D., Ph.D.
Professor of Neurology and Anatomy and Cell Biology, UCLA School of Medicine, Los Angeles

Joel P. Felmlee, Ph.D.
Department of Diagnostic Radiology, Mayo Clinic and Mayo Foundation; Assistant Professor of Radiation Physics, Mayo Medical School, Rochester, Minnesota

David R. Fish, M.D.
Institute of Neurology, National Hospital for Neurology and Neurosurgery, Queen Square, London, UK

Richard J. Friedland, M.D.
Instructor of Diagnostic Radiology, Department of
Diagnostic Imaging, Yale University School of
Medicine, New Haven, Connecticut

Andrea Halliday, M.D.
Division of Neurosurgery, University of New Mexico,
Albuquerque

Paul Hwang, M.D.
Department of Pediatrics, Hospital for Sick Children,
Toronto, Canada

Clifford R. Jack, Jr., M.D.
Department of Diagnostic Radiology, Mayo Clinic and
Mayo Foundation; Professor of Radiology, Mayo
Medical School, Rochester, Minnesota

Graeme D. Jackson, B.Sc. (Hons.), M.D., F.R.A.C.P.
Senior Lecturer in Paediatric Neurology, Institute of
Child Health, University of London, London, UK;
Senior Lecturer in Neurology, University of Melbourne,
Melbourne, Australia; and MR Neurosciences Unit,
Department of Neurology, Austin Hospital,
Heidelberg, Victoria, Australia

Neil D. Kitchen, F.R.C.S.
Institute of Neurology, National Hospital for Neurology
and Neurosurgery, Queen Square, London, UK

Ruben I. Kuzniecky, M.D.
UAB Epilepsy Center, Department of Neurology,
University of Alabama at Birmingham

Kenneth D. Laxer, M.D.
Department of Neurology, University of California,
San Francisco

Christine C. Lee, M.Sc.
Predoctoral Student in Biophysical Sciences, Mayo
Graduate School of Medicine, Rochester, Minnesota

Louis Lemieux, Ph.D.
Institute of Neurology, National Hospital for Neurology
and Neurosurgery, Queen Square, London, UK

Jeffrey David Lewine, Ph.D.
Magnetic Source Imaging Facility, Departments of
Radiology and Psychology, Veterans Affairs Medical
Center and University of New Mexico, Albuquerque

Frank Morrell, M.D.
Department of Neurology, Rush-Presbyterian St. Luke's
Medical Center, Chicago, Illinois

Mark R. Newton, M.D., F.R.A.C.P.
Department of Neurology, Austin Hospital,
Melbourne, Australia

William W. Orrison, Jr., M.D.
Magnetic Source Imaging Facility, Departments of
Radiology and Neurology, Veterans Affairs Medical
Center and University of New Mexico, Albuquerque

Stephen J. Riederer, Ph.D.
Consultant, Department of Diagnostic Radiology,
Mayo Clinic and Mayo Foundation; Professor of
Radiology, Mayo Medical School, Rochester,
Minnesota

John A. Sanders, Ph.D.
Department of Radiology, Veterans Affairs Medical
Center and University of New Mexico, Albuquerque

Cheolsu Shin, M.D.
Consultant, Department of Neurology, Mayo Clinic
and Mayo Foundation, Rochester, Minnesota

Dennis D. Spencer, M.D.
Division of Neurosurgery, Yale University School of
Medicine, New Haven, Connecticut

Susan S. Spencer, M.D.
Department of Neurology, Yale University School of
Medicine, New Haven, Connecticut

William H. Theodore, M.D.
Chief, Clinical Epilepsy Section, National Institute of
Neurological Disorders and Stroke, National Institutes
of Health, Bethesda, Maryland

Max R. Trenerry, Ph.D.
Consultant, Division of Psychology, Mayo Clinic and
Mayo Foundation; Assistant Professor of Psychology,
Mayo Medical School, Rochester, Minnesota

Kenneth P. Vives, M.D.
Division of Neurosurgery, Yale University School of
Medicine, New Haven, Connecticut

Elaine Wyllie, M.D.
Head, Pediatric Epilepsy Program, Cleveland Clinic
Children's Hospital, Cleveland, Ohio

Foreword

The obligatory introductory statement for every lecture on epilepsy to medical students—that this condition is a symptom and not a disease—remains a seminal concept of epileptology. Although epileptic seizures are transient functional events that can arise suddenly with little or no warning and disappear without a trace, they reflect a variety of enduring underlying pathophysiologic disturbances that often, but not always, are associated with structural lesions. Until recently, however, this fact was taken on faith for most patients, because such lesions usually escaped detection by imaging techniques that depended on vague shadows and that required invasive procedures for higher resolution. Furthermore, the suspicion that some epileptic disorders might be associated with enduring *functional* disruption could only be demonstrated when primary cortical areas were involved, permitting measurement by neurologic examination and neuropsychologic testing. Only electroencephalography (EEG) provided a more generalized assessment of epileptiform and nonepileptiform abnormalities. In the 1930s and 1940s, EEG data demonstrated differences between generalized convulsive, absence, and partial ictal events—distinctions that are still fundamental to modern classifications of seizures and epilepsy. However, spatial resolution of EEG signals is poor, and propagated transients are occasionally misleading, even when intracranial recording techniques are used.

A diagnostic revolution in neurology began about 20 years ago with the advent of noninvasive computerized neuroimaging methodologies capable of creating three-dimensional displays of the entire brain. This book documents the impact of modern neuroimaging on the field of epileptology and defines the current state of the art. X-ray computed tomography initially provided an unequaled opportunity to visualize small epileptogenic lesions. The yield of positive scans has not only increased

further with high-resolution magnetic resonance imaging (MRI), but important subtle pathologic changes such as atrophy, particularly of the hippocampus, and migration defects, such as focal cortical dysplasia, can now be identified with a high degree of confidence. Positron emission tomography, single-photon emission computed tomography, magnetic resonance spectroscopy, and functional MRI produce images of cerebral activity that can (or, in the case of *f*MRI, are expected to in the future) delineate the anatomical substrates of ictal and postictal disturbances and define the location, extent, and time course of persistent interictal dysfunction. Furthermore, these techniques can be used to measure specific fundamental neuronal processes such as glucose and oxygen metabolism, neurotransmitter synthesis and binding, and even antiepileptic drug pharmacokinetics in discrete areas of the human brain. Coincident with developments in neuroimaging, computer-enhanced approaches to source localization of electromagnetic signals recorded by EEG and magnetoencephalography have greatly enhanced noninvasive three-dimensional mapping of epileptiform and nonepileptiform events, which can be accurately superimposed on MRI and precisely correlated with other changes detected by functional imaging. MRI coregistration of these electrophysiologic observations and data derived from the most recent methods of *f*MRI add high temporal resolution to the spatially detailed structural and functional cerebral maps, promising unparalleled noninvasive views of neuronal substrates of human epilepsy and its consequences.

The first, and still most important, application of these revolutionary neurodiagnostic techniques to the field of epilepsy was in the arena of surgical treatment. More accurate information on the localization and extent of an epileptogenic region and adjacent essential cortical areas has resulted in an explosion of interest in surgical therapy and has greatly improved efficacy and safety of ablative procedures. Neuroimaging is also important in the diagnosis of underlying treatable causes of epilepsy and in the distinction between epilepsy and other intermittent disorders for medical and psychosocial management. It is anticipated that neuroimaging ultimately will contribute greatly to understanding basic mechanisms of the various forms of epilepsy, permitting a clinical classification that is based on anatomy and pathophysiology rather than on phenomenology. Such advances are essential to the development of more rational treatments for seizures as well as for cure and prevention of some epileptic disorders.

Neuroimaging technologies and applications to epileptology are changing rapidly, and the future appears to be limited only by the imagination of workers in the field and, unfortunately, the availability of resources for health care and research. All clinical and basic neuroscientists interested in epilepsy will need to be familiar with the current practice of neuroimaging to be prepared for what is yet to come. This is a timely volume designed to keep its readers "in the picture."

Jerome Engel, Jr.

Preface

Neuroimaging in Epilepsy reflects developments during the last two decades in the use of neuroimaging techniques to evaluate patients with seizure disorders. Arguably, the advances in imaging have equaled or surpassed any other accomplishment in epileptology during this time. The rationale for the present work is to review current information on imaging modalities in epilepsy and to discuss clinical and research applications. The organization of the textbook is somewhat unique in that the first half is devoted mainly to the specific neuroimaging techniques and the second half is concerned with the role of imaging in patient care.

Contemporary neuroimaging began with the introduction of x-ray computed tomography (CT) in the 1970s. The role of CT in evaluating patients with seizure disorders diminished markedly with the emergence of magnetic resonance imaging (MRI) nearly a decade later. The consensus is that, in patients with partial epilepsy, MRI is essential to identify the underlying epileptogenic lesion, to determine the likely site of seizure onset, and to select appropriate candidates for epilepsy surgery. Functional neuroimaging procedures—that is, single photon emission computed tomography and positron emission tomography—have proved to be sensitive indicators of cerebral perfusion and metabolism. The early promise of functional MRI is just now coming to fruition clinically. These newer techniques may alter the surgical evaluation of patients with intractable partial epilepsy. These techniques are also important investigative tools.

This work would not be possible without the efforts of our distinguished contributors. We appreciate their interest and required dedication, which have allowed this textbook to be completed in a timely manner. We would especially like to thank Dr. O. Eugene Millhouse and Roberta Schwartz, Barbara Golenzer, Dorothy Tienter, and Jen Schlotthauer from the Mayo Section of Publications who provided expert editorial assistance. We also are very grateful to our secretaries Brenda Maxwell, Karen Reinschmidt, and Elsie Sheely. Special thanks to our Mayo surgical epilepsy program colleagues who provided encouragement and shared their knowledge: Drs. Jeffrey Britton, Terrence Lagerlund, Frank Sharbrough, Cheolsu Shin, Elson So, and Mary Zupanc from the Department of Neurology; Drs. W. Richard Marsh, Frederic Meyer, and Corey Raffel from the Department of Neurologic Surgery; Dr. Max Trenerry from the Department of Psychiatry and Psychology; Drs. Glenn Forbes, Christine Lee, and Stephen Riederer from the Department of Diagnostic Radiology; and Susan Hausman and Rebecca Luckstein from the Department of Neurology. Finally, thank you to our patients with epilepsy. They are our best teachers, without whom this textbook would not have been possible.

GDC and CRJ, Jr

CHAPTER 1

Magnetic Resonance Imaging Principles

Joel P. Felmlee

The purpose of this chapter is to provide a working knowledge of the basic principles of magnetic resonance (MR) image acquisition without emphasizing the mathematics. It is intended to make the subsequent chapters on MR imaging (MRI) and spectroscopy more accessible to the reader. The following topics are considered in the chapter: MR scanner hardware, MR signal origin, radiofrequency (RF) pulses, relaxation, biologic properties of MR, spin and gradient echo acquisitions, creating the MR image, and factors affecting the image (contrast and signal-to-noise ratio). Sections on Safety in MRI and Acronyms Common to MRI are given in the Appendices.

HARDWARE

The hardware involved in producing MR images can be divided into three main categories: the magnet itself, front-end electronics, and computer (or computers).

The MR magnet consists of a long (miles) titanium alloy wire wound around a cylinder that is large enough to surround a person. The interior of the cylinder is called the "magnet bore." By being enclosed in a dewar that contains liquid helium, the titanium alloy wire is supercooled. At near absolute zero temperatures, the titanium alloy becomes superconducting; that is, resistance to the flow of electric current decreases to essentially zero. This allows the unimpeded flow of a large electric current indefinitely. Because movement of an electric charge produces a magnetic field, the case of a cylindrically wound wire produces a magnetic field directed along the long axis, or bore, of the magnet. The static magnetic field is commonly referred to as the "Bo" or "main magnetic field." The larger the current, the larger the Bo field. Field strengths common in diagnostic imaging range from 0.06 T to 2.00 T. Smaller bore magnets at higher field strength are commonly used for experimental purposes, particularly for spectroscopy. A few medical centers now have whole-body imagers with magnetic fields of 3.0 or 4.0 T. These are used predominantly for in vivo spectroscopic and functional MRI studies. The three key criteria that characterize the performance of a magnet are bore size, field strength, and field homogeneity. At higher Bo field strengths, the images produced have a greater signal-to-noise ratio, the T_1 relaxation time is increased, and the cost and complexity are increased. It is desirable to have a highly uniform magnetic field across the bore of the magnet; this is termed "homogeneity." Shimming is a process whereby standing inhomogeneities in the Bo field across the bore of the magnet are minimized. Shimming can be performed either passively (by strategic placement of steel plates outside the magnet bore) or actively (by the application of current through shim or gradient coils during the process of imaging).

The next major hardware component is the front-end electronics—gradient coils, RF coils, and their associated amplifiers. RF energy must be applied to the patient to create an MR image. This is accomplished with a transmit RF coil. Typically, the transmit coil is large and located just inside the Bo coil windings. A receiver coil is used to receive a signal from the patient. For imaging the head, a coil that fits closely around the patient's head is used.

The other coil type is the gradient coils. Three pairs of gradient coils are oriented orthogonally to the long axis of the magnet. When current is applied to the gradient coils, a small magnetic field gradient is introduced across the bore of the magnet. By activating two or three of the gradient coil pairs simultaneously, a small linear magnetic field gradient can be produced that is oriented along any oblique axis as the vector sum of the orthogonal gradients.

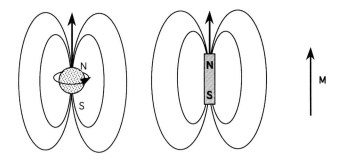

FIGURE 1-1. The spinning nuclear charge induces a net magnetic moment that acts like a small magnet. The net magnetic moment is often represented by a vector (*M*). (*N*), north; (*S*), south.

MAGNETIC RESONANCE SIGNAL ORIGIN

What Is Actually Measured?

The MR signal arises from the nucleus of the atom. All nuclei possess a property called "spin angular momentum." The following sections contain an intuitive view of nuclear spin and how it is affected by the magnetic fields.

Figure 1-1 shows how a spinning nucleus is similar to a bar magnet. The spinning, charged nucleus represents an electrical current (a charge in motion). This current sets up a magnetic field, or magnetic moment. This magnetic field acts similarly to that of a bar magnet.

The strength of the magnetic moment depends on the type of nucleus, and it determines the detection sensitivity. Sensitivity information for several nuclei of interest are given in Table 1-1. Of the nuclei shown in Table 1-1, protons (^{1}H) are used most commonly for imaging because of their high abundance and high sensitivity.

The signal in MRI is different from that of other imaging modalities, such as computed tomography, radiography, or nuclear medicine. The MR signal is caused by changes in the magnetization of the patient's body.

TABLE 1-1. Important Properties of Nuclei

Nucleus	Natural abundance, %	Gyromagnetic ratio, Hz/g	Relative sensitivity
^{1}H	99.98	4,257	1
^{2}H	0.02	653	0.000002
^{13}C	1.1	1,071	0.0002
^{19}F	100	4,005	0.83
^{23}Na	100	1,124	0.092

Data from Shaw D. Fourier transform N.M.R. spectroscopy. 2nd ed. Amsterdam: Elsevier, 1984.

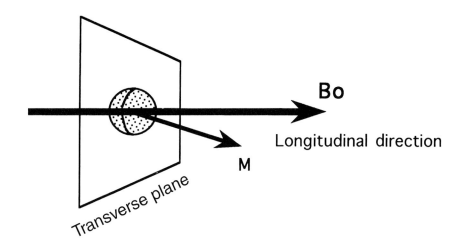

FIGURE 1-2. The magnetization (*M*) is said to point in the longitudinal direction when it points along the static magnetic field (*Bo*). The transverse plane is perpendicular to the longitudinal direction.

Recall that a magnet moving near a coil of wire causes an electric current to flow in the coil. This is the principle by which we measure the MRI signal.

Because the spin properties of the nucleus cause it to act as a small magnet, it aligns with a strong external magnetic field, just as the needle of a compass does. Figure 1-2 represents a single atom in the patient's body. The nucleus of this atom has an inherent spin quantum number and a gyromagnetic ratio and, hence, a magnetic moment. This magnetic moment means that the nucleus is affected by magnetic fields and is itself a magnet. The patient is made up of a large number of these nuclei. The vector sum of the many magnetic dipoles in the body is the net magnetization, which determines the signal used to form the image.

The Role of the External Magnetic Field (Bo)

In a person's body all the magnetic dipoles are arranged randomly (Figure 1-3). That is, the dipoles point in random directions, and a net magnetization cannot be measured. However, a strong magnetic field, Bo, tends to force these dipoles to line up along its direction, creating a net magnetization along the Bo direction in the person's body. Just as a compass needle points north in the earth's magnetic field, the magnetic dipoles point along Bo inside the magnet of an MRI scanner. To gain perspective, a 1.5-T magnet is about 30,000 times stronger than the earth's magnetic field. In fact, some of the dipoles end up pointing exactly opposite to the magnetic field. Although it is possible for a compass needle to point exactly opposite the main external field, it is a far less stable arrangement.

A large number of these dipoles occur in a patient's body, and because of the body's temperature, only slightly more dipoles line up with the field than line up against the field. Thermodynamically, this creates two distinct energy states, with the less stable conformation corresponding to the higher energy state. It is the net difference between the two energy states that gives the body a measurable magnetization and causes the MR signal.

FIGURE 1-3. A. Randomly distributed dipole moments with a net magnetization equal to zero. B. Dipole alignment in the presence of a strong external magnetic field (*Bo*).

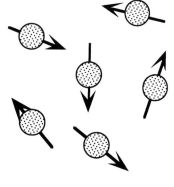

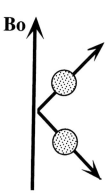

A   **B**

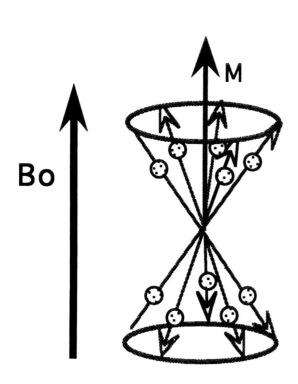

FIGURE 1-4. The net magnetic moment (M) results from the sum of a group of parallel and antiparallel spin magnetic moments.

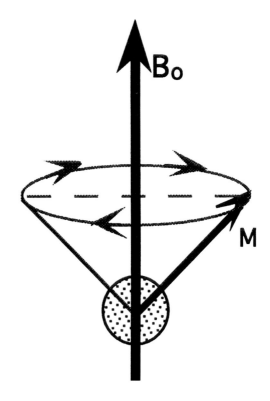

FIGURE 1-5. The nuclear magnetic moment (M) precesses about the external magnetic field (Bo) at the frequency given by the Larmor equation. The frequency of precession for a magnetic dipole is directly proportional to the strength of the external magnetic field and the gyromagnetic ratio of the nucleus ($f = \gamma$ Bo).

The net magnetic moment, or magnetization, of a given volume represents the vector sum of its individual spin magnetic moments, as shown in Figure 1-4.

How Does the Magnetization Precess?

In the classic model, shown in Figure 1-5, the individual nuclei precess about the surface of the cone. This precession frequency is given by the Larmor equation:

$$f = \gamma \, \text{Bo}$$

where f is the precessional frequency (Hz), Bo is the main magnetic field strength (G), and γ is the gyromagnetic ratio (Hz/G). For protons, $\gamma = 4{,}257$ Hz/G.

This Larmor precession is quite fast. For example, hydrogen nuclei in a 1.5-T field complete about 64 million rotations per second (that is, the resonant frequency for protons is 63.86 MHz at 1.5 T). Recall that for a given nucleus, increasing the magnetic field strength (B) causes the frequency of precession to increase. This forms the basis for MRI and can be stated as "resonant frequency is proportional to the magnetic field strength":

$$f \propto B$$

The Larmor, or resonant, frequency also depends on the inherent gyromagnetic ratio of a given nucleus; that is, resonant frequency is proportional to the gyromagnetic ratio:

$$f \propto \gamma$$

This means that different magnetic nuclei precess at different frequencies in the same magnetic field. For example, in a 1-T field, protons precess at 42.57 MHz and sodium nuclei precess at 11.26 MHz.

How Do Precessing Magnetic Moments Produce a Signal?

The actual signal arises from the rotating magnetic moments in the patient's body that induce electrical current in receiver coils placed near the patient. With the patient in the magnet of the MRI scanner, the patient's magnetic moments align with the main magnetic field Bo. RF pulses are applied to rotate the magnetization in the patient's body by 90° (Figure 1-6 A).

This RF "nutation" puts the magnetization into the transverse plane, where it precesses as it recovers to the

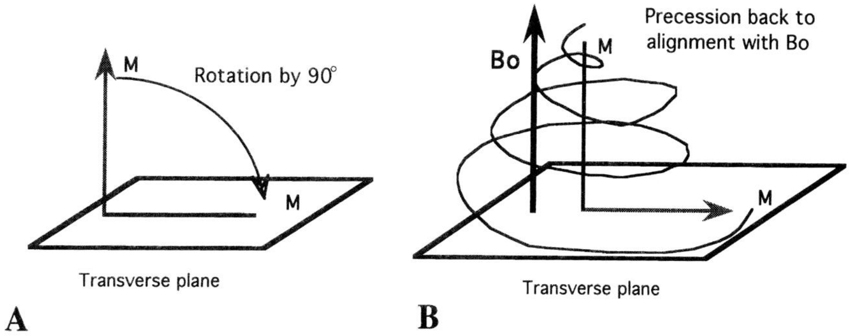

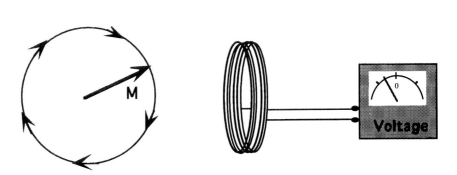

FIGURE 1-6. A. The magnetization (*M*) rotates 90° into the transverse plane, and B, precesses as it realigns with the main magnetic field (*Bo*).

FIGURE 1-7. A precessing magnet, shown by *M*, produces a voltage in a coil of wire.

longitudinal orientation (along the direction of Bo) (Figure 1-6 B). This precession causes electrical current to flow in strategically placed receiver coils (Figure 1-7). The net magnetization (precessing at the Larmor frequency $f = \gamma$ Bo) causes a changing magnetic field at the receiver coil, inducing a current in the receiver coil. This induced current is the MR signal. This signal is analyzed to get information about the patient's body and to create the final image.

Note that electrical current is induced in the receiver coil by the changing RF field (arising from magnetization precessing in the transverse plane) returning from the patient. Neither the longitudinal magnetization M (because of its orientation) nor the static magnetic field Bo (because it is static) will induce a signal in the receiver coil. Because the signals are small and in a specific frequency range, the receiver coils are specially tuned for the resonance frequency of each scanner. This is one reason why a receiver coil designed for a 0.5-T system does not work well (if at all) on a 1.5-T system.

RADIOFREQUENCY PULSES

What Is a Radiofrequency Pulse?

An RF pulse is used to rotate the magnetization into the transverse plane (Figure 1-8). To do this, a short duration of electromagnetic radiation is applied in the RF region, where the frequency of the RF is specifically set at the Larmor frequency ($f = \gamma$ Bo). In one sense, the RF coils in an MRI scanner are similar to a CB radio in which the antenna has been modified to accommodate a patient. The RF waves are the same as those used in a CB or, for that matter, in broadcast AM or FM radio, or television signals. The RF wave is an electromagnetic wave, which means that it consists of oscillating electric and magnetic fields oriented perpendicularly to each other. The frequency determines how it is classified: light, x-rays, and microwaves are examples of electromagnetic radiation of different frequencies.

How Are Radiofrequency Pulses Used to Change the Magnetization?

As shown in Figure 1-8, as the magnetization rotates away from the longitudinal direction, it precesses at the Larmor frequency. If a magnetic field is used to rotate the magnetization, the field must rotate with the precessing dipoles. This is where the idea of resonance is important: To be effective, the excitation frequency must be synchronized with the proton precession frequency given by the Larmor equation.

Imagine yourself rotating with a magnetic dipole at its precession frequency, which is analogous to standing on a merry-go-round platform. In this rotating frame of reference, the merry-go-round figures appear stationary. Analogously, a magnetic field perpendicular to the external field in the rotating frame causes the dipole to precess downward (as shown in Figures 1-8 and 1-9). In this example, the dipole rotates until it is perpendicular to the external field, and then the excitatory magnetic field is removed (Figure 1-9 A). If you had not been rotating

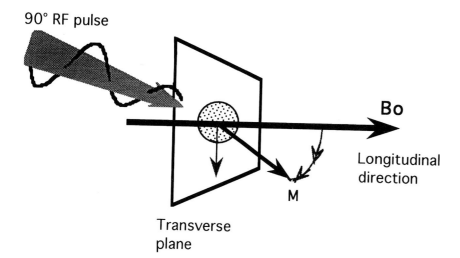

FIGURE 1-8. The RF pulse rotates the nuclear magnetization (*M*) away from alignment with Bo into the transverse plane.

with the precessing dipole, you would have seen a magnetic field oscillating at the Larmor frequency and a precessing dipole spiraling toward the transverse plane (Figure 1-9 B).

Radiofrequency Excitation

The previous section describes what is commonly referred to as the "RF excitation pulse." The 90° RF pulse is an excitation because it causes the magnetization to change to a less stable, or higher, energy state. It is a 90° pulse because the duration and amplitude of the RF pulse rotates the magnetization 90° into the transverse plane. Immediately after excitation, the magnetization in the transverse plane precesses at the Larmor frequency,

and the free induction decay signal in the receiver coils can be measured. Another commonly used RF pulse is the 180° pulse, in which the duration and amplitude of the pulse are adjusted to rotate the magnetization 180° (Figure 1-10).

RELAXATION

Relaxation is the process by which the system of spins reaches thermal equilibrium in the external magnetic field. The two types of relaxation are longitudinal and transverse. Longitudinal relaxation occurs when the magnetic magnetization aligns with or against Bo. When perturbed from this alignment, the magnetization "recovers" or realigns with Bo, and the rate of this "recovery" is identified by a time

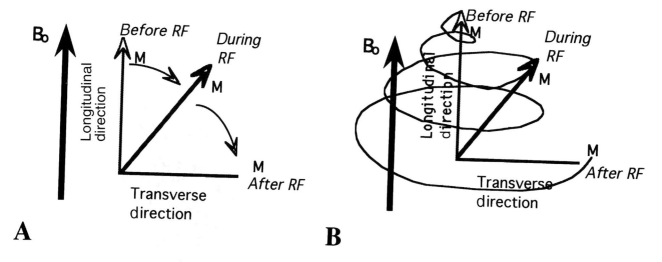

FIGURE 1-9. The effects of the 90° RF pulse, A, as seen by a rotating observer, and B, as seen by a stationary observer. *Bo*, external magnetic field; *M*, net magnetization.

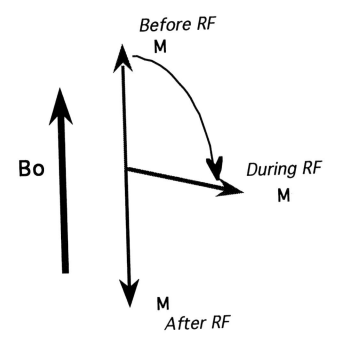

FIGURE 1-10. The 180° RF pulse produces a 180° nutation. *Bo*, external magnetic field; *M*, net magnetization.

constant T_1. Transverse relaxation occurs when components of the magnetization in the transverse plane dephase, or lose coherence. The rate of signal loss due to this dephasing is identified by a time constant T_2. Transverse relaxation causes the net magnetization to decrease, whereas longitudinal relaxation causes the net magnetization to increase. These T_1 and T_2 relaxation times are different for different tissues. The graphs in Figure 1-11 result from longitudinal (T_1) and transverse (T_2) relaxation.

Longitudinal Relaxation (T_1)

As shown in Figure 1-11, longitudinal relaxation is an exponentially increasing, or "recovering," magnetization in the direction of Bo. This recovery represents an energy exchange with the environment and is also referred to as "spin-lattice relaxation." Longitudinal relaxation is described by a time constant T_1, which is defined as the time at which 64% of the final equilibrium magnetization has recovered.

When aligned with Bo, the longitudinal magnetization represents the maximal possible signal available for each tissue and is dependent on the repetition time TR. Figure 1-12 shows how a magnetic moment relaxes or recovers after excitation by an RF pulse. The rate of this recovery is characterized by T_1.

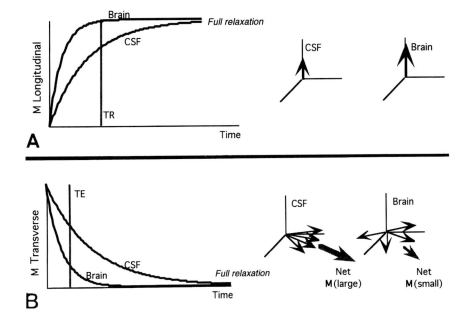

FIGURE 1-11. T_1 and T_2 relaxation diagrams showing that the rate of realignment with Bo (T_1) and the rate of dephasing (T_2) are different for different components of the body. A. At a given time, TR, the contrast between tissues in a T_1-weighted image is due to differences in how fast the longitudinal magnetization recovers toward Bo. The cerebrospinal fluid (*CSF*) has a longer T_1 relaxation time, and at the TR shown, the longitudinal magnetization is less than that of the brain. B. At a given time, TE, the contrast between tissues is due to differences in how fast the transverse signal dephases. The CSF has a longer T_2 relaxation time, and at the TE shown, the spins point in the same general direction, resulting in a large net magnetization (*M*). Brain tissue has almost completely dephased at time TE, and its spins point in different directions, resulting in a small net magnetization.

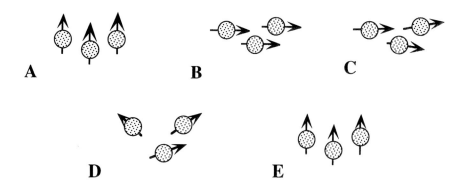

FIGURE 1-12. The T_1 relaxation cycle. A. Dipoles aligned with Bo. B. After 90° nutation. C. After a short period of time. D. After a longer period of time. E. After full relaxation.

Tissues with a short T_1 have a longitudinal magnetization that quickly realigns with Bo after excitation. Tissues with a long T_1 require a longer time for the longitudinal magnetization to realign. By re-exciting with an RF pulse before the longitudinal relaxation is complete, we can cause tissues with different T_1 values to have different intensity within the image. Ranking relevant tissue T_1 from long to short:

cerebrospinal fluid > edematous/gliotic brain lesions > gray matter > white matter > fat.

Transverse Relaxation (T_2)

Transverse relaxation is also known as "spin-spin relaxation," because this process depends on the interaction between neighboring magnetic dipoles. This effect is observed as the exponential decrease of the transverse component of the magnetization. The speed of this relaxation process is characterized by a time constant T_2, which is the time it takes for the transverse magnetization to decay to 36% of its original magnitude. In this way, the T_2 signal decay constant is similar to the decay constant of a radioisotope. On a microscopic level, the magnetic fields set up by neighboring dipoles tend randomly to add to or to subtract from the external field, causing the dipoles to precess at slightly different frequencies and, thus, to spin out of phase with each other, or dephase. In addition, dipoles are constantly tumbling around and flipping back and forth between orientations because of thermal motion, so that

the dipole magnetic field effect on any given spin (proton) is completely random.

As shown in Figure 1-13, T_2 represents a rate of signal loss. A short T_2 indicates that the signal is lost quickly, and a long T_2 indicates that it is lost slowly. The MR data acquisition technique acquires image data at discrete echo times (TE). The amount of signal lost at TE reflects the relative tissue T_2 values. Long TE values allow more T_2 relaxation to occur and influence the image contrast. The ranking of relevant tissue T_2 is:

cerebrospinal fluid > edematous/gliotic brain lesions > gray matter > white matter > fat.

To summarize tissue relaxation:

1. T_1 and T_2 represent relaxation, that is, the rate of magnetization realignment along the Bo axis (T_1) and the rate of magnetization dephasing (T_2).
2. T_1 and T_2 are properties of tissue.
3. TR and TE are times set by the image acquisition.
4. The TR and TE used to acquire the signal affect the amount of T_1 or T_2 influence on the final image contrast.

Factors Influencing Relaxation

MR images are often referred to as "weighted" by T_1, T_2, or proton density. This weighting means that the con-

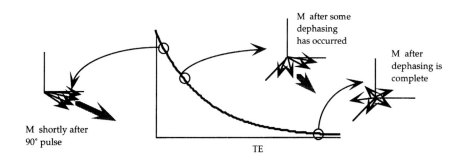

M after some dephasing has occurred

M after dephasing is complete

M shortly after 90° pulse

TE

FIGURE 1-13. T_2 decay is shown as continued dephasing of the magnetization vectors (*arrows*). This dephasing causes the magnetization vectors to cancel, resulting in decreased net magnetization (*M*) (that is, signal loss) with long TE.

TABLE 1-2. Spin Echo Image Contrast-Weighting and Imaging Variables

Image contrast-weighting	TR	TE	Example variables TR/TE (ms)
T_1-weighted	Short	Short	500/20
Proton density	Long	Short	2,000/20
T_2-weighted	Long	Long	2,000/80

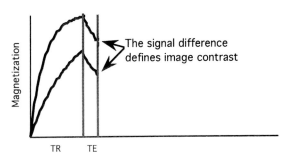

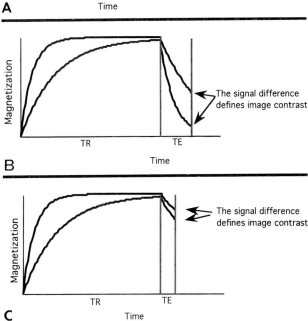

trast in the image is mainly affected by T_1, T_2, or proton density. For spin echo images, this weighting is controlled by the acquisition variables TR and TE. For gradient echo images, the contrast weighting is controlled by the TR, the TE, and the nutation angle α. Tables 1-2 and 1-3 are general summaries of image contrast-weighting for spin and gradient echoes, respectively.

Figure 1-14 gives an intuitive feel for spin echo image contrast. The acquisition TR and TE control the amount of influence T_1 or T_2 relaxation has on the final image contrast. For example, a long TR allows all longitudinal magnetization to recover and does not allow differences in T_1 to contribute to the image contrast. A long TE allows significant dephasing of transverse magnetization to occur; therefore, only tissues with long T_2 values will have signal. The signal differences (that result in image contrast) for a long TR and long TE acquisition are influenced mainly by tissue T_2. Similarly, the signal differences for a short TR and short TE acquisition are influenced mainly by tissue T_1.

The effect of imaging variables on image contrast changes when gradient echoes are acquired, as shown in Table 1-3. Gradient echo acquisitions typically use nutation angles less than 90°, which retains a large portion of the longitudinal magnetization while creating transverse magnetization using very short TE and TR times.

BIOLOGIC MAGNETIC RESONANCE PROPERTIES

Relaxation Times and Proton Density in Different Tissues

T_1 and T_2 relaxation times as well as proton density vary among different tissues and different types of lesions. These differences form the basis for contrast in the

FIGURE 1-14. Imaging variables TR and TE affect spin echo image contrast. A. A T_1-weighted image has a short TR and a short TE. The image contrast reflects how quickly the longitudinal magnetization recovers. Here, most of the signal difference is due to T_1 relaxation, and the image contrast is T_1-weighted. B. A T_2-weighted image has a long TR and a long TE. The image contrast reflects how quickly the transverse signal dephases. Here, the long TE allows T_2 relaxation to produce the signal differences, and the image contrast is T_2-weighted. C. A proton density image has a long TR and a short TE. Here, image contrast reflects the proton content of the tissue because the long TR and short TE do not allow significant T_1 or T_2 influence and the image contrast is proton density-weighted.

TABLE 1-3. Gradient Echo Image Contrast-Weighting and Imaging Variables

Image contrast-weighting	TR	TE	Nutation angle α	Example TR/TE/α (ms)
T_1-weighted	Long	Short	High	300/12/45°–90°
Proton density	Long	Short	Low	300/12/5°–20°
T_2^*-weighted	Short or long	Short or long	Medium or low	35/12/30°–60° or 300/30+/5°–20°

Note that "long" and "short" TR and TE values refer to different time ranges for gradient echo acquisitions in comparison with spin echo acquisitions.

Table 1-4. Comparison of Relaxation Times for Some Human Tissue

Tissue type	T_1, ms*	T_2, ms*
Fat	180	90
Muscle	600	40
Cerebrospinal fluid	2,000	300
Gray matter	520	100
White matter	380	90

*The data represent relaxation measurements collected at 100 MHz.

acquired image. Some values for water content and relaxation times in different tissues are shown in Table 1-4.

Proton Resonance

Clinical MRI is based on proton resonance. Much of the human body is made up of water, but fats, carbohydrates, and amino acids also contain hydrogen. The following sections describe the role that the chemical environment has in affecting the resonance frequency or relaxation characteristics of protons.

From the Larmor equation, it is known that water protons resonate at 4,257 Hz/G (63.86 MHz at 1.5 T). Water is present in all tissues throughout the body; yet, the relaxation characteristics of tissues differ. These relaxation differences are determined by the exchange mechanism described in the following sections.

Magnetization, or spins, in a rigid environment (for example, water bound to the surface of a protein) decay much more quickly. A molecule in a rigid environment is not free to diffuse through various regions and only experiences the magnetic field at a given location. Therefore, the spins in the molecule experience only the magnetic field inhomogeneities at that location, and dephasing occurs rapidly. In addition, a rigid environment allows spins in a molecule to align quickly with the main field, without the need for constant realignment.

Water in biologic tissues is in equilibrium between free and bound states (Figure 1-15) and that equilibri-

um is determined by the chemical composition of the tissue. The relaxation times of a given tissue reflect the relative proportions of bound and free water in the tissue. For example, white matter tends to have relatively fast relaxation times. The myelin basic protein in white matter binds water, and most of the water in this tissue is not free to diffuse randomly, resulting in relatively short T_1 and T_2 relaxation times. In contrast, most spins in the CSF are not bound; they diffuse and tumble freely, and CSF has long T_1 and T_2 relaxation times.

SPIN ECHO AND GRADIENT ECHO ACQUISITIONS

There are inherent differences between spin echo and gradient echo images. The mechanics of setting up the "echo" can markedly change image contrast, artifacts, and sensitivity to flow phenomena. The following sections describe how spin echo and gradient echo data are acquired.

Spin Echoes

Spin echo acquisitions use a 180° RF pulse to refocus the echo at time TE. As shown in Figure 1-16, the magnetization is placed in the transverse plane by the 90° pulse and followed by a 180° pulse at time TE/2. Once in the transverse plane, the magnetization vectors dephase somewhat during this time (TE/2), because the local magnetic environment causes some vectors to precess at a faster or slower rate. This dephasing causes a signal loss, but much of the signal can be recovered by the 180° RF pulse. The 180° pulse flips the magnetization vectors so that the fast and slow magnetization vectors exchange positions (Figure 1-16). Because the vectors are precessing in the same direction after the 180° RF as before, the fast vectors "catch up" with the slow at TE/2 after the 180° pulse (total echo time TE). The 90° and 180° RF pulses set up the magnetization to be in phase, or aligned, at time TE, resulting in maximal echo signal. The RF excitation represents only part of the story; the gradients must also be manipulated to allow the echo to form at time TE.

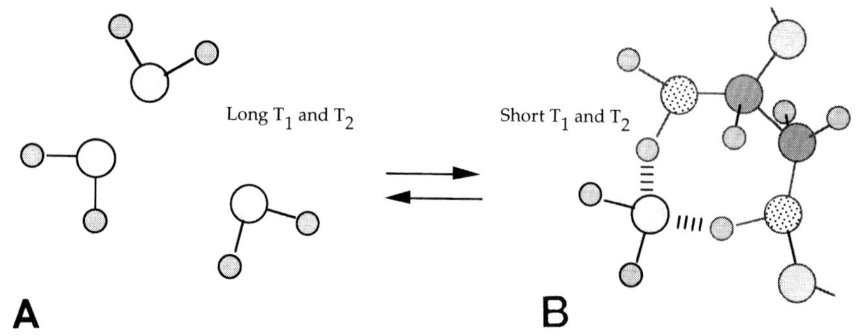

Figure 1-15. A. The protons in free, tumbling water molecules have longer T_1 and T_2 relaxation times than do (B) protons in water molecules bound to a protein. Water is in equilibrium between free and bound states, and this equilibrium determines the relaxation times of a given tissue.

Long T_1 and T_2

Short T_1 and T_2

A

B

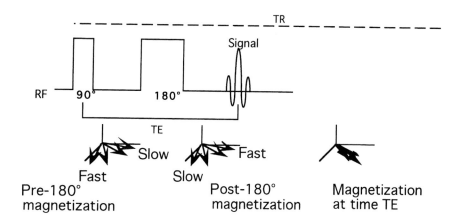

FIGURE 1-16. RF and signal diagram for a basic spin echo pulse sequence. The 90° and 180° RF pulses refocus the magnetization so that the magnetization vectors are in phase, or aligned, at time TE.

The fact that both the RF and the gradients are manipulated to allow the magnetization vector alignment at the echo time TE is an important feature that distinguishes spin echo and gradient echo acquisitions. This alignment causes spin echo acquisitions to be less sensitive to magnetic field inhomogeneity.

Multiple spin echoes can be formed, as shown in Figure 1-17. By acquiring multiple echoes at one location using progressively longer TE values, the image contrast is altered to include increased T_2 weighting. Again, the gradients must also be manipulated to allow the echo to form at each TE time.

To summarize spin echo acquisitions:

1. Spin echoes use 90° and 180° RF pulses to refocus the magnetization at time TE.
2. Multiple spin echoes can be acquired at one location to alter the image contrast, typically to increase the amount of T_2-weighting by using longer echo time (TE).
3. The magnetic field gradients must be manipulated to allow the spin echo to form at the TE times of interest.
4. Because spin echo magnetization is in phase at the echo time TE, spin echo acquisitions are

less sensitive to magnetic field inhomogeneities than gradient echo acquisitions.

Gradient Echoes

Gradient-recalled echoes differ from spin echoes in many ways. Typically, a single RF pulse (less than 90°) is used to nutate the magnetization into the transverse plane, and the magnetic field gradients are manipulated to cause an echo to form at time TE (Figures 1-18 and 1-19). The magnetization vectors dephase with time, as presented in the previous spin echo section, but they are not refocused using a 180° RF pulse (Figure 1-19).

Because the gradient echo is formed without using a 180° RF pulse, subtle magnetic field variations (inhomogeneities) can cause additional dephasing of the magnetization in the transverse plane. In spin echo imaging, local magnetic field inhomogeneities do not tend to cause signal loss (because of the realignment of the magnetization at TE), but this signal loss in gradient echo imaging can have a large effect on the image. The signal loss in gradient echo images represents T_2 relaxation as well as the magnetic field inhomogeneity. The exponential rate at which the gradient echo signal loss occurs with TE is

FIGURE 1-17. RF and signal diagram for a multiple spin echo pulse sequence. The magnetization is refocused at both times TE 1 and TE 2. Multiple echo acquisitions allow images at the same spatial location to be acquired with different contrast weighting. For example, TE 1 and TE 2 equal to 20- and 80-ms echo times acquired using a TR of 2,000 ms would reflect proton density and T_2-weighted image contrast.

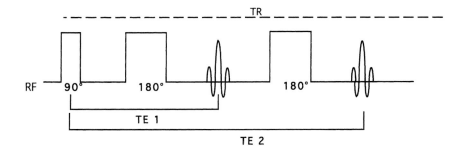

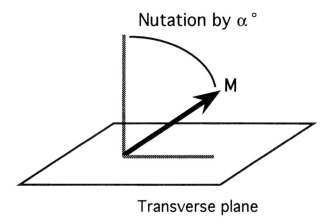

Nutation by α °

Transverse plane

FIGURE 1-18. Nutation of the magnetization (*M*) using angles less than 90°. This nutation yields magnetization in both the longitudinal (vertical) and transverse planes. Preserving the longitudinal magnetization allows for shorter TR values to be used for gradient echo acquisitions. In addition, some short TR gradient echo acquisitions preserve the transverse magnetization to increase the overall signal.

denoted by relaxation time T_2^*, which includes the effects of both T_2 and inhomogeneity.

In comparison with spin echo, gradient echo images have less signal because the RF pulse is less than 90° (putting less of the magnetization into the transverse plane) and because of the effects of magnetic field inhomogeneity. However, because a second RF pulse is not needed, the minimal TE time is less for gradient echo acquisitions, allowing less T_2 signal decay. Because a low nutation angle is often used, the residual longitudinal magnetization allows for a shorter TR. Generally, gradient echo image acquisitions take less time in comparison with spin echo image acquisitions.

To summarize gradient-recalled echo acquisitions:

1. Gradient echoes typically use low nutation angle RF pulses.
2. The amplitude of the RF pulse can markedly affect image contrast.
3. Echoes are formed at time TE by manipulation of the gradients.
4. Because gradient-recalled echoes are formed solely by manipulation of the gradients, the images are sensitive to magnetic field inhomogeneities.
5. Multiple echoes can be acquired at one location to obtain images of different contrast.
6. Because gradient echoes typically use only a single low nutation RF pulse, short TE and TR times can be used to acquire gradient echo image data.
7. Not all gradient echo acquisitions are the same. The image contrast for acquisitions using the same TE and TR can be altered greatly by the nutation angle and the extent of the gradient manipulations.

CREATING THE MAGNETIC RESONANCE IMAGE

The basis of MR image formation is that the resonant frequency is proportional to the amplitude of the magnetic field ($f = \gamma B$). The role of the magnetic field gradient in spatial encoding and slice selection is discussed in the following sections.

THE EFFECT OF MAGNETIC FIELD GRADIENTS

What Is a Magnetic Field Gradient?

The first step in creating an image is to distinguish between different locations within a patient's body. A magnetic field gradient (Figure 1-20) is applied during

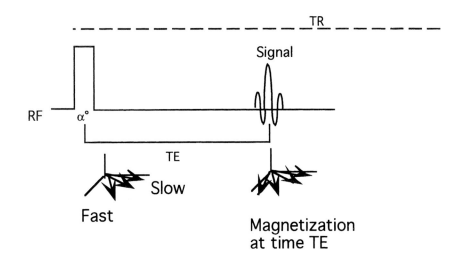

FIGURE 1-19. RF and signal diagram for a basic gradient-recalled echo pulse sequence. The α° RF pulse places the magnetization into the transverse plane, and the echo signal is formed at TE by manipulating the gradients.

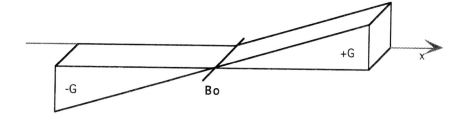

FIGURE 1-20. Representation of a gradient in the x direction. The gradient (*G*) adds to the main field (*Bo*) on the right, but subtracts from Bo on the left, creating a linear variation (gradient) in the magnetic field strength.

imaging. The gradient changes the static main field into a linear ramp. Because the resonant frequency is proportional to the magnetic field, the resonant frequency is proportional to spatial position when a gradient is present.

In practice, a gradient is usually linear (some research involves nonlinear gradients) and is on the order of 1 or 2 G/cm. Figure 1-21 shows Bo as a uniform block and the gradient field superimposed as a small wedge. The gradient can be added to Bo in any direction.

According to the Larmor equation, a magnetic dipole in a magnetic field precesses at a frequency proportional to the strength of the magnetic field. This means that when a gradient is applied, it creates a variation in the precession frequencies of magnetic dipoles in the patient. Because the frequency is different at different locations, a MR imager can distinguish between signals from different locations in the patient. The magnetic field gradient maps different locations to different frequencies. Electronically, it is a simple matter to examine different frequencies within a signal. This is a central principle of MRI: Frequency and location are related by a simple proportionality.

The relationship between an object and its frequencies (set up by the gradient) is shown in Figure 1-22.

Why Use Magnetic Field Gradients?

After the MR signal is collected, it is analyzed to find the signal intensity at different frequencies. The signal frequency and phase determine the pixel location, and the amplitude or intensity at each frequency determines the pixel gray scale value. By using a simple model, an MR image is a graph of frequency in two directions, with signal intensity as the image gray scale. The object contrast within the image is determined by the timing of the RF pulses and the type of MR signal acquisition and can be weighted by tissue proton density, T_1, or T_2 relaxation. The object position within the image is determined by the magnetic field gradients.

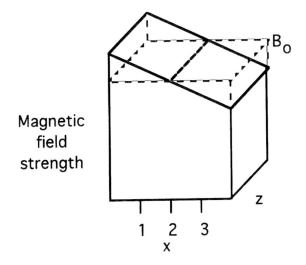

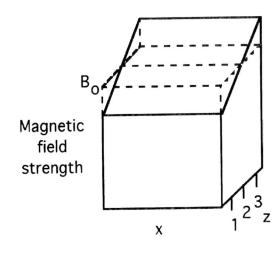

FIGURE 1-21. Representation of gradients in the x and z directions. The gradient adds to and subtracts from the main field (*dashed lines*) (*Bo*), creating a linear variation in the magnetic field strength. In each case, positions 1, 2, and 3 have different magnetic field strengths and, therefore, different resonant frequencies.

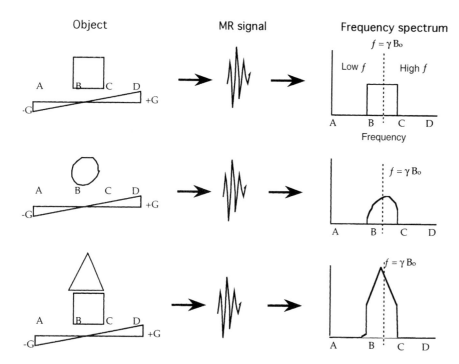

FIGURE 1-22. Representation of objects in the presence of a magnetic field gradient with the associated signal frequency components. The gradient maps the frequency spectrum to spatial position. Note the object content at positions A, B, C, and D as well as the objects' projections shown. The acquired magnetic resonance (*MR*) signal is referred to as "k-space data."

In summary, magnetic field gradients:

1. Map locations to different frequencies.
2. Can be applied along the three main axes (x, y, and z).
3. Determine the spatial location of objects within the image.

FOURIER TRANSFORMATION

The mathematical method used to determine what the MR signal contains in terms of signal amplitude and frequency is called the "Fourier transform." Because the frequency is associated with position (because of the gradient), this information can be used to form the image.

If only two or three frequencies are mixed into one signal, the composite signal looks very different from any of the original signals. By using the Fourier transform, the amplitude of each frequency is determined. In this example, the Fourier transform data would have an amplitude at only two or three frequencies (whatever is within the original signal), and all other frequencies would be zero. Other examples are shown in Figure 1-23.

Remember that the frequency contains position information and that the amplitude at each frequency ultimately determines the gray scale within the image.

In summary, the Fourier transform:

1. Is a mathematical tool used in MR image reconstruction.

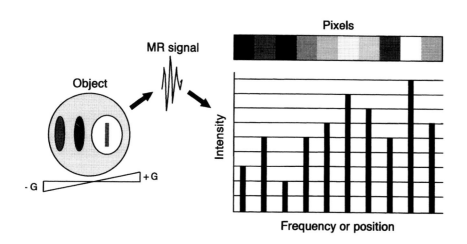

FIGURE 1-23. The Fourier transform produces a spectrum of the intensities and frequencies contained in a magnetic resonance (*MR*) signal. This information is used to generate pixels of varying gray scale value at specific locations. This diagram represents the analysis of one projection.

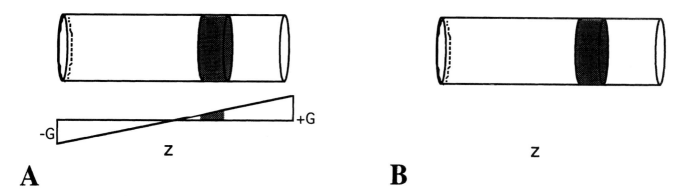

A **B**

FIGURE 1-24. Slice selection. A. RF excitation while the z gradient is present. The RF center frequency determines, along with the amplitude of the gradient, the slice position ($f = \gamma\,B$). B. After excitation, the z gradient is removed, leaving the "excited" slice. This slice can then be encoded along the x and y axes.

2. Determines the frequency content of a complex signal.
3. Can determine the amplitude of each frequency within a complex signal.
4. Is applied along two dimensions for most MR image reconstruction (two-dimensional Fourier transform).

SLICE SELECTION

To form an image, x, y, and z gradients must be applied alternately to gather information in all three directions. The most common technique for image acquisition is the two-dimensional Fourier transform method. This method acquires a tomographic slice by selectively exciting one slice and then spatially encoding the slice with frequency encoding and phase-encoding gradients. Figure 1-24 shows the slice selection process (for axial slice imaging geometry).

How Are Gradients Used to Select a Tomographic Slice?

As shown in Figure 1-24, if a gradient is applied along the patient's body (along the z direction) as the 90° RF pulse is applied, the excitation will be limited to a narrow axial slice centered at the frequency of the RF pulse. The gradient along z changed the magnetic field to allow different frequencies to correspond to different locations. The frequency content of the RF excitation pulse can be controlled, allowing excitation of individual slices. After RF excitation, only the selected slice has transverse magnetization. The magnetization at all other locations yields no signal (it is not in the transverse plane). Because gradients can be applied along x, y, or z, it is possible to select axial, sagittal, or coronal slices. Also, oblique slices can be selected because the gradients can be turned on in combination.

The width of the slice depends on the strength of the gradient and the RF bandwidth, that is, the range of frequencies contained in the RF pulse (Figure 1-25). The preceding discussion of RF pulses may have given the impression that an RF pulse contains a single frequency at one constant amplitude. This is not the case with imaging: The RF pulse contains a range of frequencies. The RF pulse frequency content (center frequency and bandwidth) along with the gradient amplitude defines the slice location and thickness.

The frequency offsets shown in Figure 1-25 for a gradient of 1 G/cm (17.028 kHz for a 4-cm offset from the isocenter) apply at any field strength. Each frequency is shown as a center frequency plus or minus some offset frequency. The main magnetic field establishes the center frequency, and the gradient amplitude establishes the offset frequency. Note that in Figures 1-25 and 1-26 the relationship between excitatory RF and bandwidth determines both the thickness of the imaging slice and its location in the brain.

SPATIAL ENCODING (PHASE AND FREQUENCY ENCODING)

After slice selection is accomplished, the x and y dimensions must be encoded. After the slice selection gradient and RF pulse are applied, the magnetization in the slice is in the transverse plane. It is this transverse magnetization that causes the MR signal. The x and y gradients are applied to make the magnetization at different locations in the slice process at different frequencies. This variation in precession frequency is used to spatially encode infor-

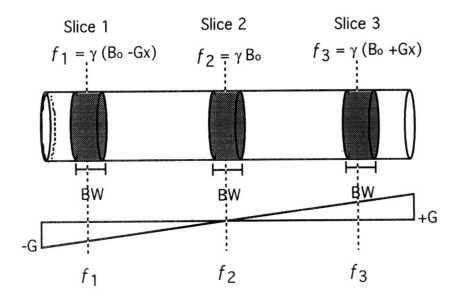

FIGURE 1-25. With the same applied gradient along z, slice location is controlled by the center frequency of the RF excitation pulse. This is the basis for multiple slice image acquisition. Using Bo = 1.5 T, G = 1 G/cm, and x = 4 cm from the isocenter, the associated frequencies for each slice are $f1 = 63.86$ MHz − 17.028 kHz, $f2 = 63.86$ MHz, and $f3 = 63.86$ MHz + 17.028 kHz. The range of frequencies centered about $f1$, $f2$, and $f3$ is the RF bandwidth (BW), which defines the thickness of each slice.

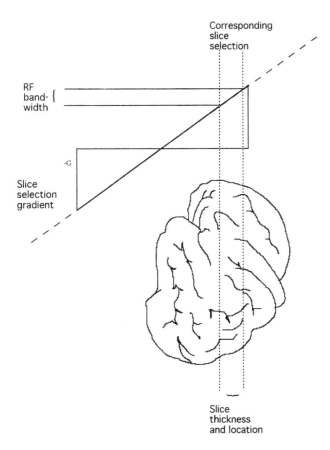

FIGURE 1-26. Slice selection as applied in brain imaging. (*RF*) radiofrequency.

mation into the signal, and the Fourier transform is used to decode this spatial information when the image is reconstructed.

Frequency Encoding

In a way, frequency encoding is the reverse of slice selection. For slice selection, a gradient is applied to map an RF excitation pulse to a specific location (via the RF pulse frequency content). For frequency encoding, the slice is excited and the transverse magnetization creates an RF signal ($f = \gamma B$). By turning on the x-direction gradient at the proper time, the MR signal (or echo) returning from the object is mapped to a range of frequencies (Figure 1-27).

While the frequency-encoding gradient causes the magnetization at different locations across the frequency encoding axis to precess at different frequencies, the signal is recorded. Because all the signals of different frequencies (from different locations) are recorded together, the recorded signal can be confusing. The Fourier transform of this signal (Figure 1-28) sorts the data into the component frequencies and shows the relative intensity of the different frequencies within the signal. Figure 1-28 shows a profile across one axis of the image, where the intensity at each frequency determines the gray scale value.

Phase Encoding

The MR image is two-dimensional. Because frequency encoding acquires information along one axis (for example, the x direction), the second direction must also be encoded. A process called "phase encoding" is used to encode the second direction (for example, the y

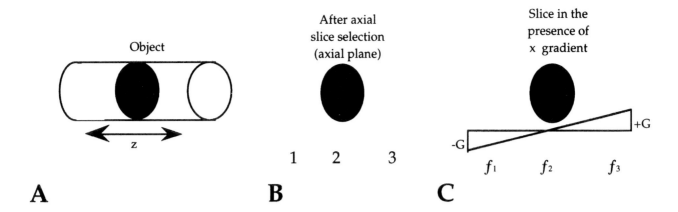

FIGURE 1-27. Frequency direction encoding. A. A cylindrical object with an "excited" slice. B. The excited slice contains magnetization in the transverse plane. C. At the TE of interest, a "readout," or frequency-encoding gradient, is applied along the x direction. This maps the spatial locations 1, 2, and 3 to the different frequencies $f1$, $f2$, and $f3$. As the magnetic resonance signal, or "echo," forms, its frequency content reflects the spatial characteristics of the object.

axis). Phase encoding for the axial slice example involves applying a y-direction gradient for some amount of time before formation of the image echo at time TE. This causes the "spins" (note that "spins" is another term for protons or magnetization) at different points along the gradient to precess at different frequencies. For example, a positive gradient amplitude causes a higher precessional frequency, and a negative gradient amplitude causes a lower precessional frequency. Spins at different frequencies precess at different rates. If the different precessional frequencies are allowed for only a short period of time, the magnetization will precess through different angles and point in slightly different directions (Figure 1-29). The net signal from the slice is affected by this phase encoding. The phase-encoding gradient amplitudes are calculated to correspond with the image field of view size and are "stepped" through a range of amplitudes to acquire a full set of image data. Phase encoding followed by fre-

quency encoding is repeated many times (for example, 128, 192, 256, . . . Ny), each time varying the strength of the phase-encoding gradient. The frequency-encoding part of the cycle remains constant throughout all the cycles. The Fourier transform of the signal along the frequency axis creates a series of projections onto the frequency-encoding axis in which each projection has different phase information. A second Fourier transform along the phase-encoding direction combines the views to form an image by decoding the magnitude and phase information in each view.

At this point, the concepts of slice selection, frequency encoding, and phase encoding have been described for the axial image plane and can be applied to other image planes. Consideration of the imaging geometry will show that if the y axis is used for slice selection, a coronal slice will result. Similarly, an x-axis slice selection gradient will result in a sagittal slice acquisition. After the slice selection axis is determined, the fre-

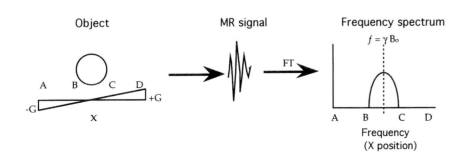

FIGURE 1-28. The frequency-encoding axis encodes each spatial position as a distinct frequency. After Fourier transformation (*FT*), the amplitude at each frequency reflects the amount of signal at the corresponding spatial position.

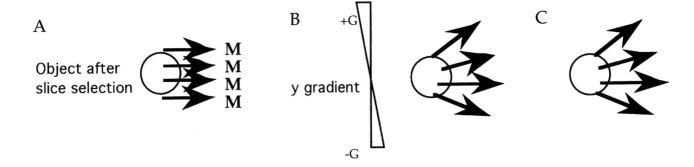

FIGURE 1-29. Phase encoding. A. Object slice after 90° nutation in which the magnetization along y is synchronized and precesses at $f = \gamma Bo$. B. The y-phase-encoding gradient is turned on, causing the magnetization to precess at different frequencies along y for a short period of time. C. After the phase-encoding gradient is turned off, the magnetization vectors again precess at one frequency ($f = \gamma Bo$), but point in different directions (that is, have different phases). The net signal from the slice is affected by this distribution of phase, a result of both the phase-encoding gradient and the object. Phase encoding of different amplitudes is applied many times (for example, 256) before the set of data required to form an image is complete.

quency-encoding and phase-encoding directions can be chosen for the particular imaging geometry.

MULTIPLE SLICE ACQUISITION

Figure 1-30 shows how the RF pulses are applied for a multiple slice acquisition. For most TR values, there is a lot of empty time spent waiting for the magnetization to relax longitudinally or for a spin echo to develop. Because any imaging slice can be excited selectively using a gradient and an RF pulse, the empty time can be used to excite more than one slice by interleaving the excitations within the TR. Often 20 or more slices are acquired during the TR time. The time savings from this are impressive; a 4-minute multiple slice acquisition would take 20 times as long without interleaving the slices.

Summary of image acquisition steps (axial image):

1. Slice selection (using RF, z gradient).

2. Phase encoding (y gradient, pulsed on during the acquisition).
3. Frequency encoding and data acquisition (at TE of interest, using x gradient).
4. Repeat steps 1 through 3 (Ny times, that is, 128, 192, 256 . . .) at the TR time of interest (change phase-encoding amplitude each time to complete phase encoding).
5. After the data are collected, transform the raw data by Fourier analysis along two dimensions (x and y) to create the image (Figure 1-31).

FACTORS AFFECTING THE IMAGE

Typically the brightness or darkness of a pixel in an MR image is determined by the magnitude of the MRI signal at that location. Areas of low signal appear dark, whereas areas of high signal appear bright. Contrast refers to how signal differences are represented by the different

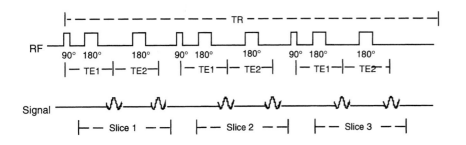

FIGURE 1-30. Multiple slice acquisition allows scanning of different tomographic sections by interleaving the respective pulse sequences of the slices into one TR period. This diagram shows how multiple echoes can be acquired for multiple slices in a single TR interval.

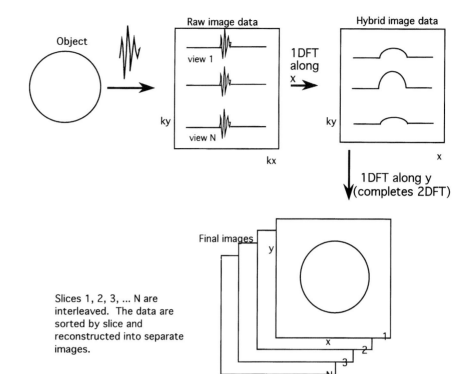

FIGURE 1-31. Summary of image acquisition and reconstruction steps for a multiple slice acquisition. *DFT*, dimensional Fourier transform.

Slices 1, 2, 3, ... N are interleaved. The data are sorted by slice and reconstructed into separate images.

gray scale values in the image. In MRI, the pulse sequence controls the acquisition so that the image contrast is based mainly on tissues T_1, T_2, or proton density.

Contrast

In MRI, image contrast depends on the density of protons at a location, the T_1 and T_2 relaxation times of the tissues being imaged, and the acquisition variables (TR, TE, and pulse sequence type). The image contrast can be weighted by proton density, T_1, T_2, or other factors, depending on the pulse sequence and imaging variables.

Brightness Is Proportional to Proton Density (Protons per Unit Volume)

The magnitude of the MR at any point in the image depends on the number of protons contributing to the signal. By keeping TR long and TE short (Table 1-5), an image reflecting proton density of various tissues can be produced without weighting the image by the respective relaxation times.

Image Contrast Is Affected by the Relaxation Times (T_1, T_2)

Image contrast can be enhanced by varying TR and TE to allow T_1 or T_2 weighting in a image (Figure 1-32). The relaxation times vary greatly throughout the body and provide for wide variations between bright and dark tissues in the image. It should be noted that T_2

TABLE 1-5. Image Contrast-Weighting* Is Determined by TE and TR

Image weighting	TE	TR
Proton density	Short	Long
T_1-weighted	Short	Short
T_2-weighted	Long	Long

*For spin echo-based acquisitions.

relaxation causes a tissue to appear dark in an image and T_1 relaxation causes a tissue to appear bright. Tissue relaxation times change with pathologic processes; thus T_1- and T_2-weighted images are very important.

Signal-to-Noise Ratio

The basic quality of an image depends on its signal-to-noise ratio. This quantity represents how clear the subject of the image (the signal) appears in comparison with the unwanted background fluctuations (the noise). The properties that affect the signal-to-noise ratio are discussed in the following sections.

The Signal-to-Noise Ratio Is Proportional to Voxel Volume

One way to improve the signal-to-noise ratio (while sacrificing resolution) is to change the size of the voxels that make up the image. A two-dimensional image of some

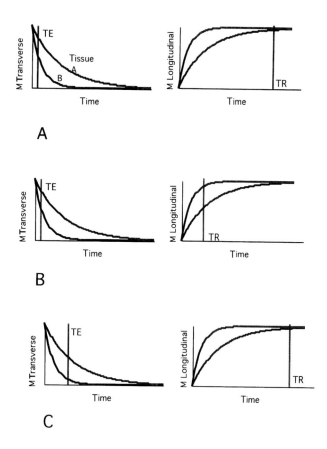

FIGURE 1-32. The choice of imaging variables (TE and TR) directly affects the image contrast. A. Short TE and long TR produce a proton-density image. B. Short TE and short TR produce T_1 weighting in the image. C. Long TR and long TE produce T_2 weighting in the image.

slice thickness is divided into volume elements (voxels). The size of these voxels is controlled by the operator via the selection of field-of-view size and imaging matrix (for example, 24-cm field of view and 256^2 matrix).

One way to increase voxel size is to increase the slice thickness. The signal-to-noise ratio is proportional to the voxel volume, so doubling the slice thickness (for example, from 5 mm to 10 mm) also doubles the ratio. Another way to increase voxel volume is to increase the field of view. As the volume of each picture element increases, the total number of spins contained in that picture element also increases. The strength of the MR signal depends on the number of spins contributing to it. Increasing the voxel volume increases the number of spins in each voxel and, thus, increases the net signal each voxel represents (Figure 1-33).

The Signal-to-Noise Ratio Is Proportional to the Square Root of the Number of Excitations per View

Signal averaging is a common way to decrease noise. Most noise is random and, therefore, tends to cancel out when averaged. In MRI, signals can be averaged by performing multiple excitations for each phase-encoding cycle (or view) and averaging the resulting signals to produce the final image. This variable is sometimes called the "number of excitations per view" (NEX). Signal averaging is often used to achieve improved image quality in MRI. The signal-to-noise ratio improves as the square root of the number of signals averaged is increased, which also increases the imaging time. For

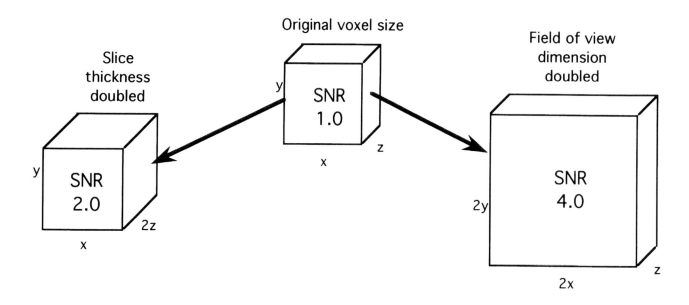

FIGURE 1-33. Signal-to-noise ratio (*SNR*) is proportional to voxel volume. Voxel volume may be increased by increasing slice thickness or the field of view.

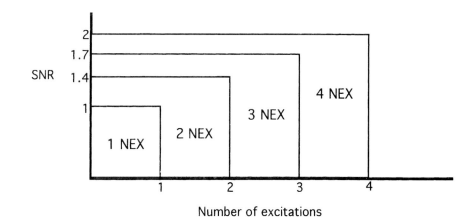

FIGURE 1-34. Signal-to-noise ratio (*SNR*) improves with the square root of the number of excitations per view (*NEX*), while acquisition time increases linearly with NEX.

example, increasing from 1 NEX to 4 NEX takes four times as long to acquire the image and improves the image signal-to-noise ratio by a factor of $\sqrt{4} = 2$. Figure 1-34 shows the relation between the signal-to-noise ratio and the image acquisition time.

The Signal-to-Noise Ratio Is Proportional to $\sqrt{N_x N_y N_z}$

For a constant field-of-view size, the SNR can be influenced by changing the number of pixels in a given direction, where Nx, Ny, and Nz represent the number of samples along the respective x and y (and z for three-dimensional acquisitions) directions. This is referred to as the "acquisition matrix size" and is controlled by the user. A typical clinical scan can use a 256×256 acquisition matrix, but other values are also common. Increasing the number of pixels in a given direction makes it easier to distinguish between objects located close together and, thus, increases the spatial resolution of the image. However, this change affects the SNR and imaging time. For example, changing from a 256×256 acquisition matrix to a 512×512 matrix results in a factor of two improvement in the resolution along x and y, but this decreases voxel size by a factor of four, which also

decreases the SNR. However, the total number of samples increases by a factor of four, which improves the SNR ratio by a factor of two because of signal averaging. As shown in Figure 1-35, changing from a 256^2 to a 512^2 matrix will change both the voxel size ($4 \times$ SNR decrease) and the number of samples $\sqrt{4} \times$ SNR gain), resulting in a net factor of two decrease in the signal-to-noise ratio.

The Signal-to-Noise Ratio Is Proportional to $\frac{1}{\sqrt{Bandwidth}}$

The acquisition bandwidth represents the range of frequencies that are sampled when an image is frequency encoded (often 16 kHz or 32 kHz). This variable is controlled by the operator and depends on the magnitude of the frequency-encoding gradient. As shown in Figure 1-36, the signal-to-noise ratio decreases as the acquisition bandwidth is increased. This signal-to-noise ratio loss remains a trade-off when acquiring image data faster using higher bandwidths.

In summary, many factors affect the image SNR. The SNR is proportional to voxel volume, $\sqrt{NEX}$, $\sqrt{N_x N_y N_z}$, and $\frac{1}{\sqrt{Bandwidth}}$.

FIGURE 1-35. SNR changes with the number of samples. A pixel within a 256^2 acquisition becomes 4 pixels within a 512^2 acquisition. Increasing the number of data samples increases SNR, but decreasing voxel volume decreases SNR. For a constant field-of-view size, changing the matrix ($N_x \times N_y$) from 256^2 to 512^2 decreases the image SNR by a factor of two.

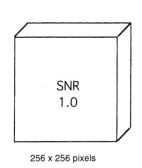

256 x 256 pixels

- SNR decreased $\frac{1}{4}$ due to decreased voxel volume

- SNR increased $\sqrt{N_x N_y}$ due to increased data sampling

- Net SNR = $\frac{1}{4}\sqrt{2 \times 2} = \frac{2}{4} = \frac{1}{2}$

- Net decrease in SNR
- Net increase in resolution

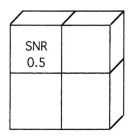

512 x 512 pixels

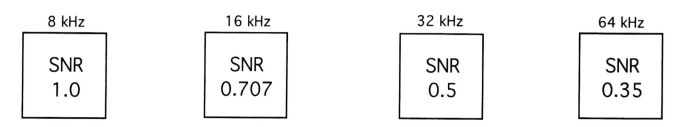

FIGURE 1-36. SNR is inversely proportional to the square root of the acquisition bandwidth. Doubling the bandwidth (that is, acquiring the data at a faster rate) degrades SNR by a factor of 0.707.

The change of one factor (for example, number of views) often will affect a number of other factors that also affect the SNR of the image. An understanding of the variables and the general effect that each one has on the SNR of the image can be important when faced with the need to improve the SNR of an examination. The following imaging variables tend to improve the SNR of the image: increased NEX, increased voxel size (field-of-view, slice thickness), decreased number of views, and decreased receiver bandwidth. Depending on the variable used, the increase in the SNR may have a "cost," such as decreased image resolution, increased chemical shift, or increased imaging time. Understanding the relevance of each variable and the image quality required to assess the particular clinical question is necessary when setting up the image acquisition.

Appendix I: Safety in Magnetic Resonance Imaging

The four main categories of safety concerns in MRI are

1. Effects of Bo
2. Effects of the changing gradient magnetic fields (dB/dt)
3. Effects of the RF field
4. Superconducting system concerns

Not all these categories are significant for clinical MRI; however each is reviewed in order to be complete and to allow assessment of the relevance of each topic to the clinical MRI environment.

BIOLOGIC EFFECTS OF Bo

The biologic effects of static magnetic fields are not fully known, although research has been conducted in this area since the 1950s. No obvious, immediate negative effect is known to be associated with clinical MRI. The results of several studies on the biologic effects of static magnetic fields can be summarized as:

1. No problems observed—no association has been found between the static magnetic field (Bo) and cancer.
2. No deleterious effect on water, basal chromosome aberration rate, sister chromatid exchange rate, spermatogenesis, cell growth, tumor survival rate, skin and body temperature, nerve conduction velocity, cardiac contractility, or behavior and memory. These data are from studies on insects, mammals, and human subjects.
3. A correlation has been shown between blood pressure and Bo, but the blood pressure values were within normal range.
4. Other results:
   a. Increased chromosomal aberrations in human lymphocyte cultures (one study).
   b. Chick and frog embryo malformations (high Bo exposure was maintained for the entire period of embryogenesis).
   c. Altered behavior in rats and growth in mice.
   d. Alterations in membrane permeability, erythrocyte shape, and bone marrow morphology.
5. Additional data to consider:
   a. Since 1983 hundreds of thousands of MRI scans have been performed in patients without causing any obvious adverse effects.
   b. Research studies have been conducted on persons exposed to MRI over extended periods of time (400+ hours for some persons since 1984).

In summary, no deleterious association has been noted for the static magnetic field strengths used for clinical MRI, although research in this area continues.

MECHANICAL ASPECTS OF Bo

The two main issues associated with the static magnetic field are the projectile effect and the torque associated with a ferromagnetic object, causing it to align with the magnetic field. The projectile effect occurs at about 300 G, at which point objects are attracted to the magnet with such force that the object can become a "projectile" as it moves into the magnet. A partial list of objects inadvertently attracted to a magnet are listed in Table I-1.

The torque on some models of aneurysm clips can be of great concern with regard to patient safety. Because some grades of stainless steel have ferromagnetic properties, the history of the surgical implant must be known before MRI is performed.

Table I-1. Objects Inadvertently Attracted to a Magnet

Badges	Metal fan
Bucket	Mop
Calculator	Nail clippers
Chest tube stand	Oxygen tank
Film magazine	Pacemaker
Forklift tines	Pager
Gurney	Pens
Hearing aid	Prosthetic devices,
Infusion pump	implants, and limbs
Intravenous stand	Shrapnel
Jewelry	Stethoscope
Keys	Tile cutter
Knife	Tile roller

To summarize the mechanical aspects of the static magnetic field:

1. The torque and projectile effect are important safety factors at the static magnetic field strengths used for clinical imaging. These effects represent the most significant safety issues at clinical MRI sites.
2. The projectile effect is more significant for magnets where the Bo shielding is placed in and around the magnet (as opposed to the shielding being placed within the walls of the room housing the magnet). The change in magnetic field as the magnet is approached (slope of the field adjacent to the magnet) is higher for these systems.

GRADIENT FIELD EFFECTS

The magnetic field gradients change during imaging to allow spatial encoding. The amplitude of these fields is small relative to Bo (perhaps 25 G maximum) but changes rapidly (from 0 to 25 G in 0.4 ms). This changing magnetic field (dB/dt) can induce an electric current in a conductor (for example, in a patient). For clinical MRI, these currents do not cause peripheral nerve stimulation or contribute significantly to patient heating. However, heating and nerve stimulation due to induced electrical currents is of interest because of the new fast-scanning sequences and hardware.

To summarize the gradient field effects in routine clinical MRI: The magnetic field gradients change rapidly during MRI, but not at a rate that would cause nerve stimulation in patients.

RADIOFREQUENCY EFFECTS

Much of the RF power used to excite protons (and produce the MR signal) is absorbed by tissues, resulting in heat. RF power limits (specific absorption rate) are based on patient weight and used to ensure that patient core temperature does not increase beyond 1°C. It is also important to ensure that no unconnected wires or loops are formed by cables in the magnet bore, because the RF can induce current in the cables, and the resulting heat can cause burns on the patient.

The RF can also affect the sensing circuitry in some models of cardiac pacemakers. The resulting synchronization of cardiac stimulation and RF excitation can lead to cardiac fibrillation. For this reason, no pacemakers should be allowed in the MR area. A second issue relevant to cardiac pacemakers is that the main magnetic field can affect an internal pacemaker switch, causing it to pace in a backup or asynchronous mode.

To summarize the RF effects:

1. The RF associated with MRI may cause mild warming of the patient, and the FDA has established tolerable limits for patient heating. On occasion, scanning variables may be limited by patient heating, but patient heating is generally not a significant factor in clinical MRI.
2. Because high RF power levels can be used for some MR examinations, it is important that no loops be formed by cables placed within the magnet bore. Furthermore, any cables must be positioned away from the bore wall.
3. The RF can also affect cardiac pacemakers; therefore, no one with a pacemaker should be imaged using MR or allowed in the MRI suite.

Overall, MR safety in a clinical MRI suite depends on the personnel training and screening techniques used. Access to the MR scan room should be limited because of the possibility of a projectile being attracted into the magnet. Furthermore, the main magnetic field can affect pacemakers. Attention should be paid to the positions of wires within the magnet bore in order to minimize the possibility of burning the patient. Diligent screening of patients and staff entering the MR scan room ensures a safe environment for all.

Appendix II: Acronyms Common to Magnetic Resonance Imaging*

TABLE II-1. Gradient-Echo Imaging Techniques

Acronym	Description	Vendor
General		
FFE	Fast field echo	Philips
GRE	Gradient-recalled echo or gradient echo	GE, Siemens
MPGR	Multiplanar gradient recalled	GE
FE	Field echo	Picker, Toshiba
PFI	Partial flip imaging	Toshiba
GE or GFE	Gradient echo or gradient field echo	Hitachi
TurboFLASH	Magnetization-prepared sub-second imaging technique	Siemens
TFE	Turbofield echo	Philips
SMASH	Short minimum-angle shot (subsecond imaging)	Shimadzu
SHORT	Short repetition techniques	Elscint
STAGE	Small tip angle gradient echo	Shimadzu
T$_1$-weighted contrast		
FLASH	Fast low angle shot	Siemens
SPGR	Spoiled gradient recalled	GE
FSPGR	Fast SPGR	GE
IR FGR	Inversion-recovery fast GRASS	GE
RF Spoiled FAST	RF-Spoiled Fourier-acquired steady-state technique	Picker
3D MP-RAGE	Three-dimensional magnetization-prepared rapid gradient echo	Siemens
T$_1$-FFE	Contrast-enhanced FFE	Philips

Acronym	Description	Vendor
Enhanced intensity (rewinding of phase-encoding gradient and no intentional spoiling)		
GRASS	Gradient-recalled acquisition in the steady state	GE
FGR	Fast GRASS	GE
FISP	Fast imaging with steady-state precession	Siemens
FAST	Fourier-acquired steady-state technique	Picker
GFEC	Gradient field echo with contrast	Hitachi
F-SHORT	Short-repetition technique based on free induction decay	Elscint
SSFP	Steady-state free precession	Shimadzu
Steady-state free precession (usually for imaging of cerebrospinal fluid)		
SSFP	Steady-state free precession	GE
CE-FAST	Contrast-enhanced FAST	Picker
True FISP	FISP with heavy T$_2$ weighting	Siemens
PSIF	Mirrored, or reverse, FISP	Siemens
ROAST	Resonant offset averaging in the steady state	Siemens
T2-FFE	Contrast-enhanced fast field echo	Philips
E-SHORT	Short-repetition technique based on echo	Elscint
STERF	Steady-state technique with refocused free induction decay	Shimadzu

*From Acronyms. J Magn Reson Imaging 1993;3 Suppl:25–26. By permission of the Society for Magnetic Resonance Imaging.

TABLE II-2. Motion-Artifact-Reduction Techniques

Acronym	Description	Vendor
Spatial presaturation to reduce magnetic resonance signal intensity in specific locations		
SAT	Saturation or presaturation	GE, Hitachi, Shimadzu, Siemens
REST	Regional saturation technique	Philips
PRE-SAT	Presaturation technique	Picker
Spectral presaturation to reduce magnetic resonance signal intensity of fat		
FATSAT	Fat saturation	GE, Siemens
SPIR	Spectral presaturation with inversion recovery	Philips
ChemSat	Chemical saturation	GE
Respiratory-ordered phase encoding		
ROPE	Respiratory ordered phase encoding	Picker
RESCOMP	Respiratory compensation	GE
RSPE	Respiratory-sorted phase encoding	GE
PEAR	Phase-encoded artifact reduction	Philips
Phase Re-ordering	Phase reordering	Hitachi
FREEZE	Respiratory selection of phase-encoding steps	Elscint
Reduction of motion-induced phase shifts during TE		
MAST	Motion-artifact suppression technique	Picker
GMR	Gradient motion rephasing	Siemens
GMN	Gradient moment nulling	GE
FLOW COMP	Flow compensation	GE, Toshiba
CFAST	Cerebrospinal fluid–artifact suppression technique	Toshiba
GMC	Gradient moment compensation	Instrumentarium
FC	Flow compensation	GE, Philips
STILL	Flow/motion compensation	Elscint
SMART	Shimadzu motion artifact reduction technique	Shimadzu
GR or GRE	Gradient rephasing	Hitachi

BIBLIOGRAPHY

Introduction and Basic Physics

Bloch F, Hansen WW, Packard M. Nuclear induction (letter to the editor). Phys Rev 1946;69:127.

Bottomley PA, Foster TH, Argersinger RE, et al. A review of normal tissue hydrogen NMR relaxation times and relaxation mechanisms from 1–100 MHz: dependence on tissue type, NMR frequency, temperature, species, excision, and age. Med Phys 1984;11:425–48.

Carlson J, Crooks L, Ortendahl D, et al. Signal-to-noise ratio and section thickness in two-dimensional versus three-dimensional Fourier transform MR imaging. Radiology 1988;166:266–70.

Cuppen JJM, Groen JP, Konijn J. Magnetic resonance fast Fourier imaging. Med Phys 1986;13:248–53.

Curry TS III, Dowdey JE, Murry RC Jr. Christensen's introduction to the physics of diagnostic radiology. 3rd ed. Philadelphia: Lea & Febiger, 1984:291–4.

Ernst RR, Anderson WA. Application of Fourier transform spectroscopy to magnetic resonance. Rev Sci Instruments 1966;37:93–102.

Hahn EL. Spin echoes. Phys Rev 1950;80:580–94.

James TL. Nuclear magnetic resonance in biochemistry: principles and applications. New York: Academic Press, 1975:3–5.

Kumar A, Welti D, Ernst RR. NMR Fourier zeugmatography. J Magn Reson 1975;18:69–78.

Lauterbur PC. Image formation by induced local interactions: examples employing nuclear magnetic resonance. Nature 1973;242:190–1.

Mansfield P. Multiplanar image formation using NMR spin echoes. J Phys 1977;10:L55–L58.

Mansfield P, Pykett IL. Biological and medical imaging by NMR. J Magn Reson 1978;29:355–373.

Parker DL, Gullberg GT. Signal-to-noise efficiency in magnetic resonance imaging. Med Phys 1990;17:250–7.

Purcelle EM, Torrey HC, Pound RV. Resonance absorption by nuclear magnetic moments in a solid (letter to the editor). Phys Rev 1946;69:37–8.

Ziedses des Plantes BG Jr, Falke THM, den Boer JA. Pulse sequences and contrast in magnetic resonance imaging. Radiographics 1984;4:869–83.

Artifacts and Artifact Reduction Techniques

Babcock EE, Brateman L, Weinreb JC, et al. Edge artifacts in MR images: chemical shift effect. J Comput Assist Tomogr 1985;9:252–7.

Bailes DR, Gilderdale DJ, Bydder GM, et al. Respiratory ordered phase encoding (ROPE): a method for reducing respiratory motion artefacts in MR imaging. J Comput Assist Tomogr 1985;9:835–8.

Cho ZH, Kim DJ, Kim YK. Total inhomogeneity correction including chemical shifts and susceptibility by view angle tilting. Med Phys 1988;15:7–11.

Constable RT, Anderson AW, Zhong J, et al. Factors influencing contrast in fast spin-echo MR imaging. Magn Reson Imaging 1992;10:497–511.

Cory DG, Reichwein AM, Veeman WS. Removal of chemical-shift effects in NMR imaging. J Magn Reson 1988;80:259–67.

Crooks LE, Mills CM, Davis PL, et al. Visualization of cerebral and vascular abnormalities by NMR imaging. The effects of imaging parameters on contrast. Radiology 1982;144:843–52.

Dixon WT. Simple proton spectroscopic imaging. Radiology 1984;153:189–94.

Felmlee JP, Ehman RL. Spatial presaturation: a method for suppressing flow artifacts and improving depiction of vascular anatomy in MR imaging. Radiology 1987;164:559–64.

Haacke EM, Lenz GW. Improving MR image quality in the presence of motion by using rephasing gradients. AJR Am J Roentgenol 1987;148:1251–8.

Henkelman RM, Bronskill MJ. Artifacts in magnetic resonance imaging. Rev Magn Reson Med 1987;2:126.

Korin H, Ehman R. Motion artifact suppression techniques. In: Higgin CB, Hricak H, Helms C, eds. Magnetic resonance imaging of the body. 2nd ed. New York: Raven Press, 1992.

Pattany PM, Marino R, McNally JM. Velocity and acceleration desensitization in 2DFT MR imaging. Magn Reson Imaging 1986;4:154–5.

Pattany PM, Phillips JJ, Chiu LC, et al. Motion artifact suppression technique (MAST) for MR imaging. J Comput Assist Tomogr 1987;11:369–77.

Perman WH, Moran PR, Moran RA, et al. Artifacts from pulsatile flow in MR imaging. J Comput Assist Tomogr 1986;10:473–83.

Wehrli FW, Perkins TG, Shimakawa A, et al. Chemical shift-induced amplitude modulations in images obtained with gradient refocusing. Magn Reson Imaging 1987;5:157–8.

Flow and Angiography

Axel L. Blood flow effects in magnetic resonance imaging. AJR Am J Roentgenol 1984;143:1157–66.

Dumoulin CL, Hart HR Jr. Magnetic resonance angiography. Radiology 1986;161:717–20.

Dumoulin CL, Souza SP, Feng H. Multiecho magnetic resonance angiography. Magn Reson Med 1987;5:47–57.

Gao J-H, Holland SK, Gore JC. Nuclear magnetic resonance signal from flowing nuclei in rapid imaging using gradient echoes. Med Phys 1988;15:809–14.

Le Bihan D, Breton E, Lallemand D, et al. MR imaging of intravoxel incoherent motions: application to diffusion and perfusion in neurologic disorders. Radiology 1986;161:401–7.

Lenz GW, Haacke EM, Masaryk TJ, et al. In-plane vascular imaging: pulse sequence design and strategy. Radiology 1988;166:875–82.

Moran PR, Moran RA, Karstaedt N. Verification and evaluation of internal flow and motion. True magnetic resonance imaging by the phase gradient modulation method. Radiology 1985;154:433–41.

Pelc NJ, Herfkens RJ, Shimakawa A, et al. Phase contrast cine magnetic resonance imaging. Magn Reson Q 1991;7:229–54.

Shimizu K, Matsuda T, Sakurai T, et al. Visualization of moving fluid: quantitative analysis of blood flow velocity using MR imaging. Radiology 1986; 159:195–9.

Wedeen VJ, Meuli RA, Edelman RR, et al. Projective imaging of pulsatile flow with magnetic resonance. Science 1985;230:946–8.

Wehrli F, Bradley W. Magnetic resonance blood flow phenomena and blood flow imaging. In: Wehrli FW, Shaw D, Kneeland JB, eds. Biomedical magnetic resonance imaging: principles, methodology, and applications. New York: VCH Publishers, 1988:465–519.

Fast Imaging

Edelman RR, Wallner B, Singer A, et al. Segmented turboFLASH: method for breath-hold MR imaging of the liver with flexible contrast. Radiology 1990;177:515–21.

Farzaneh F, Riederer SJ, Lee JN, et al. MR fluoroscopy: initial clinical studies. Radiology 1989;171:545–9.

Feinberg DA, Hale JD, Watts JC, et al. Halving MR imaging time by conjugation: demonstration at 3.5 kG. Radiology 1986;161:527–31.

Frahm J, Hanicke W, Merbolt KD. Transverse coherence in rapid FLASH NMR imaging. J Magn Reson 1987;72:307–314.

Glover G, Pelc N. A rapid-gated CINE MRI technique. In: Kressel H, ed. Magnetic resonance annual. New York: Raven Press, 1988:299–333.

Gullberg GT, Wehrli FW, Shimakawa A, et al. MR vascular imaging with a fast gradient refocusing pulse sequence and reformatted images from transaxial sections. Radiology 1987;165:241–6.

Gyngell ML. The application of steady-state free precession in rapid 2DFT NMR imaging: FAST and CE-FAST sequences. Magn Reson Imaging 1988;6:415–9.

Gyngell ML. The steady-state signals in short-repetition-time sequences. J Magn Reson 1989;81:474–83.

Haase A. Snapshot FLASH MRI. Applications to T_1, T_2, and chemical-shift imaging. Magn Reson Med 1990;13:77–89.

Haase A, Frahm J, Matthaei D, et al. FLASH imaging: rapid NMR imaging using low flip-angle pulses. J Magn Reson 1986;67:258–66.

Hennig J, Nauerth A, Friedburg H. RARE imaging: a fast imaging method for clinical MR. Magn Reson Med 1986;3:823–33.

Holsinger AE, Riederer SJ. The importance of phase-encoding order in ultra-short TR snapshot MR imaging. Magn Reson Med 1990;16:481–8.

Holsinger AE, Wright RC, Riederer SJ, et al. Real-time interactive magnetic resonance imaging. Magn Reson Med 1990;14:547–53.

MacFall JR, Pelc NJ, Vavrek RM. Correction of spatially dependent phase shifts for partial Fourier imaging. Magn Reson Imaging 1988;6:143–55.

Pauly J, Nishimura D, Macovski A. A k-space analysis of small-tip-angle excitation. J Magn Reson 1989;81:43–56.

Riederer SJ, Tasciyan T, Farzaneh F, et al. MR fluoroscopy: technical feasibility. Magn Reson Med 1988;8:1–15.

Rzedzian RR, Pykett IL. Instant images of the human heart using a new, whole-body MR imaging system. AJR Am J Roentgenol 1987;149:245–50.

Sekihara K. Steady-state magnetizations in rapid NMR imaging using small flip angles and short repetition intervals. IEEE Trans Med Imaging 1987;6:157–64.

Wehrli F. Introduction to fast-scan magnetic resonance. Milwaukee: GE Medical Systems, 1986.

Wehrli FW. Fast-scan magnetic resonance: principles and applications. Magn Reson Q 1990;6:165–236.

Wright RC, Riederer SJ, Farzaneh F, et al. Real-time MR fluoroscopic data acquisition and image reconstruction. Magn Reson Med 1989;12:407–15.

Safety

Schaefer DJ. Bioeffects of MRI and patient safety. The physics of MR imaging, No. 21. American Institute of Physics, 1993.

Shellock FG, Kanal E. Magnetic resonance: bioeffects, safety, and patient management. New York: Raven Press, 1994.

Shellock FG, Morisoli S, Kanal E. MR procedures and biomedical implants, materials, and devices: 1993 update. Radiology 1993;189:587–99.

Magnetic Resonance Imaging of Neoplastic, Vascular, and Indeterminate Substrates

Richard J. Friedland and Richard A. Bronen

OVERVIEW

The association between epilepsy and a focal lesion was first noted by Hughlings Jackson more than a century ago.[1] From a prognostic viewpoint, it makes sense to group many of the focal epileptogenic abnormalities together, because these patients have a high degree of seizure control after surgical resection.[2–6] This is true despite the fact that the pathogenesis for the epilepsy may vary from substrate to substrate.[7] This chapter considers the role of magnetic resonance (MR) imaging with respect to these focal lesions. Although focal epileptogenic lesions are sometimes referred to as "foreign tissue lesions" in the epilepsy literature, we avoid this term because "foreign tissue lesion" has an imprecise definition and is a poor term for designating a neuropathologic category. [3,5,8–12] It is best to approach these abnormalities by using a new classification scheme based on the substrate model of epilepsy, that is, grouping abnormalities by their pathologic features along with consideration of their anatomical localization.[7] In comparison with previous classifications, this method provides a more dependable clinical appraisal of a patient's diagnosis, prognosis, and treatment plan. This scheme clas-

sifies the symptomatic epilepsies (partial epilepsies with an identifiable cause) into five categories: neoplasms, vascular abnormalities, medial temporal sclerosis, nonvascular developmental disorders, and indeterminate substrates (consisting mostly of nonspecific gliosis, traumatic, atrophic, or inflammatory abnormalities). The neoplastic, vascular, and indeterminate substrates, which are essentially the focal epileptogenic lesion group plus diffuse atrophic or inflammatory abnormalities, are discussed in this chapter. These substrates have many features in common and differ substantially from the developmental and medial temporal sclerosis substrates.[7]

The incidence of focal lesions is estimated to be 15% to 25%, according to a study of the general epilepsy population as well as from surgical series of epilepsy patients.[5,13,14] Before the advent of computerized tomography (CT), a study of 516 patients receiving treatment in Rochester, Minnesota, for epilepsy showed that focal lesions were responsible for approximately 17% of cases, trauma for 5.2%, vascular lesions for 5.2%, neoplasms for 4.1%, and infections for 2.9%.[13] Lack of imaging probably resulted in underreporting the true prevalence of these lesions. The prevalence is slightly greater in patients who have had surgical treatment for medically refractory epilepsy: neoplasms, 15%; vascular lesions, 3%; trauma, 2%; hamartoma, 2%; and infections, less than 1%.[9,15–22] Preoperative detection of focal lesions in patients with intractable epilepsy is important because up to 90% are seizure-free postoperatively. In the United States, there may be 25,000 people with focal lesions who are candidates for epilepsy surgery (as extrapolated from the following: epilepsy affects 0.5% of the population; 30% of epileptic patients are refractory to medical treatment; at least one third of medically intractable epileptic patients are surgical candidates; and focal lesions account for 15% to 25% of operations for medically refractory epilepsy).[23,24] Detecting a lesion in a patient without intractable epilepsy is also important in management because surgical intervention may decrease the need for antiepileptic medications, decrease seizure frequency, alleviate the seizures, or remove a tumor that has the potential to evolve into a malignant neoplasm.[3]

Before we examine the role that MR has in the workup of an epileptogenic lesion, we must first understand the relationships among the epileptogenic zone, structural lesions, and partial epilepsy. Seizure disorders are the result of abnormal excitability and excessive discharge of neurons. The area of brain where the seizure originates, which is almost always cerebral cortex, is known as the "epileptogenic zone." The exact relationship between the lesion and seizure generation is poorly understood, but epileptogenesis probably is not due to the lesion itself but rather to its effect on the surrounding tissue.[25,26] The focus of epileptogenesis may be located at the lesion, contiguous with the lesion, or even remote from the lesion. Cytoarchitectural alterations adjacent to a lesion play a role in seizure generation. These include changes in tissue milieu due to mass effect, interstitial edema, local vascular disturbance, and prior microscopic hemorrhage that, in turn, may alter neurons or glial cells. Epileptogenesis is thought to involve biochemical mechanisms that lead to cell membrane destabilization and changes in cellular ion flux that cause abnormal depolarization of neurons. These include (1) dysfunction of the sodium-potassium pump, (2) abnormalities of axonal calcium and chloride, (3) changes in the N-methyl-D-aspartic acid (NMDA) receptor-cation channels, (4) abnormal regulation of somatostatin, (5) abnormal regulation of the inhibitory neurotransmitter gamma-aminobutyric acid, (6) lesion-induced denervation hypersensitivity, and (7) abnormal glial calcium transport.[11,25,27–30]

By definition, partial epilepsy is epilepsy that originates from a focal site (as opposed to generalized seizures). Partial seizures, in turn, must be due to a localized brain disturbance (the epileptogenic zone), which may be biochemical in nature or be due to a microscopic or macroscopic structural abnormality. This is why partial epilepsy is frequently associated with structural abnormalities of the brain. MR is ideally suited for identifying epileptogenic foci in patients with partial seizures because of its ability to depict structures, particularly the temporal lobe, in exquisite detail and its high sensitivity for detecting structural abnormalities.[9,14,31–34]

The Role of Magnetic Resonance

The primary role of preoperative MR is to locate and to define structural lesions responsible for seizure generation. MR findings may also influence whether the patient is a candidate for surgical treatment, the type of operation, invasive electroencephalographic (EEG) evaluation, and the prognosis of the surgical treatment. Patients undergo a battery of presurgical tests to determine the relationships between the MR–identified focal lesion and the epileptogenic zone and functional (eloquent) cortex. Concordance of the results of all noninvasive tests with the MR findings may preclude the need for invasive testing, which has been associated with an increased morbidity of 2% to 5%.[35–37] MR and video monitoring EEG are widely available and are the most critical noninvasive studies in the evaluation of focal lesions. Other noninvasive tests include CT, single-photon emission computed tomography (SPECT), proton emission tomography (PET), magnetoencephalography (MEG), intracarotid sodium amobarbital testing, and neurologic and neuropsychologic testing. MR is also useful in planning the placement of subdural grids or depth electrodes. MR determination of electrode position is important in the analysis of data from these electrodes.[7]

The identification of a focal lesion is predictive of surgical success and an excellent long-term outcome.[5] When the location of a lesion is identical with the epileptogenic focus, complete removal of that lesion offers an 82% to 94% chance of a seizure-free outcome.[2,4] Complete removal correlates not only with postoperative success based on seizure abatement but also with reduction of antiepileptic medication and improvement in psychologic and cognitive performance. Even incomplete lesionectomy can result in a significant rate of seizure-free outcomes (73%).[2,4] Incomplete resections may act by decreasing the critical epileptogenic mass required for seizure generation or by disrupting electrical pathways required for propagation of the seizure. If the patient's lesion is remote from the site of epileptogenesis, removal of either the lesion or the epileptogenic zone alone usually has a less favorable outcome.[38–40]

The data presented so far illustrate the potential of any tool that can accurately detect and localize a focal lesion. In the case of MR, sensitivity approaches 100%.[9,33,41,42] The experience at the Yale Medical School has been similar. MR correctly detected all 42 focal lesions in surgical epilepsy patients during a 3-year period. In comparison, CT was able to localize only 26 of the 42 lesions. The probability of positive CT findings after normal MR findings was determined to be 0%. Other advantages that MR confers over CT include the lack of ionizing radiation, multiplanar imaging capability, improved con-

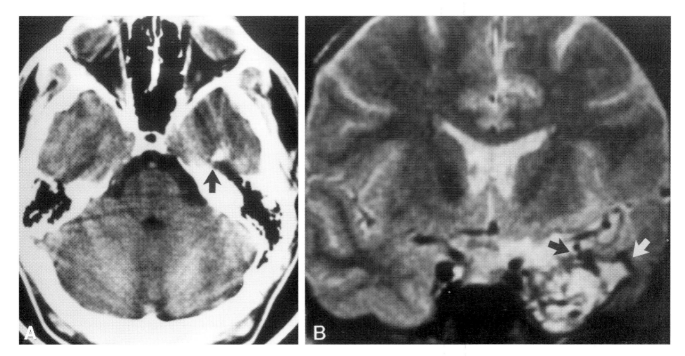

FIGURE 2-1. Mixed glioma. A. Beam-hardening artifact obscures much of the left temporal lobe on this axial CT image. The high attenuation region (*arrow*) is highly suggestive of a calcified lesion such as a glioma, but it could be an artifact. B. Coronal T$_2$-weighted MR demonstrates a heterogeneous mass larger than that suspected with CT. The heterogeneity is due to cystic changes (regions of increased signal), calcification (*black arrow*), and hemosiderin (*white arrow*). These are typical findings in patients with pure oligodendrogliomas or mixed gliomas. This patient with epilepsy had a low-grade astrocytoma with oligodendrocytic features. (From Bronen.[14] Reprinted with permission of the American Roentgen Ray Society.)

trast resolution, and the lack of beam-hardening artifacts in the temporal lobe. The routine use of CT in patients with chronic seizures is not indicated (Figure 2-1).

MR can also categorize lesions into the five substrate groups (as in the classification system proposed by Spencer[7]) with a high degree of success.[6] Generally, one can distinguish among neoplasms, arteriovenous malformations, cavernous hemangiomas, certain infections, cicatricial processes, diffuse atrophic processes, migration anomalies, hippocampal sclerosis, and, sometimes, hamartomas and cortical dysplasias.[6,14] However, MR is not very accurate in determining the histologic diagnosis within a category, such as predicting the particular type of tumor present. Whereas some groups of lesions may be difficult to distinguish from each other by MR, certain imaging characteristics may lead to the correct diagnosis (these features are discussed below). Correct categorization of a lesion can have significant impact on patient management and surgical decisions (as discussed in Chapter 16, by Vives, Al-Rodhan, and Spencer).

Epileptogenic focal lesions have several imaging features in common. Because epilepsy is usually a cortical process, epileptogenic lesions are predominantly cortical or subcortical in location. We found that more than 80% of surgical epileptogenic lesions involve either the

cerebral cortex or the junction between the gray matter and white matter.[6] These lesions are usually chronic and benign, as evidenced by lengthy seizure histories. Other features supporting their benign nature include the lack of mass effect or edema. Because most epileptogenic lesions are present for more than a decade and involve the brain periphery (cerebral cortex), it is not uncommon to discover associated calvarial remodeling[4,6,35] (Figure 2-2). This is an important caveat to remember, because calvarial changes traditionally are thought to be due to lesions outside the brain parenchyma (extra-axial); yet, epileptogenic lesions are primarily intra-axial. Most epileptogenic lesions are located in the temporal lobe.

What is the optimal imaging protocol for evaluating a patient with epilepsy? Although protocols vary widely, most include sequences useful for the detection of hippocampal sclerosis as well as focal lesions[14,42-45] (Chan S, Silver A, Hilal S, et al., *Proceedings from the American Society of Neuroradiology meeting*, Vancouver, British Columbia, May 16 to 21, 1993). We have found that long TR imaging sequences in the axial and coronal planes are the most useful for detecting focal lesions. Additional sequences that are used specifically to evaluate the hippocampus can sometimes help detect or characterize a lesion. These include spoiled gradient echo images and fast

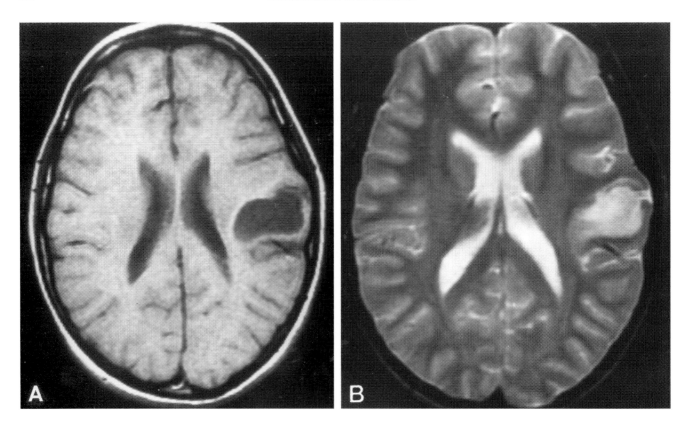

FIGURE 2-2. Low-grade glioma. A. T_1-weighted and (B) T_2-weighted axial images demonstrate a cystic subcortical mass. The mass has expanded the gyrus and caused remodeling of the overlying calvaria, a finding usually associated with an extra-axial lesion. Epileptogenic masses frequently cause calvarial remodeling because of their chronicity and peripheral location. (From Bronen.[14] Reprinted with permission of the American Roentgen Ray Society.)

spin echo images with 1.5- to 3.0-mm slice thickness. Compared with conventional spin echo imaging, fluid-attenuated inversion recovery (FLAIR) sequences appear to increase the detection rate of epileptogenic abnormalities (Chan S, Silver A, Hilal S, et al., *Proceedings from the American Society of Neuroradiology meeting*, Vancouver, British Columbia, May 16 to 21, 1993). Contrast-enhanced MR imaging has little value in routine imaging of patients with epilepsy, but it is valuable in selected cases.[46,47] After a lesion is detected with MR, contrast may: increase diagnostic confidence, improve delineation of a lesion, assist in differentiating between aggressive and nonaggressive lesions, and help direct lesion biopsy.[31] Contrast studies are extremely important in the follow-up of resected enhancing lesions in order to monitor for residual or recurrent disease. Contrast is also helpful in Sturge-Weber syndrome, because it can distinguish this entity from other forms of epilepsy-associated hemiatrophy.

Dual Pathology

Dual pathology, that is, the coexistence of hippocampal sclerosis and a focal lesion, occurs in 8% to 22% of sur-

gical epilepsy patients.[20,48] This condition should not be confused with the mild decrease in hippocampal neuronal cell density associated with temporal lobe epileptogenic lesions.[49] These patients are not considered to have "dual pathology," because they do not exhibit the axonal reorganization and immunohistochemical abnormalities that are typically seen in hippocampal sclerosis.[50] Patients with dual pathology usually have a long history of a seizure disorder that began at an early age.[20,51] Simple lesionectomy or stereotaxic surgery is often unsuccessful in controlling seizures completely. This group of patients is better served by a combination of lesionectomy and anterior temporal lobectomy.[11,30] Thus, the preoperative detection of dual pathology can have a significant impact on surgical planning and outcome. Because MR imaging has a high sensitivity for detecting hippocampal sclerosis as well as focal lesions, MR would be expected to have a high sensitivity for dual pathology (Figure 2-3). However, several issues must be considered. First, the relationship between the MR abnormality and the epileptogenic zone must be investigated. During a 3-year period, we found multiple abnormalities on MR in about 20% of our surgical epilepsy

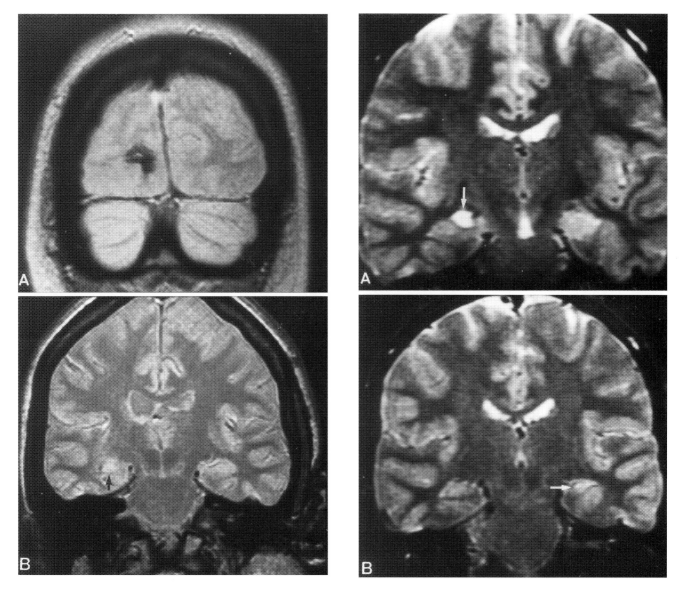

FIGURE 2-3. Dual pathology. A. Coronal proton density image demonstrates a temporal-occipital occult vascular malformation with a punctate focus of high signal surrounded by signal void of hemosiderin. B. A more anterior image through the temporal lobe reveals subtle hyperintensity in the diminutive right hippocampus (*arrow*). This second abnormality, hippocampal sclerosis, was missed by some observers. This patient underwent epilepsy surgery twice; the final diagnosis was hippocampal sclerosis and thrombosed arteriovenous malformation. A cavernous malformation has an identical imaging appearance to this thrombosed arteriovenous malformation. (From Friedland and Bronen.[150] Reprinted with permission of WB Saunders Company.)

FIGURE 2-4. Incidental finding. A. T_2-weighted coronal image demonstrates an incidental choroidal fissure cyst on the right side (*arrow*), contralateral to the patient's seizure focus. B. More posteriorly on the left side, MR shows an atrophic hyperintense hippocampus containing abnormal high signal (*arrow*), which was histologically proven to be hippocampal sclerosis. (From Bronen RA, Cheung G, Charles JT, et al. Imaging findings in hippocampal sclerosis: correlation with pathology. *AJNR Am J Neuroradiol* 1991;12:933-40. By permission of the American Society of Neuroradiology.)

patients. Most patients did not have dual pathology (that is, associated hippocampal sclerosis), and most of the secondary lesions were incidental findings (such as cysts and nonspecific focal signal abnormalities) (Figure 2-4).

Second, visual identification of hippocampal sclerosis may be underreported in patients with dual pathology. Most people viewing MR imaging studies will concentrate on the lesion without thorough assessment of the hippocampus. One needs either a high index of awareness for this entity or quantitative hippocampal data (such as volumetrics or T_2 values) (see Figures 2-3 and 2-4). Third, mass lesions may obscure the hippocampus and the MR diagnosis of hippocampal sclerosis.

NEOPLASMS

According to an epidemiologic study conducted in Rochester, Minnesota, brain tumors occur in about 4% of the general epilepsy population.[13] However, this study may have underestimated the true incidence of neoplasms, because it was performed before the advent of CT or MR. In adults with medically intractable epilepsy, the prevalence of neoplasms is 10% to 20% and may be even higher in children.[9,16,18–20,22,48,52] In studies from the Yale Medical School, the National Institutes of Health, and the Cleveland Clinic, the incidence of cerebral neoplasms in resected specimens ranged from 10% to 14%.[19,53–55] Conversely, 50% to 76% of patients with cerebral neoplasms present with seizures.[56,57] Seizures are the most common presenting symptom in patients with low-grade tumors. In the Montreal series of 230 gliomas, seizures occurred in 92% of the cases of oligodendroglioma, 70% of the cases of astrocytoma, and 35% of the cases of glioblastoma.[58]

Most patients with epilepsy due to neoplasms have normal findings on neurologic examination, and their epilepsy has been stable for at least a decade.[4,19] The phenomenology and auras produced by neoplastic lesions are indistinguishable from those due to other causes, such as hippocampal sclerosis. The type of seizure a patient manifests usually is related to the location of the lesion. Most tumors causing epilepsy are located in the cortex or subcortical regions of the temporal lobe (63%) and present with partial complex seizures.[4]

Medically intractable epilepsy is a chronic illness, usually defined as pharmacologically uncontrolled seizures for 2 years. Therefore, it is not surprising to find that most tumors are low-grade neoplasms and that long-term survival is excellent. In a recent report of 65 patients, the average seizure history was 15 years, and only 1 of 65 patients died because of the tumor.[4] The spectrum of neoplastic lesions encountered in surgical treatment of epilepsy differs from that observed in the conventional neurosurgical series. Epileptogenic lesions include astrocytomas, oligodendrogliomas, mixed tumors, pilocytic astrocytomas, pleomorphic xanthoastrocytomas, gangliogliomas, and dysembryoplastic neuroepithelial tumors. Patients with mass lesions respond well to surgical resection of the lesion.[4,5]

Some of the general imaging characteristics of epileptogenic neoplasms are mentioned above. These lesions are found predominantly within or adjacent to gray matter, have little mass effect or edema, and may produce calvarial remodeling[4,6,35] (see Figure 2-2). A recent review of neoplastic and vascular lesions demonstrated that calvarial remodeling was associated with 32% of the lesions.[6] Although subgroups of tumors usually have characteristic imaging features, these traits may not be sufficiently unique to allow a preoperative histologic diagnosis in each case. Similar imaging attributes are found in many types of tumors that cause epilepsy. A focused discussion of imaging as well as clinical and histologic features of the more common epileptogenic tumors is presented below.

Astrocytomas

Well-differentiated gliomas are the most common epileptogenic neoplasm.[4,56,58,59] The peak incidence of supratentorial astrocytomas occurs in persons 20 to 50 years old. A unique characteristic of patients with chronic epilepsy and gliomas is that they tend to have a good prognosis regardless of tumor grade.[4] The infiltrative form of fibrillary astrocytoma accounts for 75% of adult astrocytomas. Microscopic features of astrocytomas include hyperchromic angular nuclei, rare mitoses with some cellular heterogeneity, subpial and subependymal aggregation, and perivascular and perineuronal accumulations. Distant infiltration along major nerve fiber tracts is often seen. Calcification is observed in 20% of lesions, and degenerative microcysts are found in up to 20%.[4,60] Hemosiderin has been noted within macrophages adjacent to epileptogenic gliomas in 25% of cases and may have a role in epileptogenesis.[4,61]

Imaging of low-grade astrocytomas usually demonstrates a well-circumscribed lesion with little mass effect and no edema.[62] Some of these tumors show a variable pattern of enhancement with intravenously administered contrast agents. Calcification is detected in about 20% of astrocytomas by CT but can be missed with MR.[63] MR commonly demonstrates involvement of the adjacent cortex as thickening of the cortical mantle.[62] The signal intensity of most low-grade astrocytomas is decreased on T_1-weighted images and increased on T_2-weighted images (Figures 2-2, 2-5, and 2-6). High-grade gliomas may have variable mass effect, edema, and enhancement[64] (see Figure 2-6).

Oligodendrogliomas

Although oligodendrogliomas are less common than astrocytomas, they frequently are associated with seizure disorder. In the Montreal series, seizures occurred in 92% of the patients with oligodendrogliomas.[59] Oligodendrogliomas represent about 3% to 7% of all intracranial gliomas and usually present in the fourth and fifth decades. These lesions often occur in the superficial frontal and frontotemporal white matter, with extension into the cerebral cortex and leptomeninges.[60] Histologically, the tumors are

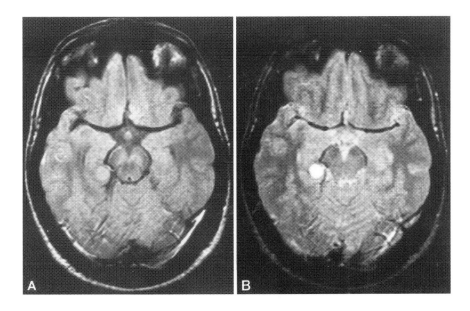

FIGURE 2-5. Low-grade glioma. A and B. A well-circumscribed lesion is demonstrated in the right parahippocampal gyrus on these axial images in a patient with a 5-year history of seizures. The signal intensity of this low-grade glioma is isointense to brain on proton density images (A) and hyperintense on T_2-weighted images (B). (From Bronen et al.[6] Reprinted with permission of Elsevier Science.)

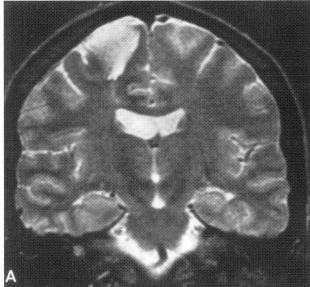

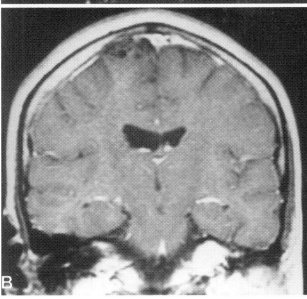

sheets of compact uniform cells with regular, central, spherical nuclei and scant cytoplasm. There is little stroma. One half of the cases are pure oligodendrogliomas, and the other half are mixed, containing an astrocytic component[65] (see Figure 2-1). Intratumoral calcification (in 90% of tumors), focal mucinous change, cystic necrosis, and hemorrhage are not uncommon, especially in larger lesions.[66,67]

Imaging may suggest a diagnosis based on location, calcification, and calvarial erosion. However, none of these findings is specific for oligodendrogliomas. On CT, these tumors appear as a round or oval mass, isodense or hypodense to gray matter. Imaging characteristics include a cystic component (20% of tumors), patchy enhancement (50%), linear or nodular calcification (30% to 40%), hemorrhage (20%), absence of edema, and calvarial erosions (17%).[64,68] MR signal characteristics of oligodendrogliomas are similar to those of other tumors: isointense to gray matter on T_1-weighted images and hyperintense on T_2-weighted images. Calcification, hemorrhage, and cystic changes are responsible for a heterogeneous appearance on MR (see Figure 2-1).

◄ FIGURE 2-6. Anaplastic glioma. A. A coronal T_2-weighted image shows a hyperintensity lesion in the right frontal lobe. B. There is no enhancement of the lesion on the gadolinium-enhanced T_1-weighted image in this patient with chronic seizures due to an anaplastic glioma. Unlike in this case, contrast agent is usually helpful in detecting high-grade gliomas and is useful for excluding residual or recurrent disease.

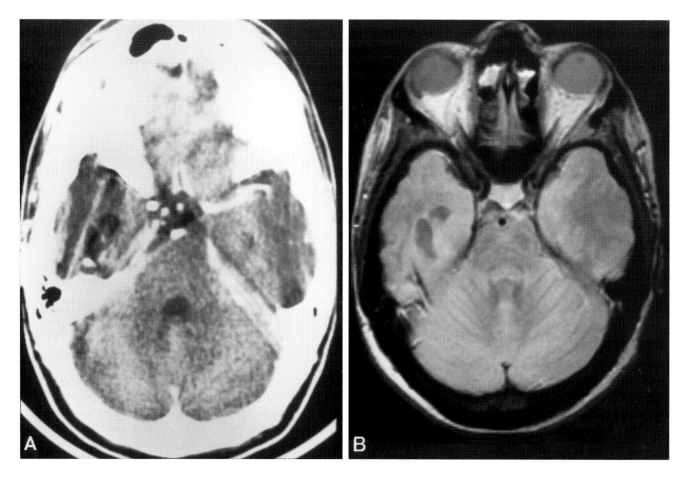

FIGURE 2-7. Ganglioglioma. A. A contrast-enhanced CT image shows a hypodense mass containing calcification in the right temporal lobe. Proton density (B), and T_2-weighted axial images (C) reveal that this is a multilobulated mass that is isointense to CSF and without associated edema. Calcification and cyst formation are typical of gangliogliomas. Note that the calcification demonstrated on CT is not visualized on MR. (B and C from Bronen et al.[6] Reprinted with permission of Elsevier Science.)

Gradient echo techniques are better than spin-echo for the detection of calcification and hemorrhage.[64]

Gangliogliomas

Gangliogliomas, like most other epileptogenic neoplasms, are slow-growing neoplasms, resulting in a prolonged clinical course. These tumors occur most frequently in the first and second decades of life; 60% to 80% of them are in persons younger than 30 years.[65,69] Although gangliogliomas are rare in the general population (0.6% of all central nervous system [CNS] neoplasms and 4% to 8% of pediatric CNS neoplasms),[70–73] they occur frequently in seizure patients. Wolf et al.[34] found that gangliogliomas were the most common intracranial tumor in the epilepsy population, occurring in 34 of 75 patients (45%). Patients commonly present with new-onset seizures or headaches.

Pathologically, the lesion is a mixed neurogliogenic tumor composed of mature ganglion and glial cells, both of which demonstrate features of neoplasia.[65] Features of these neoplastic neurons include heterotopia or cellular atypia, such as bizarre shapes or binucleation.[70] Gangliogliomas are often cystic, well circumscribed, and calcified, and they may contain a mural nodule. The temporal lobes are the most frequent site of involvement, although these tumors have been found throughout the brain.[65,69,74]

The typical CT appearance of gangliogliomas is a well-circumscribed hypodense or isodense lesion, with focal calcification (28% to 35% of tumors) and enhancement(50%).[69,74] With MR, these tumors appear as a heterogeneous mass, hypointense on T_1-weighted images and hyperintense on T_2-weighted images[74,75] (Figure 2-7). Cystic lesions may show a heterogeneous signal that is slightly hyperintense to cerebrospinal fluid (CSF) with

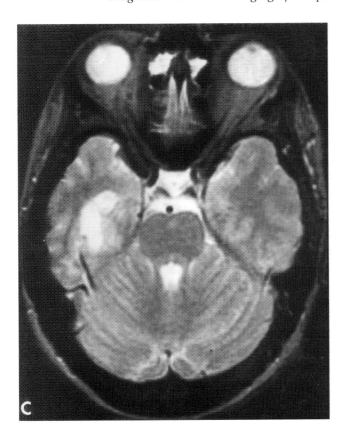

all sequences. Most gangliogliomas show some contrast enhancement on MR.[74]

Dysembryoplastic Neuroepithelial Tumors

Dysembryoplastic neuroepithelial tumor is a rare entity that was described by Daumas-Duport et al.[76] These patients usually present in childhood, have a long seizure history, and no focal neurologic deficits. Temporal lobe epilepsy was the sole presenting symptom in 37 of 39 patients. The temporal lobe was involved in 24 (62%) of the patients and the frontal lobe in 12 (31%).[76] The histologic features of these tumors are unique. The tumors are composed of astrocytes, oligodendrocytes, and neural elements, with little evidence of atypia. It is thought that the tumors arise from the secondary germinal layers, most likely the subpial granular layer. Dysembryoplastic neuroepithelial tumors have been associated with focal cortical dysplasias.[76] Grossly these lesions are multinodular, multicystic, and cortical, although they can extend to the white matter. They are thought to be distinct from gangliogliomas because of differences in the amount of various components, the cortical location, and the absence of lymphocytes.[77] Patients have an excellent prognosis after complete or even incomplete surgical excision of these tumors. Kirkpatrick et al.[78] report a long-term seizure-free rate of 81%, with an additional 10% almost seizure-free despite microscopic

evidence of incomplete tumor removal in 71% of the reported patients.

CT demonstrates a well-circumscribed hypodense cerebral lesion without edema, but the findings may be normal in 10% of cases.[76] Daumas-Duport et al.[76] documented contrast enhancement in 18% of cases and calcification in 23%. Similarly to other indolent lesions, deformity of the overlying calvarium may be seen. In lesions with this CT appearance, the differential diagnosis includes arachnoid cyst, low-grade glioma, and hamartoma. The MR appearance is primarily that of a focal cortical mass of low signal intensity on T_1-weighted images, high signal intensity on T_2-weighted images, and variable signal intensity on proton-density images[79] (Figure 2-8). In addition to their usual cortical location the lesions may demonstrate gyral thickening.[79–81] The MR appearance of dysembryoplastic neuroepithelial tumor may be indistinguishable from that of a ganglioglioma, astrocytoma, or oligodendroglioma.

Hamartomas

Hamartomas are classified as either a tumor or a developmental disorder. A hamartoma is a mass of disorganized but mature cells indigenous to the part of the brain in which the tumor occurs. The term designates a tumor-like but non-neoplastic formation or an error in tissue development.[65] The histologic and imaging characteristics of hamartomas and cortical dysplasias are similar. Although these lesions may be difficult to distinguish from neoplasms by MR or CT, certain imaging features may lead to the correct diagnosis. For instance, a mass involving the subcortical white matter that is associated with a poorly defined cortical-medullary junction, a focally thickened cortex, or other similar lesions is more likely to be a hamartoma or cortical dysplasia than a neoplasm[82–84] (Figure 2-9). A full discussion of hamartomas and cortical dysplasia is found in the chapter on developmental anomalies.

VASCULAR MALFORMATIONS

Approximately 5% of the patients in the general epilepsy population have an underlying vascular abnormality as the cause of their seizures.[13] This percentage is similar to that in surgical series for medically refractory epilepsy (2% to 7%).[9,16,19,21,22,34] These lesions include cavernous malformations, capillary telangiectasias, and arteriovenous malformations. The sensitivity of MR approaches 100% for the detection of intracranial vascular lesions.[9,17,21,31,47,85] We found MR to be 100% sensitive in localizing 8 of 8 vascular lesions that caused intractable epilepsy.[6]

Cavernous Malformations

Cavernous malformations (also known as "cavernous hemangiomas") are composed of large vascular spaces without discrete arteries or veins and in which there is

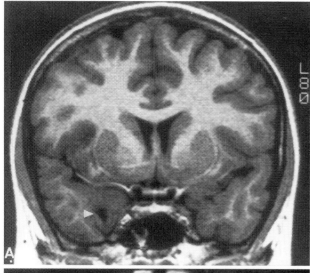

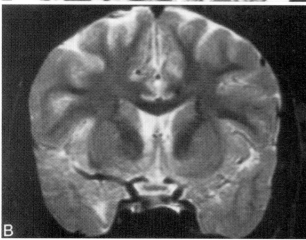

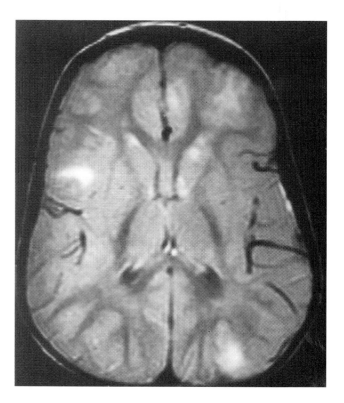

FIGURE 2-9. Hamartoma. An axial proton density image demonstrates multiple subcortical and periventricular subependymal foci of increased signal without significant mass effect. The multiplicity of the lesions suggests the correct diagnosis, that is, multiple hamartomas in a patient with tuberous sclerosis. However, if confronted with a single lesion, it may be impossible to differentiate a hamartoma from a glioma on the basis of imaging. (From Bronen.[35] Reprinted with permission of the American Roentgen Ray Society.)

FIGURE 2-8. Dysembryoplastic neuroepithelial tumor. A. Coronal T_1-weighted, and (B) T_2-weighted images showing a cystic lesion (*arrowhead*) in the subcortical white matter of the right temporal lobe. Note the associated gyral thickening indicative of an associated focal cortical dysplasia. (From Friedland and Bronen[150] Reprinted with permission of WB Saunders Company.)

no intervening neural tissue.[60,65] These lesions usually vary in size from a few millimeters to several centimeters and may contain calcification, hemorrhage, or thrombus. Although cavernous hemangiomas have no connective tissue capsule, they are usually well-defined by the surrounding gliotic and hemosiderin-stained brain tissue, which facilitates surgical removal.[86] The essential pathologic feature that distinguishes cavernous malformations from capillary telangectasias is the presence of brain parenchyma observed between the dilated vascular channels in capillary telangectasias.[65] It is debated whether cavernous malformations and capillary telangectasias are part of the spectrum of the same abnormality.[87]

The true incidence of cavernous hemangiomas within the general population is about 0.5%, as based on an MR study of 14,035 patients.[86] These lesions occur in all age groups and may be multiple (10% to 40%) and familial. They more frequently are multiple when they are familial.[30,88–91] Most cavernous malformations are located supratentorially, especially in the frontal and temporal lobes, but they may be found anywhere in the CNS.[86,89,90] Seizures are the most frequent clinical presentation, particularly with multiple hemangiomas.[92] In patients with multiple lesions, the risk of the development of seizures is higher and the seizures begin at a younger age. In comparison with arteriovenous malformations, cavernous malformations are more likely to cause medically refractory seizures.[30]

Most seizures caused by cavernous malformations can be controlled with pharmacologic treatment. Removal of the lesion may decrease the frequency and severity of the seizures, allow tapering of antiepileptic medication, and may even alleviate the seizures.[93,94]

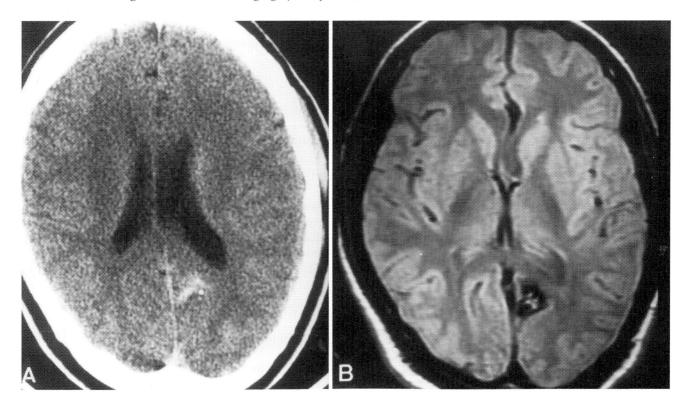

FIGURE 2-10. Cavernous hemangioma. A. CT shows a region of calcification without adjacent edema or mass effect. Either a vascular malformation or a tumor could have this appearance. B. The MR appearance is typical for an occult vascular malformation and not a tumor. The axial proton density image shows a central area containing a speckled pattern of high and low signal surrounded by hypointense rim from hemosiderin. (From Bronen.[35] Reprinted with permission of the American Roentgen Ray Society.)

Surgical resection is indicated in patients with medically intractable epilepsy that is caused by a cavernous malformation that is surgically accessible. Robinson et al.[86] reported surgical resection of hemangiomas in 14 seizure patients, 10 of whom had intractable epilepsy. One half of the patients had a good surgical outcome, with significant relief from the seizures.

Imaging has a high sensitivity for the detection of vascular malformations, but it cannot reliably distinguish among cavernous malformations, capillary telangectasias, and small, partially thrombosed arteriovenous malformations. All three lesions have a similar appearance on CT and MR. They are sometimes labeled as "occult vascular malformations" because their angiographic appearance is usually normal, and the malformation is hidden or "occult," but occasionally, a faint blush is seen. These lesions have no mass effect or edema. CT findings consist of a focal hyperdense enhancing lesion that may contain calcification. Unlike some neoplasms, mass effect and edema are not commonly associated with vascular malformations.[95] The optimal imaging modality for diagnosing occult vascular malformations is MR, because CT cannot reliably distinguish these lesions from low-grade neoplasms. Occult vascular malformations have a characteristic pattern on MR.[96] A reticulated hyperintense focus in the center of the lesion is indicative of subacute or chronic hemorrhage. This is surrounded by a rim of signal void, representing paramagnetic hemosiderin from a previous hemorrhage (Figures 2-3 and 2-10). The hemosiderin ring is best seen on gradient echo or T_2-weighted sequences. Initially, this MR appearance was thought to be pathognomonic for occult vascular malformations, but experience has shown that any hemorrhagic lesion, such as a hemorrhagic metastasis, can have these features.[97] However, a lesion with these characteristics in a seizure patient will almost always be an occult vascular malformation.[6]

Arteriovenous Malformations

Arteriovenous malformations are the most common congenital vascular malformation of the brain. The malformation consists of a group of vessels that form direct arteriovenous shunts without an intervening capillary network. Microscopically, the vessels are abnormal, thick-walled vascular channels that are neither purely arterial nor purely venous. Secondary changes such as thrombosis, calcification, hyalinosis, and fibrosis are common. Grossly, the lesion is a cluster of abnormally dilated vessels with variable amounts of ferritin and hemosiderin, and with adjacent parenchymal atrophy.[60] Several mechanisms have been proposed to explain the association of epilepsy with arteriovenous malformations, including focal cerebral ischemia due to arteriovenous shunting and steal phenomenon, gliosis of the surrounding brain tissue caused by subclinical hemorrhage or hemosiderin deposition, and secondary epileptogenesis in the temporal lobe.[30,98]

Epilepsy is second only to hemorrhage as the most common clinical presentation of arteriovenous malformations. The risk of seizure disorder in patients with arteriovenous malformations varies from 18% to 42%.[99,100] The risk of seizures developing increases with the size of the lesion, proximity to the cerebral cortex, and involvement of the frontal or temporal lobes.[99–104] Improvement in seizure control usually occurs after treatment with embolization, radiosurgery, or surgical excision.[30] Although previous reports questioned the efficacy of surgical treatment for seizure relief, recent reports indicate that surgical excision of an arteriovenous malformation is an effective method of seizure control.[30,56,99–101,105–108] In a series of 54 patients who underwent surgical excision of seizure-producing arteriovenous malformations, good to excellent seizure control was achieved in 89%. This study by Yeh et al.[106] emphasized the role of electrophysiologic testing in guiding the extent of cortical resection in patients with arteriovenous malformations. In a retrospective study of 280 patients with angiographically documented arteriovenous malformations, new seizures developed postoperatively in only 6% of 136 patients without seizures preoperatively. Surgical outcome in those with preoperative seizures was excellent: 83% were seizure-free, and 13% had a worthwhile improvement in their seizure rate.[100]

Arteriovenous malformations have a characteristic angiographic appearance. Dilated tortuous arteries are seen entering a dense nidus, with early venous drainage indicating arteriovenous shunting (Figure 2-11). Noncontrast CT findings are normal or show a region of increased attenuation. An arteriovenous malformation occasionally may be surrounded by hypodensity that represents atrophy or edema. After administration of a contrast agent, CT demonstrates dilated serpiginous structures that represent dilated vessels (in 90% of cases), with little mass effect.[109] Certain arteriovenous malformations may be difficult to detect or characterize with CT, including ones that are small, thrombosed or partially thrombosed, or have hemorrhaged. Although CT

and MR are nearly equal in their rate of detecting arteriovenous malformations, angioarchitectural features are better assessed with MR. Both T_1- and T_2-weighted sequences demonstrate a region of serpiginous flow voids that represents the nidus, dilated arterial supply, and draining veins (see Figure 2-11). Interspersed in the signal voids are areas of heterogeneous signal from calcification, hemorrhage, and gliosis. MR is often able to define the nidus of a lesion, partly because of its multiplanar imaging capability. Gradient echo sequences can help discriminate between flowing blood and calcification. Contrast enhanced MR provides little additional information and is generally not needed in the evaluation of an arteriovenous malformation. MR angiography (MRA) can identify the arterial supply and venous drainage of an arteriovenous malformation. Currently, the role of MRA is secondary to conventional catheter angiography, because MRA does not have the spatial or temporal resolution of conventional angiography. MRA is excellent for defining the relationship of an arteriovenous malformation to adjacent brain structures and for noninvasively following these lesions.[110,111]

INDETERMINATE SUBSTRATES

The indeterminate substrate group consists of epileptogenic abnormalities that do not fit into the other well-defined substrate categories (medial temporal sclerosis, developmental, neoplastic, and vascular substrates). It includes infectious, inflammatory, post-traumatic, focal atrophic, and diffuse atrophic processes. Although the mechanism of seizure generation in this diverse group of abnormalities is not well understood, these abnormalities are often associated with gliosis. Prognosis is not as clearly defined for lesions in the indeterminate substrate category as it is for the other substrate groups (for example, medial temporal sclerosis and neoplastic and vascular substrates), partly because of the diverse nature of abnormalities found in the indeterminate category.

Infections

Infections are a frequent cause of seizures worldwide but are an uncommon cause in the United States. Recently, the number of seizures caused by infections in the United States has increased because of the spread of human immunodeficiency virus (HIV) and resistance of infections to antimicrobial therapy. In a study of 630 HIV patients, new-onset seizures occurred in 70. Seizures were due to the HIV infection in 32 of these patients, and to cerebral toxoplasmosis in 11, to cerebral lymphoma in 8, to metabolic derangement in 8, to cryptococcal meningitis in 7, and to vascular infarction in 4.[112] Infections typically present as ring-enhancing lesions associated with vasogenic edema. Lymphoma usually

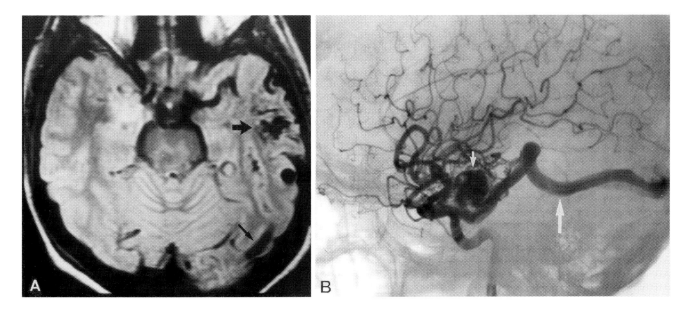

FIGURE 2-11. Arteriovenous malformation. A. A proton density-weighted axial image shows multiple serpiginous foci of signal void in the lateral aspect of the left temporal lobe. These represent flowing blood in the arteries, nidus (*large arrow*), and draining vein (*small arrow*) of an arteriovenous malformation. The left middle cerebral artery is enlarged. B. An image from a left internal carotid angiogram in the lateral projection demonstrates a round cluster of abnormal vessels (*small arrow*) with a prominent early draining vein (*large arrow*). (From Bronen et al.[6] Reprinted with permission of Elsevier Science.)

enhances homogeneously, but it may appear as a ring-enhancing lesion and be difficult to distinguish from infection.[113–115] Neurocysticercosis and tuberculosis are common causes of epilepsy in the Third World and are discussed separately.

Neurocysticercosis

Neurocysticercosis is one of the most common causes of epilepsy worldwide. In countries where the disease is endemic, cysticercosis affects 2% to 4% of the population.[116] Epilepsy is the most frequent sign of neurocysticercosis.[117] Patients may also present with focal neurologic deficits, altered mental status, movement disorders, headaches, and visual field abnormalities. Cysticercosis is caused by a pork parasite, *Taenia solium*. The immature larvae, after gaining access to the host's blood stream by penetrating the gastric mucosa, have a predilection for the CNS. Neurocysticercosis has four commonly described forms: parenchymal, meningeal, intraventricular, and mixed. In the parenchymal form, the most common form, parasites are found primarily in the gray matter. Within 2 to 3 months after the original ingestion of the parasite, mature parenchymal cysts develop. The mature parasite appears as a 3- to 30-mm

round vesicle containing a small eccentric nodule. The clear fluid in the cyst becomes turbid and gelatinous when the parasite dies.[118] The lesion eventually decreases in size, involutes, and finally calcifies. The amount of perilesional parenchymal inflammation incited by the lesion is dependent on the host response. Changes in the brain parenchyma caused by the infection include mass effect, edema, mononuclear infiltrates, and reactive gliosis.[119] The cysticidal drugs albendazole and praziquantel are effective in the treatment of neurocysticercosis and improve the prognosis of patients with seizures by either decreasing the frequency of seizures or eliminating them.[119]

CT and MR findings reflect the various forms and stages of cysticercosis (Figure 2-12). In the acute phase, imaging may show a small focus of edema or uniform enhancement. When the parasite is alive and there is little host reaction, a cystic mass that lacks significant enhancement or edema may be seen. At this stage, MR is more sensitive than CT.[120] The MR appearance is that of a cystic mass, isointense to CSF, and containing a hyperintense mural nodule best detected on long TR/short TE sequences.[120,121] Death of the larvae leads to an exuberant host reaction and a fibrous capsule. At this stage, imaging demonstrates a ring-enhancing cystic

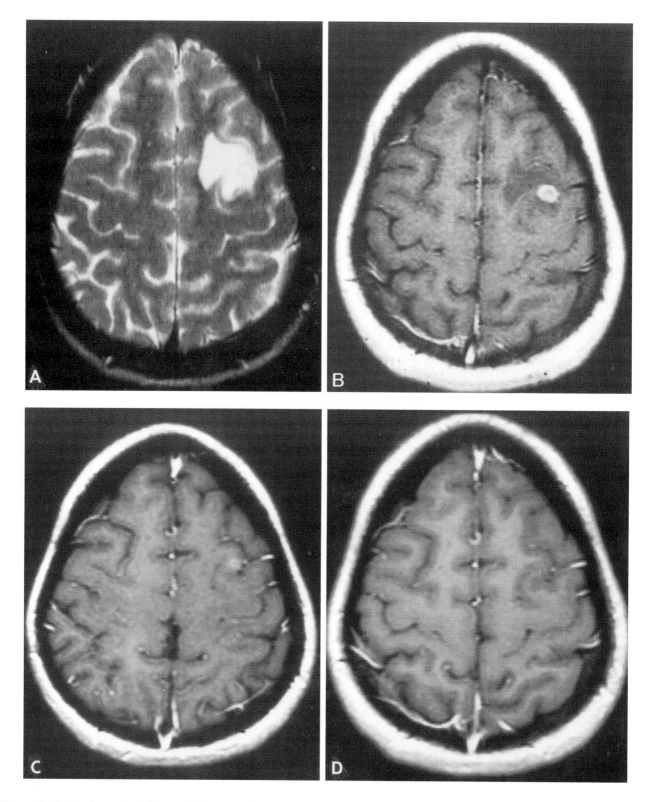

FIGURE 2-12. Cysticercosis. A 30-year-old woman who traveled extensively to Mexico as a teenager presented with seizures. A. T_2-weighted and (B) contrast-enhanced T_1-weighted axial images show a left frontal ring-enhancing lesion with considerable mass effect and edema. Although the differential diagnosis included cysticercosis, abscess, primary neoplasm, and metastatic disease, the travel history suggested cysticercosis. C. Contrast MR after 1 month of treatment with praziquantel shows the lesion has diminished in size and shows less intense contrast enhancement. The mass effect and edema associated with the lesion have also regressed. D. Nine months after treatment, the contrast-enhanced image shows no residual abnormalities. (From Friedland and Bronen.[150] Reprinted with permission of WB Saunders Company.)

mass associated with edema. As the host inflammatory response diminishes, lesion enhancement and surrounding edema also decrease. The lesion eventually involutes, leaving residual focal calcification or normal parenchyma. CT demonstrates parenchymal calcifications better than MR.[121]

Tuberculomas

Tuberculomas are focal granulomatous nodules of chronic inflammatory tissue containing areas of caseous necrosis caused by acid-fast bacilli.[60] Although tuberculomas are uncommon in the United States, they constitute between 10% and 40% of intracranial mass lesions in people in developing nations.[122–124] Tuberculomas are most common in children and young adults. CNS involvement with tuberculosis is believed to occur through hematogenous spread from the lung or gut, although at presentation only a small percentage of patients have positive findings on chest radiographs.[125] Patients with intracranial tuberculomas may present with focal seizures or increased intracranial pressure, but otherwise, they often are neurologically intact. In a series of 30 pathologically proven intracranial tuberculomas, 28 presented with focal seizures.[126]

The CT appearance of parenchymal tuberculomas is nonspecific. They may be solid or ring-enhancing and solitary or multiple (10% to 34% of cases).[127] The thickness of ring enhancement and associated edema varies considerably. Calcification is rare, occurring in only 1% to 6% of tuberculomas.[128] The MR appearance is also variable, depending on the amount of macrophages, fibrosis, and gliosis.[129] As the amount of these components increases, the granulomas tend to become more hypointense on T_2-weighted sequences.[126] Tuberculomas and adjacent edema are usually hypointense on T_1-weighted images. After the intravenous administration of gadolinium, a nodular or ring-like enhancement is observed. The MR features of these lesions are nonspecific, and the differential diagnosis includes many space-occupying lesions, such as neoplasms and other infections.[124]

Atrophic Processes

Tissue loss, which may be focal or diffuse, is the result of many phenomena, including infections, infarctions, and trauma. Most focal atrophic processes associated with epilepsy are the result of trauma. Diffuse atrophy involves large sections of the brain or an entire cerebral hemisphere. It is usually due to perinatal insults but can be caused by such entities as Sturge-Weber syndrome, Rasmussen's encephalitis, and infantile spasms.[130,131] Diffuse atrophic entities associated with medically refractory epilepsy may be amenable to surgical treatment, usually functional hemispherectomy or corpus calloso-

tomy.[130] Hippocampal sclerosis is a specialized atrophic process that is discussed in chapters 4, 5, and 6.

Trauma

Head trauma has been recognized as a cause of epilepsy for thousands of years.[58] In our society, the large number of head injuries that occur makes the prevalence of post-traumatic epilepsy significant.[132] Motor vehicle accidents alone account for 500,000 head injuries annually in the United States.[133] However, post-traumatic epilepsy develops in only a small proportion of patients with head injuries. Commonly accepted risk factors for the development of late-onset seizures include severe head trauma (especially missile injuries that pierce the dura mater), early post-traumatic seizures (seizures occurring within the first week after the event), intracranial hemorrhage, and depressed skull fractures.[134,135] Acutely, CT may document post-traumatic hemorrhages such as intracerebral bleeding and may identify extra-axial collections of blood. Months after the injury, cortical and subcortical atrophy may be detected with CT or MR.[136]

Perinatal/Neonatal Insults

Perinatal and neonatal causes of epilepsy represent a diverse group of insults rather than a discrete disease entity. These processes commonly include birth hypoxia, metabolic disorders, infections, and intracranial hemorrhage. Focal, hemispheric, or global injury to the brain may result. Seizure foci arise from partially viable tissue, regions that are hyperintense on long TR images (Figure 2-13). Areas isointense to CSF on all pulse sequences usually represent areas of complete tissue loss or macrocystic changes. The role of MR is to assess accurately the location and extent of tissue damage in patients deemed to be surgical candidates.[137]

Sturge-Weber Syndrome

Sturge-Weber syndrome (encephalotrigeminal angiomatosis) is a neurocutaneous syndrome characterized by the association of a facial capillary angioma with ipsilateral leptoangiomatosis. This disease is believed to be due to the persistence of embryonic vasculature.[138] Most cases are considered sporadic, without a sex predilection.

The clinical hallmarks of the disease are unilateral cutaneous facial nevus, epilepsy, mental retardation, hemiplegia, and ocular abnormalities. Like other neurocutaneous syndromes, there is wide variability in the clinical manifestations of Sturge-Weber syndrome. Epilepsy is a prominent feature of this disease and is the most common and usually the first neurologic manifestation of the disorder. Seizures occur in 71% to 89% of affected children, usually before 2 years of age.[139–141] Patients with

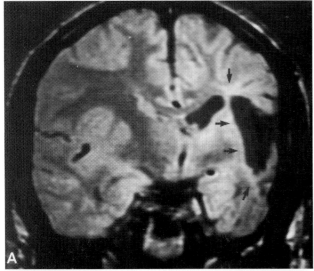

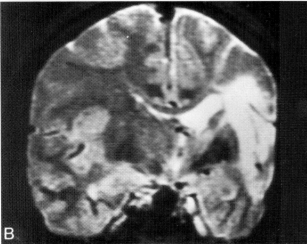

FIGURE 2-13. Diffuse atrophic process. A. Coronal proton density and (B) T$_2$-weighted images demonstrate a small left cerebral hemisphere with complete tissue loss adjacent to the sylvian fissure. The findings are consistent with perinatal infarction of the middle cerebral artery. The vague hyperintense rim (*arrows*) surrounding the area of complete tissue loss represents gliosis and is usually responsible for multifocal seizure generation in patients with perinatal insults. (From Bronen.[35] Reprinted with permission of the American Roentgen Ray Society.)

bihemispheric involvement (15%) are more likely to present earlier with seizures.[139]

CT and MR findings in Sturge-Weber syndrome usually include hemiatrophy, cortical calcification, and enhancement of the pial angioma (Figure 2-14). Unilateral cerebral atrophy is frequently accompanied by secondary changes such as thickening of the ipsilateral hemicranium and enlargement of the frontal sinus and petrous bone. The cortical calcification, commonly found in the parietal and occipital lobes, has been described as serpiginous, gyriform, or "tram-track–like" in appearance. It appears to be due to cortical hypoxia related to lack of normal cortical draining veins. The characteristic cortical calcifications are seen best with CT but can be imaged with MR by using gradient echo imaging techniques.[142] Cortical calcification may not be as conspicuous in younger children as in older children whose disease has progressed. Enlargement and calcification of the ipsilateral choroid plexus may also be seen.[143] Although the above findings are all part of the spectrum of Sturge-Weber syndrome, demonstration of the pial angioma (adjacent to cerebral atrophy) on contrast MR is the most important criterion for making the diagnosis on the basis of imaging findings. Marked enhancement of the leptomeninges and choroid plexus occurs after gadolinium injection[144] (see Figure 2-14). The differential diagnosis of patients with cortical calcification associated with epilepsy includes a syndrome of folate deficiency associated with celiac disease, epilepsy, and occipital calcifications.[145,146]

Rasmussen's Encephalitis

Intractable seizures due to chronic encephalitis were first described by Rasmussen et al. in 1958.[147] The hallmark of Rasmussen's (chronic) encephalitis is intractable epilepsy beginning in childhood and leading to severe neurologic and mental impairment. The onset of seizures begins before the age of 11 years in 85% of patients. An antecedent history of an infectious or inflammatory episode involving the patient or a family member is present in two thirds of the patients.[148] Medically refractory epilepsy, hemiparesis, dysphasia, and hemianopia develop in the patient. Although the disease is self-limited and rarely fatal, only 10% of patients are left with no permanent neurologic deficit.[149] Rasmussen's encephalitis tends to localize in one hemisphere, but it can be bilateral.[149] Early microscopic changes parallel those identified in viral infections. These include perivascular cuffing most prominent in the cerebral cortex, scattered glial nodules, and diffuse proliferation of microglia. Late pathologic changes of cortical atrophy, scattered spongy degeneration, and neuronal cell loss without evidence of inflammatory cells are observed. Research results raise the possibility that autoantibodies to a glutamate receptor (glutamate is an excitatory neurotransmitter) may increase neuronal excitation and lead to seizures.[150]

At the onset of symptoms, CT and MR examination results are often normal.[149] CT scans performed later in the course of the disease show marked unihemispheric atrophy with ipsilateral ventriculomegaly. Some atrophic changes may be seen in the contralateral hemisphere, although these changes may be due to the chronic anoxia and trauma produced by the seizures.[24] MR experience with Rasmussen's encephalitis is limited.

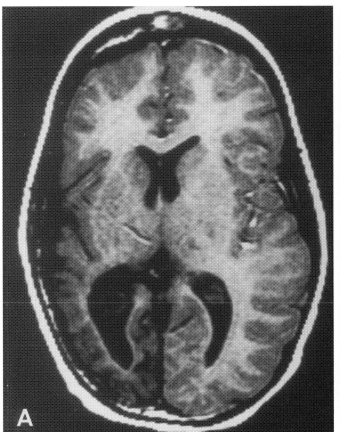

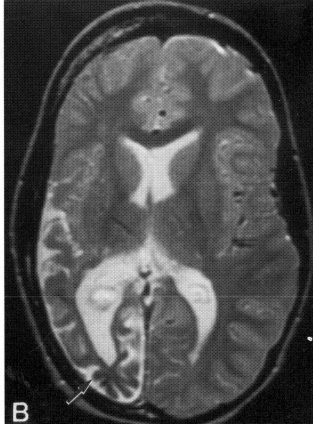

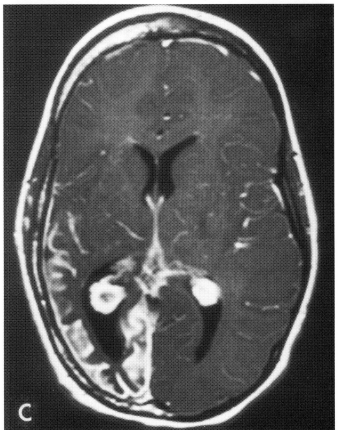

FIGURE 2-14. Sturge-Weber syndrome. A. T_1-weighted axial image demonstrates right hemiatrophy with localized parieto-occipital volume loss and enlargement of the adjacent lateral ventricle. B. Gyriform hypointensity (*arrow*) is seen on the T_2-weighted image and is indicative of either dystrophic calcification or hemosiderin. C. A contrast-enhanced T_1-weighted image shows the classic meningeal enhancement and ipsilateral enlargement of the choroid plexus. (From Friedland and Bronen.[150] Reprinted with permission of WB Saunders Company.)

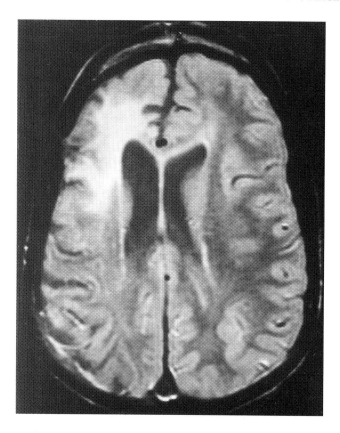

FIGURE 2-15. Rasmussen's encephalitis. This child had persistent seizures for years. A proton density axial image shows abnormal high signal throughout the white matter of the right frontal lobe. In patients with long-standing Rasmussen's encephalitis, there is often volume loss involving an entire hemisphere, as in this patient. (From Friedland and Bronen.[150] Reprinted with permission of WB Saunders Company.)

Findings of the involved hemisphere on T_2-weighted images include significant unilateral atrophic changes and hyperintensity, which may represent edema, in the periventricular region and basal ganglia[149,151,152] (Figure 2-15). This syndrome is often refractory to medical treatment. Antiepileptic medication may contribute to a decline in a patient's overall deteriorating condition. Hemispherectomy is often necessary to control the patient's seizures.

CONCLUSION

MR has a prominent and often pivotal role in the evaluation of epilepsy due to focal lesions. It is the best imaging modality for detecting and categorizing focal lesions. Decisions about surgical treatment of epileptogenic lesions depend on MR findings about lesion location and identity. When MR reveals an underlying focal structural abnormality in a patient with medically refractory epilepsy, the probability that the seizure disorder is amenable to surgical treatment and cure is increased.

Acknowledgments

We wish to thank Ann Wrider and Janice Weinstein, M.D., for their editorial comments.

REFERENCES

1. Jackson JH, Beevor CE. Case of tumour of the right temporo-sphenoidal lobe bearing on the localisation of the sense of smell and on the interpretation of a particular variety of epilepsy. Brain 1889–1890;12:346–57.

2. Awad IA, Rosenfeld J, Ahl J, et al. Intractable epilepsy and structural lesions of the brain: mapping, resection strategies, and seizure outcome. Epilepsia 1991;32:179–86.

3. Cascino GD, Boon PAJM, Fish DR. Surgically remediable lesional syndromes. In: Engel J Jr, ed. Surgical treatment of the epilepsies. 2nd ed. New York: Raven Press, 1993:77–86.

4. Fried I, Kim JH, Spencer DD. Limbic and neocortical gliomas associated with intractable seizures: a distinct clinicopathological group. Neurosurgery 1994;34:815–23.

5. Kuzniecky R, Burgard S, Faught E, et al. Predictive value of magnetic resonance imaging in temporal lobe epilepsy surgery. Arch Neurol 1993;50:65–9.

6. Bronen RA, Fulbright RK, Spencer DD, et al. MR characteristics of neoplasms and vascular malformations associated with epilepsy. Magn Reson Imaging 1995;13:1153–62.

7. Spencer DD. Classifying the epilepsies by substrate. Clin Neurosci 1994;2:104–9.

8. Kuzniecky RI, Cascino GD, Palmini A, et al. Structural neuroimaging. In: Engel J Jr, ed. Surgical treatment of the epilepsies. 2nd ed. New York: Raven Press, 1993:197–209.

9. Kuzniecky R, de la Sayette V, Ethier R, et al. Magnetic resonance imaging in temporal lobe epilepsy: pathological correlations. Ann Neurol 1987;22:341–7.

10. Babb TL, Brown WJ, Pretorius J, et al. Temporal lobe volumetric cell densities in temporal lobe epilepsy. Epilepsia 1984;25:729–40.

11. Cascino GD, Jack CR Jr, Parisi JE, et al. Operative strategy in patients with MRI-identified dual pathology and temporal lobe epilepsy. Epilepsy Res 1993;14:175–82.

12. Cendes F, Andermann F, Gloor P, et al. Atrophy of mesial structures in patients with temporal lobe epilepsy: cause or consequence of repeated seizures? Ann Neurol 1993;34:795–801.

13. Hauser WA, Kurland LT. The epidemiology of epilepsy in Rochester, Minnesota, 1935 through 1967. Epilepsia 1975;16:1–66.

14. Bronen RA. Epilepsy: the role of MR imaging. AJR Am J Roentgenol 1992;159:1165–74.

15. Mathieson G. Pathology of temporal lobe foci. Adv Neurol 1975;11:163–85.

16. Heinz ER, Crain BJ, Radtke RA, et al. MR imaging in patients with temporal lobe seizures: correlation of results with pathologic findings. AJR Am J Roentgenol 1990;155:581–6.

17. Dowd CF, Dillon WP, Barbaro NM, et al. Magnetic resonance imaging of intractable complex partial seizures: pathologic and electroencephalographic correlation. Epilepsia 1991;32:454–9.

18. Currie S, Heathfield KW, Henson RA, et al. Clinical course and prognosis of temporal lobe epilepsy. A survey of 666 patients. Brain 1971;94:173–90.

19. Boon PA, Williamson PD, Fried I, et al. Intracranial, intraaxial, space-occupying lesions in patients with intractable partial seizures: an anatomo-clinical, neuropsychological, and surgical correlation. Epilepsia 1991;32:467–76.

20. Babb TL, Brown WJ. Pathological findings in epilepsy. In: Engel J Jr, ed. Surgical treatment of the epilepsies. New York: Raven Press, 1987:511–40.

21. Brooks BS, King DW, el Gammal T, et al. MR imaging in patients with intractable complex partial epileptic seizures. AJNR Am J Neuroradiol 1990;11:93–9.

22. Bruton CJ. The neuropathology of temporal lobe epilepsy. Oxford: Oxford University Press, 1988.

23. Spencer SS. Surgical options for uncontrolled epilepsy. Neurol Clin 1986;4:669–95.

24. Engel J Jr, Van Ness PC, Rasmussen TB, et al. Outcome with respect to epileptic seizures. In: Engel J Jr, ed. Surgical treatment of the epilepsies. 2nd ed. New York: Raven Press, 1993:609–21.

25. Engel J Jr. Seizures and epilepsy. Philadelphia: FA Davis Company, 1989:71–111.

26. Gloor P. Approaches to localization of the epileptogenic lesion. In: Engel J Jr, ed. Surgical treatment of the epilepsies. New York: Raven Press, 1987:97–100.

27. Canapicchi R, Padolecchia R, Puglioli M, et al. Heterotopic gray matter. Neuroradiological aspects and clinical correlations. J Neuroradiol 1990;17:277–87.

28. Echlin F. The supersensitivity of chronically "isolated" cerebral cortex as a mechanism in focal epilepsy. Electroencephalogr Clin Neurophysiol 1959;11:697–722.

29. Ketz E. Brain tumours and epilepsy. In: Vinken PJ, Bruyn GW, eds. Handbook of clinical neurology. Vol. 16. Tumours of the brain and skull. Amsterdam: North-Holland, 1974:254–69.

30. Kraemer DL, Awad IA. Vascular malformations and epilepsy: clinical considerations and basic mechanisms. Epilepsia 1994;35 Suppl 6:S30–S43.

31. Cascino GD, Jack CR Jr, Hirschorn KA, et al. Identification of the epileptic focus: magnetic resonance imaging. Epilepsy Res Suppl 1992;5:95–100.

32. Dowd CF, Dillon WP, Barbaro NM. Intractable complex partial seizure: correlation of magnetic resonance imaging with pathology and electroencephalography. Epilepsy Res Suppl 1992;5:101–10.

33. Sperling MR, Wilson G, Engel J Jr, et al. Magnetic resonance imaging in intractable partial epilepsy: correlative studies. Ann Neurol 1986;20:57–62.

34. Wolf HK, Campos MG, Zentner J, et al. Surgical pathology of temporal lobe epilepsy. Experience with 216 cases. J Neuropathol Exp Neurol 1993;52:499–506.

35. Bronen RA. Evaluation of the seizure patient. In: Huckman MS, Harwood-Nash DC, Forbes GS, eds. ARRS: Neuroradiology categorical course syllabus. Reston, Virginia: American Roentgen Ray Society, 1992:147–57.

36. Spencer SS, Spencer DD, Schwartz SS. The treatment of epilepsy with surgery. Merritt-Putnam Q 1988;5:3–17.

37. Van Buren JM. Complications of surgical procedures in the diagnosis and treatment of epilepsy. In: Engel J Jr, ed. Surgical treatment of the epilepsies. New York: Raven Press, 1987:465–75.

38. Sperling MR, Cahan LD, Brown WJ. Relief of seizures from a predominantly posterior temporal tumor with anterior temporal lobectomy. Epilepsia 1989;30:559–63.

39. Olivier A, Gloor P, Andermann F, et al. Occipitotemporal epilepsy studied with stereotaxically implanted depth electrodes and successfully treated by temporal resection. Ann Neurol 1982;11:428–32.

40. Fish D, Andermann F, Olivier A. Complex partial seizures and posterior temporal or extratemporal lesions: surgical management. Neurology 1991;41:1781–4.

41. Bergen D, Bleck T, Ramsey R, et al. Magnetic resonance imaging as a sensitive and specific predictor of neoplasms removed for intractable epilepsy. Epilepsia 1989;30:318–21.

42. Jack CR Jr. Epilepsy: surgery and imaging. Radiology 1993;189:635–46.

43. Bergin PS, Fish DR, Shorvon SD, et al. FLAIR imaging in partial epilepsy: improving the yield of MRI (abstract). Epilepsia 1993;34 Suppl 6:121.

44. Jackson GD, Berkovic SF, Duncan JS, et al. Optimizing the diagnosis of hippocampal sclerosis using MR imaging. AJNR Am J Neuroradiol 1993;14:753–62.

45. Tien RD, Felsberg GJ, Campi de Castro C, et al. Complex partial seizures and mesial temporal sclerosis: evaluation with fast spin-echo MR imaging. Radiology 1993;189:835–42.

46. Cascino GD, Hirschorn KA, Jack CR, et al. Gadolinium-DTPA–enhanced magnetic resonance imaging in intractable partial epilepsy. Neurology 1989;39:1115–8.

47. Elster AD, Mirza W. MR imaging in chronic partial epilepsy: role of contrast enhancement. AJNR Am J Neuroradiol 1991;12:165–70.

48. Drake J, Hoffman HJ, Kobayashi J, et al. Surgical management of children with temporal lobe epilepsy and mass lesions. Neurosurgery 1987;21:792–7.

49. Kim JH, Guimaraes PO, Shen MY, et al. Hippocampal neuronal density in temporal lobe epilepsy with and without gliomas. Acta Neuropathol (Berl) 1990;80:41–5.

50. de Lanerolle NC, Kim JH, Robbins RJ, et al. Hippocampal interneuron loss and plasticity in human temporal lobe epilepsy. Brain Res 1989;495:387–95.

51. Jay V, Becker LE, Otsubo H, et al. Pathology of temporal lobectomy for refractory seizures in children. Review of 20 cases including some unique malformative lesions. J Neurosurg 1993;79:53–61.

52. Duchowny M, Levin B, Jayakar P, et al. Temporal lobectomy in early childhood. Epilepsia 1992;33:298–303.

53. Morris HH, Estes ML, Gilmore W, et al. Primary brain tumors in patients with chronic epilepsy: EEG, neuroimaging, neuropathologic, and clinical findings (abstract). Epilepsia 1989;30:660.

54. Spencer DD, Spencer SS, Mattson RH, et al. Intracerebral masses in patients with intractable partial epilepsy. Neurology 1984;34:432–6.

55. Theodore WH, Katz D, Kufta C, et al. Pathology of temporal lobe foci: correlation with CT, MRI, and PET. Neurology 1990;40:797–803.

56. Rasmussen T. Surgery of epilepsy associated with brain tumors. Adv Neurol 1975;8:227–39.

57. Hirsch JF. Epilepsy and brain tumours in children. J Neuroradiol 1989;16:292–300.

58. Le Blanc FE, Rasmussen T. Cerebral seizures and brain tumors. In: Vinken PJ, Bruyn GW, eds. Handbook of clinical neurology. Vol 15. The epilepsies. Amsterdam: North-Holland, 1974: 295–301.

59. Penfield W, Erickson T, Tarlov I. Relation of intracranial tumors and symptomatic epilepsy. Arch Neurol Psychiatry 1940;44:300–15.

60. Okazaki H. Fundamentals of neuropathology. New York: Igaku-Shoin, 1983.

61. Spencer SS, Spencer DD, Kim JH, et al. Gliomas in chronic epilepsy. In: Wolf P, Janz D, Dreifuss FE, eds. Advances in epileptology. New York: Raven Press, 1987:39–41.

62. Atlas SW. Intraaxial brain tumors. In: Atlas SW, ed. Magnetic resonance imaging of the brain and spine. New York: Raven Press, 1991:223–326.

63. Holland BA, Kucharcyzk W, Brant-Zawadski M, et al. MR imaging of calcified intracranial lesions. Radiology 1985;157:353–6.

64. Masters LT, Zimmerman RD. Imaging of supratentorial brain tumors in adults. Neuroimaging Clin North Am 1993;3:649–69.

65. Russell DS, Rubinstein LJ. Pathology of tumors of the nervous system. 5th ed. Baltimore: Williams & Wilkins, 1989.

66. Burger PC, Scheithauer BW, Vogel FS. Surgical pathology of the nervous system and its coverings. 3rd ed. New York: Churchill Livingstone, 1987.

67. Mork SJ, Lindegaard KF, Halvorsen TB, et al. Oligodendroglioma: incidence and biological behavior in a defined population. J Neurosurg 1985;63:881–9.

68. Lee YY, Van Tassel P. Intracranial oligodendrogliomas: imaging findings in 35 untreated cases. AJR Am J Roentgenol 1989;152:361–9.

69. Dorne HL, O'Gorman AM, Melanson D. Computed tomography of intracranial gangliogliomas. AJNR Am J Neuroradiol 1986;7:281–5.

70. Johannsson JH, Rekate HL, Roessmann U. Gangliogliomas: pathological and clinical correlation. J Neurosurg 1981;54:58–63.

71. Demierre B, Stichnoth FA, Hori A, et al. Intracerebral ganglioglioma. J Neurosurg 1986;65:177–82.

72. Sutton LN, Packer RJ, Rorke LB, et al. Cerebral gangliogliomas during childhood. Neurosurgery 1983;13:124–8.

73. Ventureyra E, Herder S, Mallya BK, et al. Temporal lobe gangliogliomas in children. Childs Nerv Syst 1986;2:63–6.

74. Castillo M, Davis PC, Takei Y, et al. Intracranial ganglioglioma: MR, CT, and clinical findings in 18 patients. AJNR Am J Neuroradiol 1990;11:109–14.

75. Chamberlain MC, Press GA. Temporal lobe ganglioglioma in refractory epilepsy: CT and MR in three cases. J Neurooncol 1990;9:81–7.

76. Daumas-Duport C, Scheithauer BW, Chodkiewicz JP, et al. Dysembryoplastic neuroepithelial tumor: a surgically curable tumor of young patients with intractable partial seizures. Report of thirty-nine cases. Neurosurgery 1988;23:545–56.

77. Armstrong DD. The neuropathology of temporal lobe epilepsy. J Neuropathol Exp Neurol 1993; 52:433–43.

78. Kirkpatrick PJ, Honavar M, Janota I, et al. Control of temporal lobe epilepsy following en bloc resection of low-grade tumors. J Neurosurg 1993;78:19–25.

79. Koeller KK, Dillon WP. Dysembryoplastic neuroepithelial tumors: MR appearance. AJNR Am J Neuroradiol 1992;13:1319–25.

80. Vali AM, Clarke MA, Kelsey A. Dysembryoplastic neuroepithelial tumour as a potentially treatable cause of intractable epilepsy in children. Clin Radiol 1993;47:255–8.

81. Kuroiwa T, Kishikawa T, Kato A, et al. Dysembryoplastic neuroepithelial tumors: MR findings. J Comput Assist Tomogr 1994;18:352–6.

82. Chugani HT, Shields WD, Shewmon DA, et al. Infantile spasms: I. PET identifies focal cortical dysgenesis in cryptogenic cases for surgical treatment. Ann Neurol 1990;27:406–13.

83. Byrd SE, Osborn RE, Radkowski MA. The MR evaluation of pachygyria and associated syndromes. Eur J Radiol 1991;12:53–9.

84. Kuzniecky R, Garcia JH, Faught E, et al. Cortical dysplasia in temporal lobe epilepsy: magnetic

resonance imaging correlations. Ann Neurol 1991;29:293–8.

85. Duncan R, Patterson J, Hadley DM, et al. CT, MR and SPECT imaging in temporal lobe epilepsy. J Neurol Neurosurg Psychiatry 1990;53:11–5.

86. Robinson JR, Awad IA, Little JR. Natural history of the cavernous angioma. J Neurosurg 1991;75:709–14.

87. Rigamonti D, Johnson PC, Spetzler RF, et al. Cavernous malformations and capillary telangiectasia: a spectrum within a single pathological entity. Neurosurgery 1991;28:60–4.

88. Clark JV. Familial occurrence of cavernous angiomata of the brain. J Neurol Neurosurg Psychiatry 1970;33:871–6.

89. Voigt K, Yasargil MG. Cerebral cavernous haemangiomas or cavernomas. Incidence, pathology, localization, diagnosis, clinical features and treatment. Review of the literature and report of an unusual case. Neurochirurgia (Stuttg) 1976;19:59–68.

90. McCormick WF, Hardman JM, Boulter TR. Vascular malformations ("angiomas") of the brain, with special reference to those occurring in the posterior fossa. J Neurosurg 1968;28:241–51.

91. Rigamonti D, Hadley MN, Drayer BP, et al. Cerebral cavernous malformations. Incidence and familial occurrence. N Engl J Med 1988;319:343–7.

92. Fortuna A, Ferrante L, Mastronardi L, et al. Cerebral cavernous angioma in children. Childs Nerv Syst 1989;5:201–7.

93. Cascino GD, Kelly PJ, Hirschorn KA, et al. Stereotactic resection of intra-axial cerebral lesions in partial epilepsy. Mayo Clin Proc 1990;65:1053–60.

94. Schneider RC, Liss L. Cavernous hemangiomas of the cerebral hemispheres. J Neurosurg 1958;15:392–9.

95. Kucharczyk W, Lemme-Pleghos L, Uske A, et al. Intracranial vascular malformations: MR and CT imaging. Radiology 1985;156:383–9.

96. Gomori JM, Grossman RI, Goldberg HI, et al. Occult cerebral vascular malformations: high-field MR imaging. Radiology 1986;158:707–13.

97. Sze G, Krol G, Olsen WL, et al. Hemorrhagic neoplasms: MR mimics of occult vascular malformations. AJR Am J Roentgenol 1987;149:1223–30.

98. Yeh HS, Tew JM. Management of arteriovenous malformations of the brain. Contemp Neurosurg 1988;9:1–8.

99. Crawford PM, West CR, Chadwick DW, et al. Arteriovenous malformations of the brain: natural history in unoperated patients. J Neurol Neurosurg Psychiatry 1986;49:1–10.

100. Piepgras DG, Sundt TM Jr, Ragoowansi AT, et al. Seizure outcome in patients with surgically treated cerebral arteriovenous malformations. J Neurosurg 1993;78:5–11.

101. Crawford PM, West CR, Shaw MD, et al. Cerebral arteriovenous malformations and epilepsy: fac-

tors in the development of epilepsy. Epilepsia 1986;27:270–5.

102. Heros RC, Tu YK. Is surgical therapy needed for unruptured arteriovenous malformations? Neurology 1987;37:279–86.

103. Ondra SL, Troupp H, George ED, et al. The natural history of symptomatic arteriovenous malformations of the brain: a 24-year follow-up assessment. J Neurosurg 1990;73:387–91.

104. Trussart V, Berry I, Manelfe C, et al. Epileptogenic cerebral vascular malformations and MRI. J Neuroradiol 1989;16:273–84.

105. Aminoff MJ. Treatment of unruptured cerebral arteriovenous malformations. Neurology 1987;37:815–9.

106. Yeh HS, Tew JM Jr, Gartner M. Seizure control after surgery on cerebral arteriovenous malformations. J Neurosurg 1993;78:12–8.

107. Parkinson D, Bachers G. Arteriovenous malformations. Summary of 100 consecutive supratentorial cases. J Neurosurg 1980;53:285–99.

108. Forster DM, Steiner L, Hakanson S. Arteriovenous malformations of the brain. A long-term clinical study. J Neurosurg 1972;37:562–70.

109. Heinz ER, Dubois P, Osborne D, et al. Dynamic computed tomography study of the brain. J Comput Assist Tomogr 1979;3:641–9.

110. Atlas SW. Intracranial vascular malformations and aneurysms. In: Atlas SW, ed. Magnetic resonance imaging of the brain and spine. New York: Raven Press, 1991:379–409.

111. Smith HJ, Strother CM, Kikuchi Y, et al. MR imaging in the management of supratentorial intracranial AVMs. AJR Am J Roentgenol 1988;150:1143–53.

112. Wong MC, Suite NDA, Labar DR. Seizures in human immunodeficiency virus infection. Arch Neurol 1990;47:640–2.

113. Orron DE, Kuhn MJ, Malholtra V, et al. Primary cerebral lymphoma in acquired immunodeficiency syndrome (AIDS)—CT manifestations. Comput Med Imaging Graph 1989;13:207–14.

114. Namasivayam J, Teasdale E. The prognostic importance of CT features in primary intracranial lymphoma. Br J Radiol 1992;65:761–5.

115. Tan EC, Wakabayashi S, Kanai H, et al. Ring-enhanced primary intracranial malignant lymphoma—report of two cases. Neurol Med Chir (Tokyo) 1991;31:214–8.

116. Del Brutto OH, Sotelo J. Neurocysticercosis: an update. Rev Infect Dis 1988;10:1075–87.

117. Sotelo J, Guerrero V, Rubio F. Neurocysticercosis: a new classification based on active and inactive forms. A study of 753 cases. Arch Intern Med 1985;145:442–5.

118. Escobar A. The pathology of neurocysticercosis. In: Palacios E, Rodríguez-Carbajal J, Taveras JM, eds. Cysticercosis of the central nervous system. Springfield, Illinois: Charles C Thomas, 1983:27–54.

119. Vazquez V, Sotelo J. The course of seizures after treatment for cerebral cysticercosis. N Engl J Med 1992;327:696–701.

120. Suss RA, Maravilla KR, Thompson J. MR imaging of intracranial cysticercosis: comparison with CT and anatomopathologic features. AJNR Am J Neuroradiol 1986;7:235–42.

121. Teitelbaum GP, Otto RJ, Lin M, et al. MR imaging of neurocysticercosis. AJR Am J Roentgenol 1989;153:857–66.

122. Bhargava S, Tandon PN. Intracranial tuberculomas: a CT study. Br J Radiol 1980;53:935–45.

123. Ramamurthi B, Ramamurthi R, Vasudevan MC. Changing concepts in the treatment of tuberculomas of the brain. Childs Nerv Syst 1986;2:242–3.

124. Salgado P, Del Brutto OH, Talamas O, et al. Intracranial tuberculoma: MR imaging. Neuroradiology 1989;31:299–302.

125. Draouat S, Abdenabi B, Ghanem M, et al. Computed tomography of cerebral tuberculoma. J Comput Assist Tomogr 1987;11:594–7.

126. Gupta RK, Pandey R, Khan EM, et al. Intracranial tuberculomas: MRI signal intensity correlation with histopathology and localised proton spectroscopy. Magn Reson Imaging 1993;11:443–9.

127. Jinkins JR. Computed tomography of intracranial tuberculosis. Neuroradiology 1991;33:126–35.

128. Whelan MA, Stern J. Intracranial tuberculoma. Radiology 1981;138:75–81.

129. Bowen BC, Donovan Post MJ. Intracranial infection. In: Atlas SW, ed. Magnetic resonance imaging of the brain and spine. New York: Raven Press, 1991:501–38.

130. Andermann F, Freeman JM, Vigevano F, et al. Surgically remediable diffuse hemispheric syndromes. In: Engel J Jr, ed. Surgical treatment of the epilepsies. New York: Raven Press, 1993:87–101.

131. Cusmai R, Ricci S, Pinard JM, et al. West syndrome due to perinatal insults. Epilepsia 1993;34:738–42.

132. Dinner DS. Posttraumatic epilepsy. In: Wyllie E, ed. The treatment of epilepsy: principles and practice. Philadelphia: Lea & Febiger, 1993:654–8.

133. Kalsbeek WD, McLaurin RL, Harris BSH III, et al. The National Head and Spinal Cord Injury Survey: major findings. J Neurosurg 1980;53 Suppl:S11–9.

134. Jennett WB, Lewin W. Traumatic epilepsy after closed head injuries. J Neurol Neurosurg Psychiatry 1960;23:295–301.

135. Caveness WF. Onset and cessation of fits following craniocerebral trauma. J Neurosurg 1963;20:570–83.

136. Heikkinen ER, Ronty HS, Tolonen U, et al. Development of posttraumatic epilepsy. Stereotact Funct Neurosurg 1990;54–55:25–33.

137. Dietrich RB, el Saden S, Chugani HT, et al. Resective surgery for intractable epilepsy in children: radiologic evaluation. AJNR Am J Neuroradiol 1991;12:1149–58.

138. Roizin L, Gold G, Berman HH, et al. Congenital vascular anomalies and their histopathology in Sturge-Weber-Dimitri syndrome. J Neuropathol Exp Neurol 1959;18:75–97.

139. Bebin EM, Gomez MR. Prognosis in Sturge-Weber disease: comparison of unihemispheric and bihemispheric involvement. J Child Neurol 1988;3:181–4.

140. Peterman AF, Hayles AB, Dockerty MB, et al. Encephalotrigeminal angiomatosis (Sturge-Weber disease). Clinical study of thirty-five cases. JAMA 1958;167:2169–76.

141. Alexander GL. Sturge-Weber syndrome. In: Vinken PJ, Bruyn GW, eds. Handbook of clinical neurology. Vol 14. Amsterdam: North-Holland Publishing Company, 1972:223–40.

142. Atlas SW, Grossman RI, Hackney DB, et al. Calcified intracranial lesions: detection with gradient-echo-acquisition rapid MR imaging. AJNR Am J Neuroradiol 1988;9:253–9.

143. Wasenko JJ, Rosenbloom SA, Duchesneau PM, et al. The Sturge-Weber syndrome: comparison of MR and CT characteristics. AJNR Am J Neuroradiol 1990;11:131–4.

144. Benedikt RA, Brown DC, Walker R, et al. Sturge-Weber syndrome: cranial MR imaging with Gd-DTPA. AJNR Am J Neuroradiol 1993;14:409–15.

145. Gobbi G, Bouquet F, Greco L, et al. Coeliac disease, epilepsy, and cerebral calcifications. The Italian Working Group of Coeliac Disease and Epilepsy. Lancet 1992;340:439–43.

146. Gobbi G, Ambrosetto P, Zaniboni MG, et al. Celiac disease, posterior cerebral calcifications and epilepsy. Brain Dev 1992;14:23–9.

147. Rasmussen T, Olszweski J, Lloyd-Smith D. Focal seizures due to chronic localized encephalitis. Neurology 1958;8:435–45.

148. Rasmussen T, Andermann F. Update on the syndrome of "chronic encephalitis" and epilepsy. Cleve Clin J Med 1989;56 Suppl 2:S181–4.

149. Zupanc ML, Handler EG, Levine RL, et al. Rasmussen encephalitis: epilepsia partialis continua secondary to chronic encephalitis. Pediatr Neurol 1990;6:397–401.

150. Friedland RJ, Bronen RA. Magnetic resonance imaging of epilepsy. In: Edelman RR, Hesselink JR, Zlatkin MI, eds. Clinical magnetic resonance imaging. 2nd ed. Philadelphia: WB Saunders Company (in press).

151. English R, Soper N, Shepstone BJ, et al. Five patients with Rasmussen's syndrome investigated by single-photon–emission computed tomography. Nucl Med Commun 1989;10:5–14.

152. Tien RD, Ashdown BC, Lewis DV Jr, et al. Rasmussen's encephalitis: neuroimaging findings in four patients. AJR Am J Roentgenol 1992;158:1329–32.

Magnetic Resonance Imaging in Cerebral Developmental Malformations and Epilepsy

Ruben I. Kuzniecky

The development of magnetic resonance imaging (MRI) has permitted a previously undreamed of level of diagnosis in neurologic disorders and has significantly modified our understanding of epilepsy. It is well established that a multitude of neocortical lesions that are not only associated with epilepsy but directly responsible for it can be recognized in vivo with MRI.

Developmental cortical malformations are increasingly recognized as a major cause of epilepsy.[1-7] Recognition of these malformations during life is important because they are often associated with variable degrees of neurodevelopmental delay and intractable epilepsy. Recent studies have suggested that adequate recognition and classification of these disorders in patients with intractable epilepsy have important implications for surgical treatment and prognosis.[6,8,9]

Developmental malformations of the neocortex encompass various congenital entities that can be classified according to etiologic, pathologic, or morphologic features.[3,10] Although various cortical malformations have been recognized among these patients, epilepsy may not be the most relevant clinical problem in some of them. However, clinical and laboratory data indicate that developmental cortical malformations in general are intrinsically highly epileptogenic.

Although this chapter is not intended to provide a comprehensive review of normal cortical development, some of the essential events of fetal neuronal and cortical development are described (for additional details, see reference 11).

DEVELOPMENT OF THE CEREBRAL CORTEX

The development of the human nervous system begins with the formation of the notochord, which in turn induces the neural plate, a thickened area of embryonic ectoderm. The neural plate forms the neural tube, from which the spinal cord and brain develop. Shortly after this occurs, the prosencephalon and various cerebral and cerebellar structures develop. Development of the telencephalon results in two hemispheres and two lateral ventricles. This process occurs between the fifth and tenth weeks of gestation.

After the essential framework of the brain is established, complex processes of neuronal proliferation, differentiation, migration, and organization occur. The vast majority of neurons and a large number of glial cells are generated in the germinal zone,[11] which in the early phases of development is located at the ventricular surface.

The process of differentiation and migration of the cerebral cortex occurs in different stages, each one closely related to the next. In the first two stages, cell proliferation occurs. In the following stages, the major portions of the cerebral cortex (layers II to VI) develop in an inside-out fashion, with cells of layer VI migrating first and cells of layer II migrating last. There are two exceptions to this pattern: (1) neurons destined to migrate to the first layer (they may be the first ones generated and the first to arrive in the cortex) and (2) neurons destined to occupy layer VII (subplate layer), which is a transient layer.

The migration of cells from the germinal plate to their final destination in the cortex is a complex process that begins during the eighth gestational week. Studies have indicated that the neurons destined for the deepest layers leave the mitotic cycle first and migrate to form the cortical plate.[12] The correlation between the time of cell generation and the ultimate location of the cell in the cortex suggests that the time of generation (cell cycle) determines the position and function of the cell in the cortex.[13] Although experiments have suggested that environmental perturbations can alter the final position of cortical neurons, it appears that the cell cycle may be the determining factor. Most of the neurons that migrate into the cerebral cortex do so along specialized radial glial fibers. In the early stages of cortical development, radial glial fibers span the entire thickness of the hemisphere from the ventricle to the pia mater. The mechanism of migration may depend on surface proteins on the radial glial fibers, such as laminin, cytotactin, astrotactin, and integrins.[14] Other structures, such as thalamocortical axon bundles, may also be important in neuronal migration.

After completion of neuronal migration, radial glial fibers are transformed into astrocytes. The major cell migration activity begins at approximately the eighth fetal week and lasts about 2 months (that is, until about week 16). However, some migration continues up to the twenty-fifth week; therefore, any injury to the brain during this period will result in migration defects (Table 3-1).

DISORDERS OF CORTICAL DEVELOPMENT

With a basic understanding of the normal mechanisms of brain development, one can appreciate that developmental malformations result from variations in the processes of cell generation, proliferation, differentiation, and migration into the cerebral cortex. There probably are multiple genetic and acquired causes of developmental malformations of the central nervous system (Table 3-2). Also, these malformations may occur in conjunction with other congenital anomalies.

The major disorders discussed in this chapter include those related to neuronal proliferation, differentiation, and histogenesis, and postmigratory congenital malformations. A pathologic classification of these disorders has been available for many years, but MRI has made it possible to diagnose some of these conditions in vivo; it has also facilitated the recognition of distinctive syndromes.

TABLE 3-1. Classification of Cerebral Malformations According to Time of Onset

Induction (3 to 4 weeks)
Anencephaly
Encephalocele
Arnold-Chiari malformation
Ventral induction (5 to 10 weeks)
Holoprosencephaly
Septo-optic dysplasia
Lobar aplasia
Agenesis of septum pellucidum
Neuronal proliferation, differentiation, and so forth (2 to 5 months)
Megalencephaly
Tuberous sclerosis
Sturge-Weber syndrome
Ataxia telangiectasia
Hydranencephaly
Migration (2 to 5 months)
Schizencephaly
Lissencephaly
Pachygyria
Polymicrogyria
Heterotopias
Focal cortical dysplasia

Cortical malformations can be divided into generalized, lateralized, and focal types, depending on the characteristic features and distribution of the lesions. However, this classification does not take into consideration the different pathogenic mechanisms underlying these malformations (Table 3-3). (Although tuberous sclerosis is listed in Table 3-3, it is not discussed in this chapter.)

Generalized Developmental Disorders

1. *Lissencephaly (Agyria).* "Lissencephaly," or "agyria," is the term used to describe *smooth* brains or brains with poor sulcation. Two clinicopathologic types of lissencephaly have been identified.[15] Type I lissencephaly usually has both agyria and pachygyric regions. The characteristic histologic feature is that of four-layered cortex, consisting of a molecular layer, a disorganized outer cellular layer, a cell-sparse layer, and a thick inner cellular layer. The cell-sparse layer may be the result of laminar necrosis, which may have prevented further migration of neurons. Timing for the occurrence of

TABLE 3-2. Causes and Conditions Associated with Migration and Postmigration Disorders of the Central Nervous System

Metabolic

    Zellweger syndrome

    Menkes' kinky-hair disease

    GM_2 gangliosidosis

    Glutaric aciduria II

Chromosomal

    Miller-Dieker syndrome

    Trisomy 13, 18, 21

    Deletion 4p

Neurocutaneous

    Incontinentia pigmenti

    Neurofibromatosis I

    Hypomelanosis of Ito

    Tuberous sclerosis

    Epidermal nevus

Neuromuscular

    Walker-Warburg syndrome

    Fukuyama muscular dystrophy

    Myotonic dystrophy

Environmental

    Cytomegalovirus infection

    Toxoplasmosis

    Syphilis

    Toxins

    Radiation

TABLE 3-3. Classification of Cortical Developmental Malformations Based on Magnetic Resonance Imaging

Generalized or diffuse disorders

    Lissencephaly

    Pachygyria

    Band heterotopia

    Subependymal heterotopia

    Megalencephaly

Unilateral disorders

    Hemimegalencephaly

Focal disorders

    Focal cortical dysplasia

    Polymicrogyria

    Schizencephaly

    Focal subcortical heterotopia

Diffuse or focal

    Tuberous sclerosis

these malformations is related to an arrest of migration at approximately 3 to 4 months of gestation. The exact mechanism underlying lissencephaly is not clear. In type I lissencephaly, other malformations are often present, including cerebellar or callosal agenesis, enlarged ventricles, and heterotopias.

Clinically, patients with type I lissencephaly may present with variable but closely similar phenotypes, including Miller-Dieker syndrome (associated with deletion of the short arm of chromosome 17) and Norman-Roberts syndrome, or with isolated lissencephaly. However, there is controversy among investigators about the usefulness of these subclassifications. Clinical characteristics in some patients include bitemporal hollowing, mild telecanthus, and micrognathia. Most of them have mild microcephaly and severe hypotonia. Also, infantile spasms usually develop during the first year.

MRI studies of type I lissencephaly have demonstrated a thickened cortex, diminished white matter, and vertical sylvian fissures, giving the brain the figure-eight shape typical of this condition (Figure 3-1). The cortex is 11- to 20-mm thick (normal, 3.5 mm). Regions of pachygyric cortex are also seen in some patients. Barkovich et al.[16] have also reported the presence of incomplete inversion of the hippocampi, a marker of the arrest of neuronal migration.

Type II lissencephaly[17] is characterized pathologically by disorganized unlayered cortex that is penetrated by vessels and fibroglial bundles. This condition has also been called "Walker's lissencephaly." There is controversy about the relationship of Walker's lissencephaly and Fukuyama's congenital muscular dystrophy, which have overlapping features. Hydrocephalus is commonly seen, and the clinical presentation is often typical of that of patients with Walker-Warburg syndrome. Congenital hypotonia, eye malformations, and severe developmental delay are common. The MRI features in this condition— that is, thick cortex, hydrocephalus, and hypomyelination—are different from those of type I lissencephaly.

Some authors have also included three other conditions with the lissencephalies: microcephalia vera, radial microbrain, and diffuse polymicrogyria. Although the MRI features are somewhat similar to those of lissencephaly types I and II, the pathogenic and histologic abnormalities are different.[2]

2. *Pachygyria.* Pachygyria can be considered a less severe form of lissencephaly.[18] Although the cortex in pachygyria may have a more organized structure than in lissencephaly, the clinical and imaging features of patients with pachygyria often depend on the extent of pachygyria relative to agyria. Those with

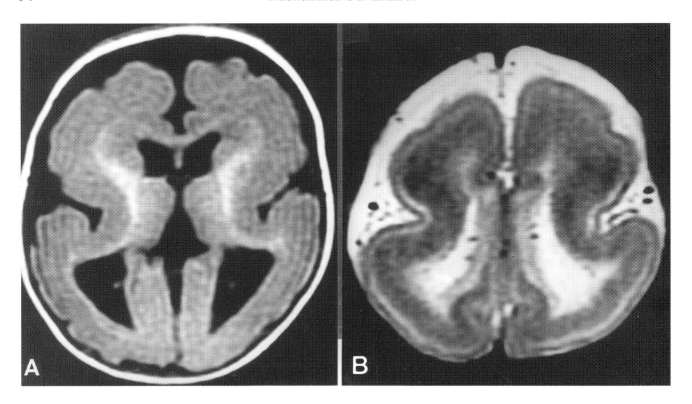

Figure 3-1. Type I lissencephaly. A. Axial T_1 magnetic resonance image showing thick, smooth cortex and shallow sylvian fissures, which give the brain a figure-eight–shaped appearance. B. Axial T_2 magnetic resonance image showing a thin outer layer of gray matter representing neurons. The high intensity rim represents the area of laminar necrosis, the cell-sparse layer, and the underlying thick zone represents arrested neurons. Note enlargement of occipital horns and the myelination pattern, which is normal for this age. (Courtesy of Dr. J. Barkovich.)

a predominance of pachygyric cortex have a lesser degree of neurodevelopmental dysfunction. It is also clear in many cases that lissencephaly and pachygyria coexist in the same patient. MRI in pachygyria shows a thick cortex, but the figure-eight image typical of lissencephaly is not seen (Figure 3-2). The sylvian fissures are closed in comparison with those in lissencephaly, and the cortex is approximately 15-mm thick. In some patients, the distribution of abnormalities may be localized to certain regions, but it is usually bilateral and symmetrical as compared with polymicrogyric cortex, in which asymmetrical lesions may be observed. The clinical presentation includes developmental delay and tonic and generalized tonic-clonic seizures; half of the patients have microcephaly. The electroencephalographic (EEG) features are different in agyria and pachygyria. Fast, high-amplitude rhythms are seen in almost 80% of the patients with agyria but are present in only 50% of those with pachygyria.[17]

3. *Band Heterotopia, or Double Cortex Syndrome.* Band heterotopia occurs more frequently in females than in males (all but one patient thus far

reported have been female). Patients have mild-to-severe developmental delay, pyramidal tract signs, and, in some cases, dysarthria. Full-scale intelligence quotients, ranging from severely low to normal, have been reported. EEG investigations usually demonstrate generalized spike and wave discharges or multifocal EEG abnormalities.[19]

The classic MRI finding is a circumferential band of subcortical gray matter heterotopia separated from the cortical mantle by a thin rim of white matter.[19] This is usually more obvious over the frontocentral parietal region (Figure 3-3). Pathologic specimens have shown normal lamination of cortical layers I to IV. Layers V and VI usually cannot be seen, and layer VI is merged with the U fibers of the white matter. Underneath, clusters of ganglion cells are present below the cortex. The thickness of the cortex overlying the heterotopia is mildly increased or normal, and the temporal lobes, particularly the hippocampal structures, are normal, as opposed to their appearance in lissencephaly. Barkovich and Kjos[20] have suggested that the thickness of the heterotopic gray matter is correlated with the severity of the clinical syndrome.

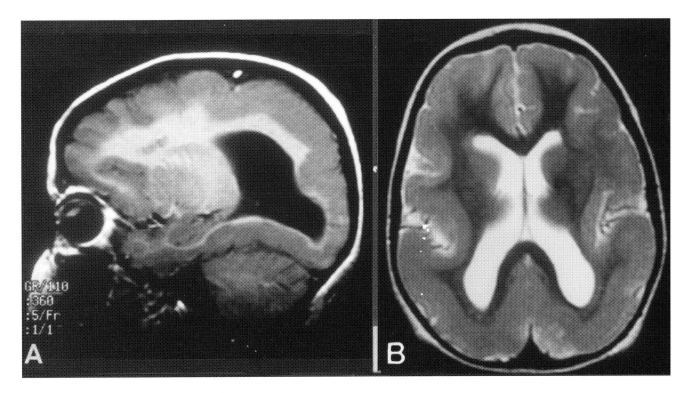

FIGURE 3-2. Pachygyria. A. Sagittal magnetic resonance image showing thick cortex and poor sulcation. Note white matter heterotopia. B. Axial magnetic resonance image showing thick cortex with closed sylvian fissures. Compared with lissencephaly, pachygyria has more sulcation.

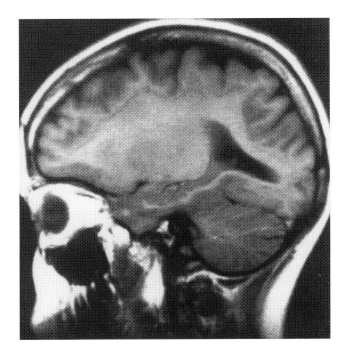

FIGURE 3-3. Band heterotopia. Sagittal T_1 magnetic resonance image showing a band of gray matter separated from the cortex by white matter.

Lissencephaly, pachygyria, and band heterotopia probably share pathogenetic mechanisms. In lissencephaly, there is almost a complete absence of gyration, with a large number of heterotopic neurons. At the other end of the spectrum, the cortex in band heterotopia is almost normal, with a few cells located in the subcortical mantle. Further evidence supporting a similar pathogenetic, and possibly genetic, mechanism for these conditions is the recent report of several families in which the mothers had band heterotopia and some of the children were born with classic lissencephaly (Pinard et al., personal communication, 1993).

4. *Subependymal Heterotopias.* Subependymal heterotopias, or periventricular nodular heterotopias, belong to one of the most common forms of developmental disorders. They are due to a failure of a group of neurons to either initiate or complete the migration process toward the cortical mantle. Depending on the number of cells that do not migrate, gray matter heterotopias are classified as periventricular nodular heterotopias, focal subcortical heterotopias, and bilateral corticosubcortical heterotopias. Subependymal heterotopias can range from a few nodular clusters of neurons to a diffuse lining of the ependymal regions. A recent study reported that 90% of the patients with subependy-

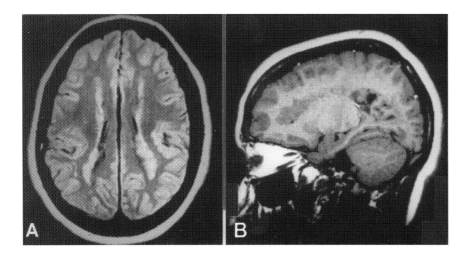

FIGURE 3-4. Diffuse subependymal heterotopias. A. Axial T_2 (TE: 30) magnetic resonance image showing multiple ovoid heterotopias lining the lateral ventricles. B. Sagittal T_1 image showing nodules isointense to gray matter.

mal heterotopias had diffuse, narrow involvement of all subventricular regions.[1]

Clinically, patients with subependymal heterotopias usually have normal neurologic development. The majority have normal intellectual and motor functions or mild mental retardation. However, seizures are common, and almost 80% of patients have epilepsy. Of interest, the seizures develop in the second decade of life. In those with seizures, temporal and parieto-occipital symptoms are common.

The MRI features typical of subependymal heterotopias consist of multiple smooth ovoid nodules of cortical gray matter lining the lateral ventricles (Figure 3-4). The third and fourth ventricles are spared. Approximately 75% of patients have bilateral lesions, and 30% also have focal subcortical heterotopias. Callosal and cerebellar malformations may be present in 25% of patients. Signal intensity from the nodules is isointense with gray matter in all sequences, and no enhancement occurs with contrast medium, which distinguishes them from the subependymal hamartomas seen in tuberous sclerosis. In 20% of patients, other cortical malformations may be detected.

Unilateral Hemispheric Disorders

Hemimegalencephaly

Hemimegalencephaly, or unilateral megalencephaly, refers to an enlargement of all or part of a cerebral hemisphere. In most cases, the ipsilateral ventricular system is also enlarged. In some patients, this condition is associated with contralateral somatic hypertrophy. Hemimegalencephaly is more common than megalencephaly.

Pathologic changes in hemimegalencephaly vary from mildly hypertrophic neurons and gliosis to pachygyria and heterotopias.[21] However, polymicrogyria, with or without preservation of the junction between the gray matter and white matter, and multiple heterotopias are probably more frequent. Lissencephalic or agyric malformations may also be present in some cases. The mechanisms underlying hemimegalencephaly are not known. Some authors have reported an increased neuronal content of DNA and RNA in the affected hemisphere.[22] Barkovich and Chuang[23] have suggested that an insult to the developing brain in the middle-to-late second trimester could account for both polymicrogyria and overgrowth of the hemispheric white matter as the result of alterations in the cell membrane receptors and molecules that guide developing axons. This would result in the disorganized axonal migration that has been reported in these patients.

An interesting correlation found in imaging studies is the inverse relationship between the severity of the cortical and white matter abnormalities and the size of the cerebral hemisphere. In patients with agyria and in those with more severe injury and marked gliosis, the enlargement of the hemisphere is less marked. Conversely, those with polymicrogyria and a normal pattern of white matter tend to have larger hemispheres. This supports the suggestion that severe injuries result in a less severe degree of enlargement.

Focal seizures are often the initial clinical problem in patients with hemimegalencephaly.[24] In most patients, seizures start within the first 6 months of life and are unilateral and often partial, with secondary generalization. They are frequently intractable to medical therapy. Infantile spasms and drop attacks may occur in early childhood. Unilateral neurologic signs are common (for example, hemiparesis and hemianopia). However, minimal neurologic dysfunction and normal intelligence quotients have been reported in some patients.

Hemimegalencephaly has characteristic CT and MRI findings. Enlargement of at least one lobe, ranging from mild to severe, is present in all the patients. In more than half of the patients, the entire hemisphere appears to be enlarged, but in some, the enlargement may be localized to the frontal or temporoparietal region. Careful review of the underlying gray matter reveals thick, broad,

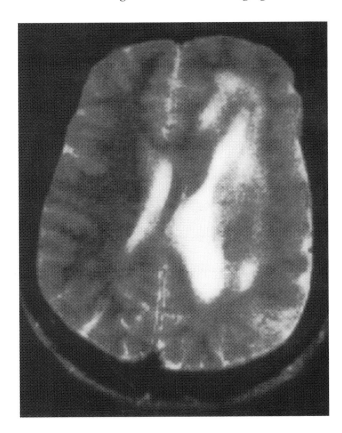

FIGURE 3-5. Hemimegalencephaly. Axial magnetic resonance image demonstrating an enlarged hemisphere and increased signal from white matter. Note that the ventricle in the affected hemisphere is also enlarged.

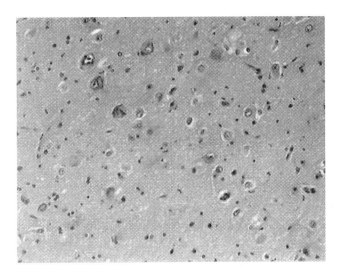

FIGURE 3-6. Focal cortical dysplasia. Note the cluster of abnormal cells, large poorly defined cell bodies, and lack of cortical lamination. (Hematoxylin-eosin stain, × 150.)

and flat gyri and shallow sulci (Figure 3-5). The underlying hemispheric white matter is usually abnormal, with diminished white matter in some patients. Heterotopias are commonly seen, and in most patients, the ventricular system is enlarged. Angiographic studies have revealed abnormal vascular patterns, with arterial-venous shunting in the regions of neuronal migration.

Focal Developmental Disorders

Focal abnormalities are probably the most common malformation among patients with developmental abnormalities studied for intractable seizures. Focal abnormalities can be divided into cortical, subcortical, and corticosubcortical lesions. Focal cortical malformations can be subdivided into focal, unilateral, and bilateral types, depending on their distribution.

Focal Cortical Dysplasia

Focal cortical dysplasia is probably the most common form of focal developmental disorder diagnosed in patients referred for intractable epilepsy. The pathologic character-

istic of these lesions is the disruption of cortical lamination by giant neurons and large astrocytes. The most prominent histologic feature is the great number of large and abnormal cells, with the loss of cortical architecture (Figure 3-6). Since the original description of Taylor et al.,[7] focal cortical dysplasia has been recognized to encompass a spectrum of histologic changes. This spectrum ranges from mild cortical disruption without giant neurons to the most severe forms in which cortical dyslamination, large bizarre cells (neuronal and glial elements), and astrocytosis occur.[8,25] These lesions have been divided into type I and type II on the basis of the degree of change (Figure 3-7).

From a pathogenic point of view, one can postulate that in mild cortical dysplasia (type I) the cortex has the expected number of cells, but they are disorganized because of disrupted neuronal organization. In type II cortical dysplasia, there are, in addition, excessive and abnormal cells (neuronal and/or glial) and disorders of proliferation, migration, and organization. From a pathologic perspective, these two types suggest a spectrum of changes, but the underlying mechanisms may not be the same in both types.

The clinical manifestations of patients with cortical dysplasia vary. Patients who present with seizures may have partial motor or partial-complex seizures or secondary generalized attacks. Drop attacks occur in some patients with centrally located lesions.[26] The location of the lesion determines the clinical presentation.[9]

In my experience, most patients have extratemporal cortical dysplasias. The frontal lobes and the precentral and postcentral gyri particularly appear to be more involved than other regions (Figures 3-8 and 3-9). Correlative studies in children with intractable partial seizures have shown that 25% of them have cortical dys-

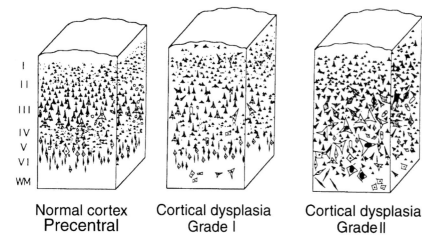

FIGURE 3-7. Cortical architecture in normal cortex and in grade I and grade II cortical dysplasia. Grade II cortical dysplasia is characterized by increased cellularity, giant cells, and cortical chaos. (*I-VI*) cortical layers, (*WM*) white matter.

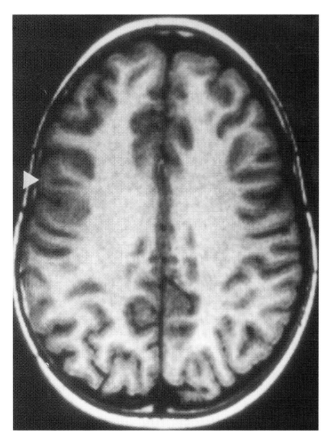

FIGURE 3-8. Focal cortical dysplasia. Axial magnetic resonance image demonstrating small gyral malformation of the right precentral and postcentral gyri (*arrowhead*) in a 9-year-old child with intractable focal epilepsy.

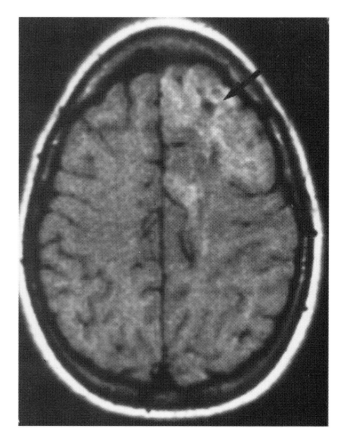

FIGURE 3-9. Focal cortical dysplasia. Axial T₁ image demonstrating abnormal left frontal gyration (*arrow*), with mixed signal abnormality. The patient had relatively well-controlled simple-partial seizures.

plastic lesions.[9,27] Of those patients with these lesions, the central cortex was involved in almost half. The reasons for this involvement stem from the propensity of the precentral and postcentral gyri for ischemic injury, as observed in other developmental disorders such as polymicrogyria and schizencephaly.

Cortical dysplasia may be subdivided according to the patterns of gyral involvement. It may be difficult to differentiate multifocal dysplasia from hemimegalencephaly in some cases. The typical MRI findings in these patients consist of focal areas of cortical thickening, with poor gray-white matter differentiation, and shallow sulci.

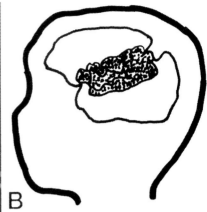

FIGURE 3-10. Congenital bilateral perisylvian syndrome. A. Sagittal magnetic resonance image showing abnormal opercula with polymicrogyria. Polymicrogyria involves subcentral, superior, temporal, and angular gyri. B. Diagram of abnormal opercula.

Focal dysplasia of the temporal lobes has also been reported,[8,25,28] but this appears to be less frequent than extratemporal lobe dysplasias. The exact frequency varies with the pathologic classification; in different studies of temporal lobe resection, it ranges from 6% to 20%. Involvement of both mesial and lateral neocortical structures has been reported, but in some cases, the lesions may be restricted to the neocortex. The clinical behavior of these patients appears to be similar to that of those with temporolimbic epilepsy, but the EEG localization is generally less circumscribed. In temporal lobe cases without involvement of the hippocampus, the most definite abnormality is cortical thickening of temporal convolutions associated with poor differentiation between gray matter and white matter. With higher resolution MRI, it is likely that the sensitivity of this method for detecting these lesions will increase.

Polymicrogyria

The term "polymicrogyria" refers to an abnormal macroscopic appearance of brain gyration characterized by too many abnormal small gyri. In some cases, the gyri are shallow, small, and separated by shallow sulci, but in other cases, the gyri are wider.[29]

The histologic changes in polymicrogyria include ischemic laminar necrosis in cortical layer V. Cortical layers II, III, and IV are normal. Because late migrating neurons reach their normal positions before laminar necrosis occurs, this type of malformation may originate in some cases after the twentieth fetal week and be considered postmigratory in origin.[11]

Histologically, polymicrogyria is divided into four-layered and unlayered types. Although most of the experimental and human fetal pathologic data suggest that polymicrogyria results from a postmigratory ischemic mechanism, some investigators have postulated a premigratory mechanism for some forms of polymicrogyria.[3,30]

Clinically, the presentation of polymicrogyria is extremely variable and depends on the location and extent of the malformation and whether both cerebral hemispheres are involved. Diffuse polymicrogyria may present with severe developmental delay, microcephaly, and hypotonia. It can be localized to one hemisphere and may be one of the underlying pathologic changes in patients with hemimegalencephaly.

MRI findings demonstrate a thick cortex that can be interpreted as pachygyria. However, cortical thickness is less than that observed in pachygyria. The sulci are shallow and the underlying white matter may show an abnormal T_2 signal.

In view of the ischemic nature of the lesions, polymicrogyria may often present on imaging studies with bilateral perisylvian malformations. The presence of these lesions is usually correlated with a homogeneous syndrome described as "congenital bilateral perisylvian syndrome,"[31] which consists of congenital pseudobulbar paresis, developmental delay, and characteristic bilateral lesions seen on CT or MRI. Almost 90% of patients present with seizures, and half of them have intractable epilepsy. The imaging findings are quite characteristic, with involvement of the sylvian and perisylvian regions (Figure 3-10). The opercular region is most affected.[32] EEG abnormalities consist of generalized slow spike and wave discharges, but 20% of the patients may have localized epileptogenic abnormalities.

In some patients, bilateral polymicrogyria may occur in regions other than the perisylvian ones. These lesions may be located posteriorly and involve the occipitoparietal junction or occipital lobes.

Schizencephaly

The term "schizencephaly" is used to describe clefts lined with gray matter which extend through the cerebral hemispheres from the pia mater to the ependymal lining.[33] The clefts may be in apposition (closed lip, or type I, schizencephaly) or separated (open lip, or type II, schizencephaly).[34] The cerebral cortex around the clefts may be normal or have polymicrogyria. The gray matter that lines the clefts usually consists of polymicrogyric cortex. The mechanism underlying schizencephaly is

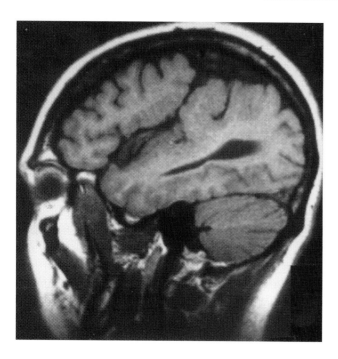

FIGURE 3-11. Unilateral schizencephaly. Cleft is lined by polymicrogyric cortex.

probably similar to the one that causes polymicrogyria and porencephaly. The extent of cortical injury determines whether a lesion is polymicrogyric or schizencephalic. Injuries that extend more deeply into the cortex and that destroy the superficial portions of the glial fibers will produce cortical infoldings lined by polymicrogyria. If the injury involves the entire thickness of the developing hemisphere, the result will be schizencephaly.

Patients with schizencephaly may have features resembling those of polymicrogyria. Similar to polymicrogyria, schizencephaly can also be divided into bilateral and unilateral types. Furthermore, bilateral lesions can be either symmetrical or asymmetrical.

Bilateral schizencephaly is less common than unilateral schizencephaly (Figure 3-11). In my experience, approximately 30% to 40% of patients with schizencephaly have bilateral lesions, which are often asymmetrical, with type I schizencephalic lesions in one hemisphere and type II lesions in the other.

Clinical correlations indicate that patients with bilateral schizencephaly often have moderate-to-severe motor dysfunction that is characterized as spastic quadriparesis. Marked developmental delay, severe mental retardation, and language disorders are common. Infantile spasms may be the presenting seizure type; focal motor seizures, with or without secondary generalization, are common. In a small proportion of patients with bilateral lesions, the seizure disorder is controlled with drugs.

Unilateral schizencephalies appear to be evenly distributed between the two hemispheres (Figure 3-12). The relative frequencies of type I and type II lesions appear to be similar to those seen with bilateral lesions. Developmental delay and intellectual impairment are also common in these patients. Hemiparesis contralateral to the side of the cleft is also common. I have not observed significant differences in speech dysfunction between left and right dominance in patients with schizencephaly. It is likely that in these patients speech function is transferred to the other hemisphere. Seizures are usually focal motor ones, but sensory attacks as well as partial-complex seizures are seen. EEG investigations may reveal unilateral focal discharges, often in the temporal lobe when the lesions are localized to the temporoparietal convexity. On MRI, the lesions appear to be evenly distributed, with the majority in the precentral and postcentral regions.

An interesting issue about patients with unilateral polymicrogyria or schizencephaly is the subtle cortical developmental malformations in the opposite hemisphere, usually in "mirror regions" of the hemisphere. This may explain why some patients with apparent unilateral lesions present with severe developmental delay. These findings underscore a possible pathogenic mechanism for cortical dysplasia, polymicrogyria, and schizencephaly.

On MRI, schizencephalies are characterized by unilateral or bilateral clefts lined with gray matter; the clefts extend from the calvarium (inner table) to the ventricle. Subependymal heterotopias are common, and the cortical pattern is usually abnormal. Also, the septum pellucidum is absent in 70% to 90% of patients.[1]

Focal Subcortical Heterotopias

Although most patients with subependymal heterotopias have diffuse nodular lesions, some occasionally present with a few focal lesions in one hemisphere. According to a recent review,[20] the frequency of focal subcortical subependymal heterotopias is less than 20%. These lesions may be only coincidental findings in a patient without neurologic symptoms. If seizures occur, they may start in the second decade; they may be controlled easily with drugs.

More commonly, subcortical heterotopias present with focal lesions, which usually appear as clusters of nodules of gray matter with irregular margins.

Patients with subcortical heterotopias may develop normally, but, depending on the size of the lesions, pyramidal signs may be present on the opposite side of the body. Developmental delay has been reported in some patients who have concomitant callosal agenesis. Speech appears to be normal in some patients, but when the lesions are extensive and involve the dominant hemisphere, speech development is delayed. Seizures in these patients are a mixture of focal motor and secondary generalized convulsions. Infantile spasms have also been described.

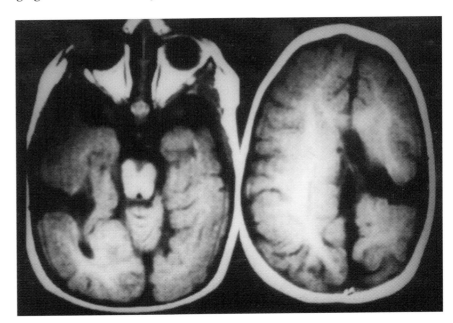

FIGURE 3-12. Bilateral schizencephaly. Axial T_1 images showing open clefts (type II). Note abnormal cortex lining the clefts. (Courtesy of Dr. J. Barkovich.)

Imaging features in patients with subcortical heterotopias are quite characteristic. Heterotopias appear as clusters of nodules of gray matter with irregular margins (Figure 3-13). The surrounding white matter is usually normal and has a normal intensity signal. At times, the heterotopias may appear as masses that cause ventricular compression. Corpus callosum abnormalities have been reported.[34]

According to the type of lesions, one can state that patients with subependymal heterotopias, even if diffuse, have a relatively late onset of seizures, mild cognitive impairment, and usually normal neurologic findings. In contrast, patients with focal subcortical heterotopias have a significantly greater chance of having developmental and cognitive delay.

The ultimate neurologic and seizure outcomes depend not only on the type, location, and size of the lesion but also on the type of developmental disorder. Patients with subependymal heterotopias usually have a normal cortical thickness and convolutional pattern. Conversely, patients with focal subcortical heterotopias have abnormalities of the white matter. In the regions of neuronal malformation, the cerebral cortex is usually thin and neuron poor.

Magnetic Resonance Imaging Examination in Developmental Malformations

It would be most useful if there was a single MRI study protocol that provided complete anatomical and diagnostic information about the pathologic substrate with high sensitivity and specificity. It is difficult to obtain all this information in a cost-effective and reliable way with MRI techniques, and compromise is often necessary in

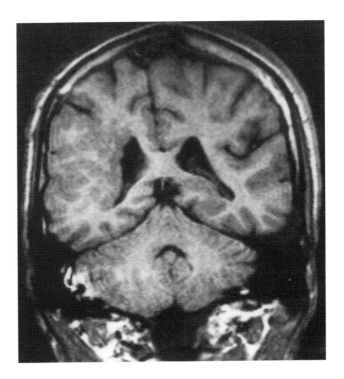

FIGURE 3-13. Focal subcortical heterotopias. Coronal T_1 magnetic resonance image showing abnormal heterotopic gray matter extending from the ventricle to the cortex.

planning an MRI study. This may be directly related to the inherent characteristics of MRI. However, choosing the appropriate imaging variables on the basis of the suspected diagnosis is the most cost-effective and sensitive way to decide on the best imaging sequences for a particular patient.

A guiding principle in the MRI evaluation of patients with epilepsy is the concept of individualization of the MRI study. By this, I mean that each patient has a potential diagnosis and that the MRI study should help substantiate the clinical hypothesis. This concept is a useful one, but it is important to recognize that it is highly dependent on the correct clinical hypothesis being put forward by the clinician.

The approach to MRI studies in patients with epilepsy is in many ways the same as the method of using EEG to investigate patients with seizures. As in the electrophysiologic investigations, the MRI study should be individualized according to the relevant clinical question being asked. In turn, the appropriate imaging variables must be selected depending on the question being asked clinically. It must be emphasized that this approach does not mean that appropriate protocols should not be applied to each level of investigation. The issue is: Which protocols and what information do we seek?

In our experience, patients being investigated for developmental malformations should first undergo a T_1-weighted sagittal pulse sequence. This is used for subsequent "landmarking" as well as for examining midline structures such as the corpus callosum, cerebellum, and brain stem. A double spin echo pulse sequence providing T_2 and spin density contrast should also be performed to reveal areas with abnormal T_2 signal. A T_1-weighted three-dimensional acquisition with thin-slice thickness (1 to 1.5 mm) is obtained in the coronal plane through the entire brain. These images are reformatted in three planes so they can be analyzed simultaneously. I also prefer to include a nonangulated coronal study with inversion recovery sequences because of the high contrast between the gray matter and white matter. Although this sequence increases scanning time, it is particularly useful in the investigation of patients with focal dysplastic lesions and may have greater accuracy in demonstrating small subcortical white matter heterotopias. Recently, three-dimensional reconstruction and gray matter and white matter segmentation have been used in patients with developmental malformations, but it is not clear whether these methods provide significant advantages over two-dimensional reconstructions.

RELEVANCE OF MAGNETIC RESONANCE IMAGING TO SURGICAL STRATEGIES

Epilepsy is a common manifestation of cerebral developmental malformations and an increasing number of patients with intractable epilepsy and developmental malformations are being selected for surgical treatment. The detection of these lesions by MRI is relevant not only to diagnosis but also to surgical planning and ultimate outcome.

Dysplastic abnormalities are probably among the most epileptogenic of the structural lesions. The high incidence of intractable epilepsy and episodes of status epilepticus is compelling evidence of this fact. Also, the common presence of highly epileptogenic discharges in the form of continuous spiking and ictal-like activity recorded directly at operation indicates that these lesions are intrinsically epileptogenic.[26]

Many focal dysplastic lesions, including cortical dysplasia, polymicrogyria, and schizencephaly, are in the precentral and postcentral regions.[4,9,16,26,35] However, temporal lobe dysplasia is also seen in isolation and, in some cases, in association with hippocampal lesions. This distribution is important because it may affect surgical outcome; temporal lobe dysplasia responds better to surgical treatment than does a centrally located lesion, unless the lesion can be resected in toto. Conversely, patients with a unigyral occipital, frontal, or parietal lesion may respond well to focal resections.

The detection of bilateral lesions usually is correlated with bilateral epileptogenic abnormalities and signs of diffuse brain dysfunction. However, some patients may demonstrate asymmetrical lesions and give the impression of having a unilateral abnormality. This is sometimes seen in patients with unilateral polymicrogyria who may have subtle dysplastic lesions in the contralateral hemisphere. Recognition of such patients is important because the surgical treatment needs to be tailored on the basis of these findings.

SUMMARY

Developmental disorders of the cerebral cortex are a complex group of congenital malformations that often present with variable neurodevelopmental dysfunction. Epilepsy is a common manifestation of these disorders and, in some cases, may be associated with specific clinical syndromes. MRI is a powerful imaging technique for investigating these congenital disorders. The information provided by MRI in conjunction with the clinicoelectrographic features is extremely important in recognizing these syndromes and in treating them appropriately with medical and surgical means.

REFERENCES

1. Barkovich AJ, Kjos BO. Nonlissencephalic cortical dysplasias: correlation of imaging findings with clinical deficits. AJNR Am J Neuroradiol 1992;13:95–103.

2. Barkovich AJ, Gressens P, Evrard P. Formation, maturation, and disorders of brain neocortex. AJRN Am J Neuroradiol 1992;13:423–46.

3. Barth PG. Disorders of neuronal migration. Can J Neurol Sci 1987;14:1–16.

4. Guerrini R, Dravet C, Raybaud C, et al. Epilepsy and focal gyral anomalies detected by MRI: electroclinico-morphological correlations and follow-up. Dev Med Child Neurol 1992;34:706–18.

5. Kuzniecky RI, Cascino GD, Palmini A, et al. Structural neuroimaging. In: Engel J Jr, ed. Surgical treatment of the epilepsies. 2nd ed. New York: Raven Press, 1993:197–209.

6. Palmini A, Andermann F, Olivier A, et al. Neuronal migration disorders: a contribution of modern neuroimaging to the etiologic diagnosis of epilepsy. Can J Neurol Sci 1991;18 Suppl 4:580–7.

7. Taylor DC, Falconer MA, Bruton CJ, et al. Focal dysplasia of the cerebral cortex in epilepsy. J Neurol Neurosurg Psychiatry 1971;34:369–87.

8. Kuzniecky R, Garcia JH, Faught E, et al. Cortical dysplasia in temporal lobe epilepsy: magnetic resonance imaging correlations. Ann Neurol 1991;29:293–8.

9. Kuzniecky R, Murro A, King D, et al. Magnetic resonance imaging in childhood intractable partial epilepsies: pathologic correlations. Neurology 1993;43:681–7.

10. Evrard P, Gaddisseux J, Lyon G. Les malformations du systeme nerveux. In: Royer P, ed. Naissance du cerveau. Paris: Lafayette, 1982:49–74.

11. Caviness VJ. Normal development of the cerebral cortex. In: Evrard P, Minkowski A, eds. Developmental neurobiology. New York: Raven Press, 1989:1–10.

12. Austin CP, Cepko CL. Cellular migration patterns in the developing mouse cerebral cortex. Development 1990;110:713–32.

13. McConnell SK, Kaznowski CE. Cell cycle dependence of laminar determination in developing neocortex. Science 1991;254:282–5.

14. Rakic P, ed. Contact regulation of neuronal migration. In: Edelman GTJ, ed. The cell in contact: adhesions and junctions as morphogenetic determinants. New York: Neuroscience Research Foundation, 1985:67–91.

15. Dobyns WB, Stratton RF, Greenberg F. Syndromes with lissencephaly. I: Miller-Dieker and Norman-Roberts syndromes and isolated lissencephaly. Am J Med Genet 1984;18:509–26.

16. Barkovich AJ, Chuang SH, Norman D. MR of neuronal migration anomalies. AJNR Am J Neuroradiol 1987;8:1009–17.

17. Aicardi J. The agyria-pachygyria complex: a spectrum of cortical malformations. Brain Dev 1991;13:1–8.

18. Crome L. Pachygyria. J Pathol Bacteriol 1956; 71:335–52.

19. Palmini A, Andermann F, Aicardi J, et al. Diffuse cortical dysplasia, or the 'double cortex' syndrome: the clinical and epileptic spectrum in 10 patients. Neurology 1991;41:1656–62.

20. Barkovich AJ, Kjos BO. Gray matter heterotopias: MR characteristics and correlation with developmental and neurologic manifestations. Radiology 1992;182:493–9.

21. Townsend JJ, Nielsen SL, Malamud N. Unilateral megalencephaly: hamartoma or neoplasm? Neurology 1975;25:448–53.

22. Manz HJ, Phillips TM, Rowden G, et al. Unilateral megalencephaly, cerebral cortical dysplasia, neuronal hypertrophy, and heterotopia: cytomorphometric, fluorometric cytochemical, and biochemical analyses. Acta Neuropathol (Berl) 1979;45:97–103.

23. Barkovich AJ, Chuang SH. Unilateral megalencephaly: correlation of MR imaging and pathologic characteristics. AJNR Am J Neuroradiol 1990;11:523–31.

24. Vigevano F, Bertini E, Boldrini R, et al. Hemimegalencephaly and intractable epilepsy: benefits of hemispherectomy. Epilepsia 1989;30:833–43.

25. Hardiman O, Burke T, Phillips J, et al. Microdysgenesis in resected temporal neocortex: incidence and clinical significance in focal epilepsy. Neurology 1988; 38:1041–7.

26. Palmini A, Andermann F, Olivier A, et al. Focal neuronal migration disorders and intractable partial epilepsy: a study of 30 patients. Ann Neurol 1991; 30:741–9.

27. Kuzniecky R, Powers R. Epilepsia partialis continua due to cortical dysplasia. J Child Neurol 1993;8:386–8.

28. Hopkins IJ, Klug GL. Temporal lobectomy for the treatment of intractable complex partial seizures of temporal lobe origin in early childhood. Dev Med Child Neurol 1991;33:26–31.

29. Friede RL. Developmental neuropathology. 2nd revised edition. Berlin: Springer-Verlag, 1989.

30. Dvorak K, Feit J, Jurankova Z. Experimentally induced focal microgyria and status verrucosus deformis in rats—pathogenesis and interrelation. Histological and autoradiographical study. Acta Neuropathol (Berl) 1978;44:121–9.

31. Kuzniecky R, Andermann F, Guerrini R. Congenital bilateral perisylvian syndrome: study of 31 patients. The CBPS Multicenter Collaborative Study. Lancet 1993;341:608–12.

32. Kuzniecky R, Andermann F. The congenital bilateral perisylvian syndrome: imaging findings in a multicenter study. CBPS Study Group. AJNR Am J Neuroradiol 1994;15:139–44.

33. Yakovlev PI, Wadsworth RC. Schizencephalies: a study of the congenital clefts in the cerebral mantle. I. Clefts with fused lips. J Neuropathol Exp Neurol 1946;5:116–30.

34. Byrd SE, Osborn RE, Bohan TP, et al. The CT and MR evaluation of migrational disorders of the brain. Part II. Schizencephaly, heterotopia and polymicrogyria. Pediatr Radiol 1989;19:219–22.

35. Guerrini R, Dravet C, Battaglia A, et al. Focal anomalies of the cortical development and epilepsy: electroclinical features in the bilateral opercular malformations. Boll Lega Ital Epilessia 1990;71:109–11.

Functional Neuropathology of Temporal Lobe Epilepsy

Cheolsu Shin

Partial or localization-related epilepsy is the most frequently occurring type of seizure disorder.[1] The ictal manifestations in patients with partial epilepsy include simple partial, complex partial, and secondarily generalized tonic-clonic seizures.[1] The distinction between simple partial and complex partial seizures is that an impairment of consciousness occurs during the latter.[1,2] Complex partial seizures originate in the temporal lobe in nearly 80% of patients.[1] Seizures emanate from the amygdala or hippocampus, or both, in more than 90% of patients with temporal lobe epilepsy.[2]

Pharmacoresistant seizures (that is, seizures refractory to maximally tolerated antiepileptic drug therapy) develop in about 50% of patients with partial epilepsy.[1] Poorly controlled partial epilepsy may be psychosocially disabling because of difficulty working, attending school, or operating a motor vehicle safely.[3] Medically refractory partial seizures of temporal lobe origin may be associated with a decline in neurocognitive performance.[2] The diagnosis of intractable partial epilepsy is established when the seizures are medically refractory *and* a person's quality of life is impaired.[1,2] The most effective treatment for intractable partial epilepsy of temporal lobe origin is anterior temporal lobe cortical resection with amygdalohippocampectomy, that is, anterior temporal lobectomy.[2,3]

The abnormality most commonly identified in patients with intractable partial epilepsy of temporal lobe origin is mesial temporal sclerosis.[4] Mesial temporal sclerosis is associated with a specific pattern of neuronal loss in the hippocampus, amygdala, parahippocampal gyrus,

and entorhinal cortex.[4] The pathologic features of mesial temporal sclerosis include hippocampal formation atrophy and gliosis. Recently, magnetic resonance imaging (MRI) has been shown to be highly sensitive and specific in detecting mesial temporal sclerosis in patients with temporal lobe epilepsy.[5] Furthermore, MRI findings are of prognostic importance in patients undergoing anterior temporal lobectomy.[5] MRI may serve as a preoperative surrogate for the diagnosis of mesial temporal sclerosis in patients with intractable partial epilepsy.[5] This chapter reviews the functional neuropathologic changes that occur in temporal lobe epilepsy.

NEUROPATHOLOGY

Historical Background

Study of the histopathologic features of the temporal lobe in patients with partial epilepsy did not begin until en bloc resection was introduced, enabling detailed histologic examination. Margerison and Corsellis[6] described various degrees of histologic abnormalities that ranged from normal to severe bilateral mesial temporal sclerosis in autopsy specimens from institutionalized patients with chronic epilepsy. Although classic mesial temporal sclerosis was found in many of these specimens, some had only mild unilateral gliosis in the dentate hilus, termed "end-folium sclerosis." However, on the basis of this information, it was not clear whether the sclerosis was the result of many seizures over the lifetime of the patient or whether the sclerosis per se was the cause of the chronic seizure disorder.

Bruton[4] examined the specimens from temporal lobectomies performed by Falconer and found that 43% of 249 patients had histologic findings of sclerosis of Ammon's horn that were similar in pattern to the mesial temporal sclerosis Margerison and Corsellis[6] described in their autopsy series.

Over the years, many terms have been used to describe the specific pattern of sclerosis found in the temporal lobe of patients with complex partial epilepsies, including "incisural sclerosis," "pararhinal sclerosis," "Ammon's horn sclerosis," "hippocampal sclerosis," and "mesial temporal sclerosis" as well as the subtype "end-folium sclerosis." The most appropriate term for this pathologic entity is "mesial temporal sclerosis," because the neuronal cell loss extends beyond the hippocampus proper into the amygdala, subiculum, and parahippocampal gyrus.

Histologic Features of Mesial Temporal Sclerosis

"Ammon's horn," or "cornu ammonis" (CA), is the classic anatomical term describing the hippocampus proper and is the term used most widely to describe the subfields of the hippocampus: CA1, CA2, CA3, and CA4 (or dentate hilus) (Figure 4-1A). Most of the neuropathologic features of mesial temporal sclerosis are concentrated in this region (Figure 4-1B). There is loss of hippocampal pyramidal neurons and gliosis and shrinkage of the neuropil. This is marked especially in the most susceptible subfield, CA1 and the dentate hilus (or CA4). Less severe damage occurs in the dentate gyrus and CA3, and minimal damage occurs in CA2. The CA2 subfield tends to be resistant to damage, even from ischemia. With gliosis and atrophy (that is, sclerosis), the volume of the hippocampus is decreased, resulting in an atrophic appearance and altered signal characteristics on MRI. In the most severe cases, the gliosis may be overwhelming, with minimal neuronal survival, thus raising the question of how seizures can be sustained without a minimum number of neurons to form a network. Most likely, the seizure activity in these instances is generated and sustained in a surrounding region, such as the amygdala, subiculum, entorhinal cortex, or parahippocampal gyrus. In cases with severely atrophic hippocampus seen on MRI, it would be of interest to determine whether the surrounding limbic structures have any MRI abnormalities.

Milder forms of mesial temporal sclerosis may involve only the dentate hilus/CA4 region and may represent an earlier stage of hippocampal epileptogenesis, as explained below. This has been termed "end-folium sclerosis" by Margerison and Corsellis.[6] Whether this kind of mild mesial temporal sclerosis is even detectable with MRI as volume loss or as T_2 signal change has not been studied systematically.

In the mildest recognizable form of mesial temporal sclerosis, neuronal loss (as determined by actual cell counts) without significant gliosis may be the only abnormality. It could be argued that in such cases the hippocampus is not likely to be the focus of epilepsy. Clinical experience corroborates this argument, because surgical results are much less favorable in these cases. The corollary is that the outcome for patients with normal MRI findings is less favorable after temporal lobectomy than for those with findings of atrophy on MRI. This kind of mild abnormality has been recognized more in cases in which there is an extrahippocampal foreign tissue lesion.[7] Fried et al.[7] reported that the younger the age at the onset of seizures and the more mesial the lesion, the smaller the neuronal cell count in all regions of hippocampus. This finding suggests that seizures early in life, when neuronal development is still occurring, may be more detrimental to neuronal survival than seizures in later life.

A decrease in the number of neurons in mesial temporal sclerosis may partly explain the decreased uptake of 2-deoxyglucose seen in interictal positron emission tomography, because neurons account for much of the energy consumption and, thus, glucose uptake in the brain.

Immunohistochemistry

Interneurons in the hippocampus contain peptides, including dynorphin, enkephalin, somatostatin, neuropeptide Y, vasoactive intestinal peptide, cholecystokinin, and substance P, whose functions are unknown. Dynorphin is localized to the terminals of the mossy fibers (the axons of the dentate granule cells) and, thus, coexists with the excitatory neurotransmitter glutamate. Many g-aminobutyric acid-containing (GABAergic) interneurons in the hippocampus are immunoreactive for GABA per se or for glutamic acid decarboxylase, which is the synthesizing enzyme for GABA. All of these interneurons presumably are inhibitory and provide local feedback or feed-forward inhibition to the principal excitatory neurons of the hippocampus (that is, the pyramidal cells and dentate granule cells).

GABAergic neurons appear to be preserved in mesial temporal sclerosis despite the presumed loss or reduction of their inhibitory function (see below). There appears to be a selective loss of somatostatin, neuropeptide Y, and substance P immunoreactive neurons in the dentate hilus but not in CA1.[8] The explanation for this selective loss of neurons is not clear. The presence of immunoreactivity to calcium-binding proteins that may buffer intracellular calcium and, thus, may protect from N-methyl-D-aspartate (NMDA)–mediated excitotoxicity

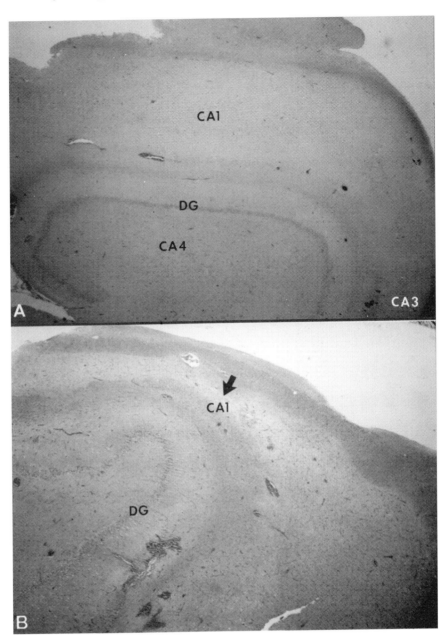

FIGURE 4-1. A. Photomicrograph of histologically normal hippocampus from a patient with nonlesional temporal lobe epilepsy. B. Photomicrograph showing changes consistent with mesial temporal sclerosis. Note the prominent hippocampal neuronal loss (*arrow*) in the subicular complex and CA1 subfield. (*DG*) dentate gyrus. (A and B. Hematoxylin and eosin.)

is not always correlated with preservation of neurons in experimental models of neuronal injury.

As mentioned above, dynorphin immunoreactivity is localized to the mossy fiber terminals, and this pattern correlates with that seen with Timm staining, which stains heavy metal zinc that is also present in the mossy fiber terminals. Both Timm staining and dynorphin immunohistochemistry demonstrate "mossy fiber sprouting" into the inner molecular layer of the dentate gyrus in mesial temporal sclerosis in humans and experimental animals. These "sprouting fibers" appear to synapse on dendrites, but it is not certain whether they are the dendrites of granule cells or inhibitory GABAergic basket neurons. The results of electrophysiologic studies indicate that the correlation between the degree of mossy fiber sprouting, as

indicated by the aberrant pattern of Timm staining, and the hyperexcitability of dentate granule neurons from human epileptic hippocampus is significant.[9]

Receptor Biochemistry

Neurotransmitter receptor systems are integral to synaptic mechanisms, and neuronal hyperexcitability may be reflected in changes in receptor systems. Because receptor proteins do not turn over rapidly and are well preserved in surgical specimens (and even in postmortem tissue), receptor-binding studies with radioactive ligands can be performed in these specimens. GABA and glutamate are the principal inhibitory and excitatory neurotransmitters, respectively, and benzodiazepines augment

GABA receptor function. Their respective receptor systems have been examined in mesial temporal sclerosis with in vitro receptor autoradiographic techniques.

Although the density of ligand binding was decreased in mesial temporal sclerosis, after correction for neuronal loss, benzodiazepine receptor density per surviving neuron appears to be unchanged.[10] Results of studies of glutamate receptor systems with various ligands for subtypes NMDA and α-amino-3-hydroxy-5-methylisoxazole-4-propionate (AMPA)/quisqualate are not consistent. Increases and decreases in the binding of these ligands were found in mesial temporal sclerosis when corrected for neuronal density. However, because different investigators reported different anatomical distributions, the interpretation of these results is difficult.[8,11,12] One of the many explanations for these conflicting results may be differences in the selection of controls.

Electrophysiology

In addition to the in vivo electrophysiologic studies performed with depth electrodes intraoperatively and extraoperatively, excised hippocampus can be sliced into thin sections and perfused with oxygenated, artificial cerebrospinal fluid. The neurons survive temporarily in these slices, thus allowing more detailed in vitro electrophysiologic studies. Masukawa et al.[13] reported an increase in synaptic hyperexcitability of dentate granule neurons in cases of mesial temporal sclerosis, as compared with cases of foreign tissue lesions outside the hippocampus. This hyperexcitability was in the form of an increased tendency for burst firing in response to afferent stimulation, which appears to be NMDA-receptor mediated. These findings appear to be consistent with the results of experimental studies in animals, lending support to the validity of the animal models.

The results of many of the biochemical and physiologic studies are difficult to interpret because of the inability to obtain ideal human control tissue. Most anatomical studies use autopsy controls, which tend to be from an older population. In addition, chronic antiepileptic drug therapy cannot easily be controlled for in clinical situations. Because most antiepileptic drugs control neuronal excitability, many of the receptor systems that modulate the excitability (GABA receptors or glutamate receptors) may well be altered simply from the down-regulation or up-regulation due to the administration of agonists/antagonists. Even in cases in which the control "normal" hippocampus was resected as part of the resection of an adjacent tumor or vascular malformation, the hippocampus could be susceptible to some possible unknown effect of the nearby foreign tissue lesion. Thus, the ability to study noninvasively (for example, with new MRI technology) the functional biochemical and physiologic properties would be a big step

toward correlating many of the experimental results from animal studies with the pathophysiologic features of human epilepsy.

FUNCTIONAL IMPLICATIONS OF NEUROPATHOLOGY

Experimental work in animals has shown that repeated or prolonged seizures, as in status epilepticus, is sufficient to cause mesial temporal sclerosis, even without hypoxia or hypoperfusion. This effect likely is caused by excitotoxicity.[14,15] Surgical removal of sclerotic hippocampus by temporal lobectomy produces marked improvement in or "cure" of the epileptic condition in humans, suggesting that the sclerotic hippocampus or the surrounding region included in the resection margin is the cause of the epilepsy. Many of these patients have a history of complicated febrile seizures or status epilepticus in childhood, with later development of temporal lobe epilepsy.[4,16] One possibility is that a perinatal ischemic injury (perhaps subclinical) may produce a certain degree of mesial temporal sclerosis that, in turn, makes the person susceptible to complicated febrile convulsions or status epilepticus, which further damages the hippocampus and surrounding region. In the absence of a definitely known perinatal insult, it seems equally plausible that intense seizures themselves can cause hippocampal sclerosis, and that, once it has developed, hippocampal sclerosis can cause epilepsy. Thus, the question is: which occurs first, mesial temporal sclerosis or temporal lobe epilepsy? From the current experimental evidence, the answer appears to be that either one can precede the other (that is, both can occur).

By what process does neuronal death and gliosis, with accompanying functional and morphological rearrangements, lead to epileptogenesis in the hippocampus and the eventual emergence of temporal lobe epilepsy? Status epilepticus in animals causes a loss of recurrent, GABA-mediated inhibition of the dentate granule cells.[17] Although it was assumed that the neurons that were damaged in the hippocampus were GABAergic inhibitory neurons, detailed immunohistochemical studies of sclerotic hippocampi from experimental animals (models of partial epilepsy) and from humans have shown that GABAergic interneurons are generally preserved. However, the mossy cells and somatostatin/neuropeptide Y immunoreactive neurons are damaged and lost in the dentate hilus (CA4).[18–20] The mossy *cells* (not to be confused with mossy *fibers*, which are the axons of the dentate granule cells) are the most numerous neurons in the hilus of the dentate gyrus[21] to receive synaptic input from both dentate granule cells (via mossy fibers) and entorhinal cortex (through the perforant path, the major afferent pathway to the hippocampus).[22] Mossy cells project ipsilaterally and contralaterally to the molecular layer of the

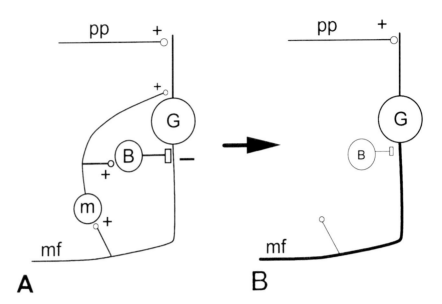

FIGURE 4-2. Dormant basket cell hypothesis. A. When mossy cell (*m*) is damaged, tonic activation of the basket cell (*B*) is eliminated, producing disinhibition of dentate granule cell (*G*). B. Even physiologic input through perforant path (*pp*) to *G* may result in hyperactive output through mossy fiber (*mf*). (+) excitatory; (-) inhibitory.

dentate gyrus, where the dendrites of the granule cells are located.[23] Electrophysiologically, mossy cells are activated at a lower threshold than dentate granule cells and appear to have an excitatory effect on their targets.[24] Intense synaptic activation, as in repetitive seizures or status epilepticus, can damage mossy cells through excitotoxicity by activation of the NMDA subtype of glutamate receptor. Activation of these receptors produces an excessive increase in intracellular calcium.[25]

Preservation of GABAergic neurons in the face of functional loss of GABA-mediated recurrent inhibition of the dentate granule cells after intense seizures appeared paradoxical, leading to the "dormant basket cell hypothesis" (Figure 4-2).[26–28] According to this hypothesis, the seizure-induced death of the most susceptible mossy cells in the hilus removes a tonic excitatory input to the GABAergic inhibitory basket cells in the dentate gyrus. This results in disinhibition, because the basket cells lie dormant without their usual tonic excitatory input from the mossy cells. Thus, a partial loss of this inhibition in combination with excitatory synaptic input from otherwise physiologic stimuli may lead to excessive firing by the granule cells, the death of more mossy cells, further loss of GABAergic inhibition, and, ultimately, the emergence of an epileptic condition, even many years after the initial injury. Similar anatomical and synaptic arrangements are found in the CA3/CA1 region of the hippocampus proper.[24]

An alternative to the "dormant basket cell hypothesis" is the "mossy fiber sprouting hypothesis" (Figure 4-3). According to this hypothesis, the observed hyperexcitability of the dentate granule cells is a consequence of a pathologic neuronal rearrangement in which the excitatory granule cells innervate themselves, thus establishing a recurrent excitatory circuit. This hypothesis proposes that the death of neurons in the dentate hilus that normally project to the dendrites of the granule cells results in the loss of synaptic contacts on these dendrites, and these synaptic contacts are replaced by the mossy fibers of the dentate granule cells themselves, presumably through the process of sprouting. A marked increase in this projection in the molecular layer of the dentate gyrus has been demonstrated with Timm staining after seizures were induced with a neurotoxin, kainate (in kindling model of epilepsy), and in surgical specimens from patients with medically intractable epilepsy.[29,30] The usual paired pulse inhibition (a physiologic indicator of recurrent GABAergic inhibition) obtained from normal animals was not only eliminated but changed to paired pulse facilitation in animals with intense sprouting, as demonstrated anatomically, thus supporting the argument for the emergence of functional recurrent excitatory synapses.[31] However, the functional consequences of these aberrant projections are still a matter of controversy because of evidence that suggests that sprouting actually may be promoting inhibition, perhaps in response to the abnormal hyperexcitability.

Both the dormant basket cell and the mossy fiber sprouting hypotheses may be correct and both mechanisms may cooperate to promote epileptogenesis. Of interest is that in a fluid percussion model of closed head injury, similar damage is observed in the dentate hilus.[32] This may be an explanation of the mesial temporal sclerosis found in post-traumatic epilepsy. Regardless of how the damage occurs initially, once the process of self-perpetuating hyperexcitability is established, even in a

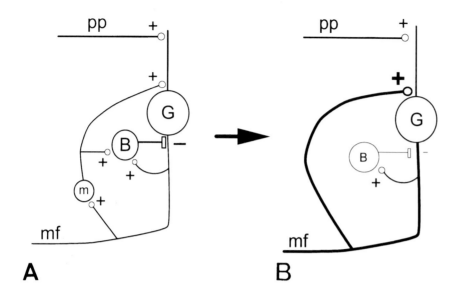

FIGURE 4-3. Mossy fiber sprouting hypothesis. A. Normal circuit. (*m*) mossy cell; (*B*) basket cell; (*G*) granule cell; (*mf*) mossy fiber; (*pp*) perforant path; (+) excitatory; (-) inhibitory. B. After m is eliminated, mf sprouts terminals that synapse on G, "filling in the gap" caused by loss of m terminals. This establishes a recurrent excitatory circuit that results in hyperactive output through mf, even after physiologic input from pp.

limited area of hippocampus, it could spread throughout the hippocampus. This process of self-perpetuating hyperexcitability then will inevitably influence the synaptically downstream structures with similar circuitry. If the local protective inhibitory system is overcome by constant hyperexcitable afferent input, CA3/CA1 hippocampus, subiculum, and entorhinal cortex could be recruited in a sequential fashion into the seizure network, each with its own intrinsic hyperexcitability. When the synaptically affiliated network develops to the point that hyperexcitability can be synchronized throughout the network, then a spontaneous paroxysmal expression of seizures may occur whenever the brain's inhibitory control of the seizure network falls below a certain threshold.

CONCLUSION

Understanding of the pathophysiology of temporal lobe epilepsy has come a long way. First, with the empirical observation that surgical resection of the temporal lobe cured epilepsy, second, with careful analysis of the neuropathologic features of mesial temporal sclerosis, and, third, with the use of various animal models and experimental techniques, tremendous insight has been gained into the possible mechanisms of epileptogenesis. Furthermore, the technological revolution, with advances such as the advent of MRI, has refined the evaluation of patients with partial epilepsy and has improved the care of those with medically intractable complex partial seizures.

However, many questions remain, and answering them will require further developments in basic science and continued improvement in clinical tools. Through the collaboration of basic research and clinical investigation, it should be possible to devise novel strategies for preventing and effectively treating, even curing, epilepsy.

REFERENCES

1. Dreifuss FE. Goals of surgery for epilepsy. In: Engel J Jr, ed. Surgical treatment of the epilepsies. New York: Raven Press, 1987:31–49.

2. Cascino GD. Surgical treatment of epilepsy. Neurology Chronicle 1993;3:1–8.

3. Walczak TS, Radtke RA, McNamara JO, et al. Anterior temporal lobectomy for complex partial seizures: evaluation, results, and long-term follow-up in 100 cases. Neurology 1990;40:413–8.

4. Bruton CJ. The neuropathology of temporal lobe epilepsy. Oxford: Oxford University Press, 1988.

5. Cascino GD, Jack CR Jr, Parisi JE, et al. Magnetic resonance imaging-based volume studies in temporal lobe epilepsy: pathological correlations. Ann Neurol 1991;30:31–6.

6. Margerison JH, Corsellis JA. Epilepsy and the temporal lobes. A clinical, electroencephalographic and neuropathological study of the brain in epilepsy, with particular reference to the temporal lobes. Brain 1966; 89:499–530.

7. Fried I, Kim JH, Spencer DD. Hippocampal pathology in patients with intractable seizures and temporal lobe masses. J Neurosurg 1992;76:735–40.

8. de Lanerolle NC, Brines M, Williamson A, et al. Neurotransmitters and their receptors in human temporal lobe epilepsy. Epilepsy Res Suppl 1992;Suppl 7:235–50.

9. Masukawa LM, Uruno K, Sperling M, et al. The functional relationship between antidromically evoked field responses of the dentate gyrus and mossy fiber reorganization in temporal lobe epileptic patients. Brain Res 1992;579:119–27.

10. Johnson EW, de Lanerolle NC, Kim JH, et al. "Central" and "peripheral" benzodiazepine receptors:

opposite changes in human epileptogenic tissue. Neurology 1992;42:811–5.

11. Geddes JW, Cahan LD, Cooper SM, et al. Altered distribution of excitatory amino acid receptors in temporal lobe epilepsy. Exp Neurol 1990;108:214–20.

12. Hosford DA, Crain BJ, Cao Z, et al. Increased AMPA-sensitive quisqualate receptor binding and reduced NMDA receptor binding in epileptic human hippocampus. J Neurosci 1991;11:428–34.

13. Masukawa LM, Higashima M, Kim JH, et al. Epileptiform discharges evoked in hippocampal brain slices from epileptic patients. Brain Res 1989;493:168–74.

14. Meldrum BS, Brierley JB. Prolonged epileptic seizures in primates. Ischemic cell change and its relation to ictal physiological events. Arch Neurol 1973;28:10–7.

15. Olney JW. Inciting excitotoxic cytocide among central neurons. Adv Exp Med Biol 1986;203:631–45.

16. Sagar HJ, Oxbury JM. Hippocampal neuron loss in temporal lobe epilepsy: correlation with early childhood convulsions. Ann Neurol 1987;22:334–40.

17. Sloviter RS. "Epileptic" brain damage in rats induced by sustained electrical stimulation of the perforant path. I. Acute electrophysiological and light microscopic studies. Brain Res Bull 1983;10:675–97.

18. Sloviter RS. Decreased hippocampal inhibition and a selective loss of interneurons in experimental epilepsy. Science 1987;235:73–6.

19. Babb TL, Pretorius JK, Kupfer WR, et al. Glutamate decarboxylase-immunoreactive neurons are preserved in human epileptic hippocampus. J Neurosci 1989;9:2562–74.

20. Houser CR. GABA neurons in seizure disorders: a review of immunocytochemical studies. Neurochem Res 1991;16:295–308.

21. Amaral DG. A Golgi study of cell types in the hilar region of the hippocampus in the rat. J Comp Neurol 1978;182:851–914.

22. Scharfman HE, Schwartzkroin PA. Responses of cells of the rat fascia dentata to prolonged stimulation of the perforant path: sensitivity of hilar cells and changes in granule cell excitability. Neuroscience 1990;35:491–504.

23. Ribak CE, Seress L, Amaral DG. The development, ultrastructure and synaptic connections of the mossy cells of the dentate gyrus. J Neurocytol 1985; 14:835–57.

24. Schwartzkroin PA, Scharfman HE, Sloviter RS. Similarities in circuitry between Ammon's horn and dentate gyrus: local interactions and parallel processing. Prog Brain Res 1990;83:269–86.

25. Scharfman HE, Schwartzkroin PA. Protection of dentate hilar cells from prolonged stimulation by intracellular calcium chelation. Science 1989;246: 257–60.

26. Sloviter RS. Permanently altered hippocampal structure, excitability, and inhibition after experimental status epilepticus in the rat: the "dormant basket cell" hypothesis and its possible relevance to temporal lobe epilepsy. Hippocampus 1991;1:41–66.

27. Sloviter RS. The functional organization of the hippocampal dentate gyrus and its relevance to the pathogenesis of temporal lobe epilepsy. Ann Neurol 1994;35:640–54.

28. Bekenstein JW, Lothman EW. Dormancy of inhibitory interneurons in a model of temporal lobe epilepsy. Science 1993;259:97–100.

29. Sutula T, Cascino G, Cavazos J, et al. Mossy fiber synaptic reorganization in the epileptic human temporal lobe. Ann Neurol 1989;26:321–30.

30. Cavazos JE, Golarai G, Sutula TP. Mossy fiber synaptic reorganization induced by kindling: time course of development, progression, and permanence. J Neurosci 1991;11:2795–803.

31. Tauck DL, Nadler JV. Evidence of functional mossy fiber sprouting in hippocampal formation of kainic acid-treated rats. J Neurosci 1985;5:1016–22.

32. Lowenstein DH, Thomas MJ, Smith DH, et al. Selective vulnerability of dentate hilar neurons following traumatic brain injury: a potential mechanistic link between head trauma and disorders of the hippocampus. J Neurosci 1992;12:4846–53.

Visual Analysis in Mesial Temporal Sclerosis

Graeme D. Jackson

The role of visual analysis in the investigation of patients with epilepsy is considered in this chapter. The features in the magnetic resonance (MR) studies that need to be optimized to facilitate sensitive interpretation of the structures important in epilepsy are considered. The interpretation of these studies and the criteria by which individual diagnoses can be made are discussed. Emphasis is on the diagnosis of hippocampal sclerosis, because damage to the hippocampus is the most common lesion in intractable epilepsy and is thought to be particularly important in the genesis of intractable seizures. Usually, it is not diagnosed with any sensitivity on routine imaging studies not focused on the question of intractable epilepsy. Despite this appropriate emphasis on the hippocampus, the mesial temporal region does not consist of only the hippocampus but also of the dentate gyrus, subiculum, parahippocampal gyrus, amygdala, and entorhinal area. All these structures can be evaluated visually. The mesial temporal region is distinct in its development (archicortex) in comparison with the rest of the cerebral cortex (neocortex). It is also special in its importance in intractable partial epilepsy.

In many ways, visual analysis is the most important technique for the interpretation of neuroimaging studies, even of the hippocampus, because it is the most common technique and the most usual source of clinical information. Generally, there is little that cannot be seen on optimized imaging (in expert hands) that quantitative interpretation or other derived analytic measures can

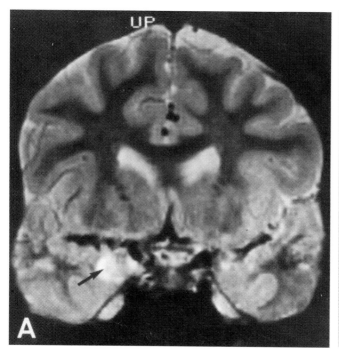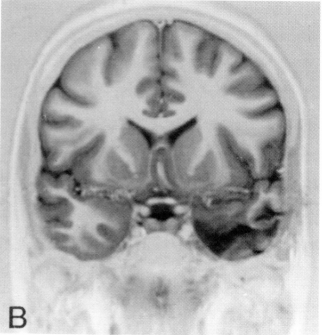

Figure 5-1. Foreign tissue lesions in the temporal lobes account for about 20% of all cases of temporal lobe epilepsy seen in an epilepsy clinic. Before MRI, about only half of these were diagnosed on x-ray CT scans. Often, small uncalcified lesions were not detected. A. T_2-weighted image in which the cerebrospinal fluid (CSF) appears white (long T_2), and the lesion (*arrow*) in the right mesial temporal region also has bright signal. This is a dysembryoplastic neuroepithelial tumor in a 25-year-old woman. It originally was diagnosed as a low-grade astrocytoma on pathologic examination. B. T_1-weighted image with CSF appearing black (long T_1). The extensive lesion in the left temporal lobe appears dark, and the excellent contrast between the gray and white matter allows anatomical features to be identified (compare with A). On a proton density image (not shown), the CSF still appeared dark, but the temporal lobe tissue had the signal characteristics of gray matter, indicating that this black area was not CSF in an atrophied region. The lesion is gliosis in a 26-year-old man who sustained a head injury in a motorcycle accident.

detect, although quantitation gives the confidence to interpret the subtle features that are seen and can set a standard for visual analysis. Whereas quantitation is important for research purposes, visual analysis must first be optimized for clinical practice.

BACKGROUND

Routine magnetic resonance imaging (MRI) studies can noninvasively detect virtually all foreign tissue lesions (tumors) such as hamartomas, gliomas, oligodendrocytomas, dysembryoplastic neuroepithelial tumors, and other developmental lesions.[1–3] MR has enabled these lesions to be diagnosed with sensitivity and good specificity (Figure 5-1). In itself, this is an advance over previously available imaging methods. Compared with MR, x-ray computed tomography (CT) detects about only 50% of the small foreign tissue lesions (for example, tumors and hamartomas) present in the temporal lobes of patients with intractable partial epilepsy presenting to

epilepsy clinics. These foreign tissue lesions usually have altered free water in the tissues and, thus, show an increased signal on a T_2-weighted image (Figure 5-1 A) and a decreased signal on a heavily T_1-weighted image (Figure 5-1 B).

More impressive has been the ability of optimized structural imaging techniques to detect less distinct abnormalities of gray matter, in particular lesions such as cortical dysplasias (Figure 5-2), minor abnormalities of gray matter, and especially hippocampal sclerosis (Figure 5-3).[3–44] Hippocampal sclerosis is important in epilepsy because it (1) is the most common lesion found in patients with intractable seizures, (2) is epileptogenic, and (3) identifies the group of patients with a good outcome from surgical treatment of their epileptic condition (for an overview of epilepsy surgery, see ref. 45). In this important group of patients with hippocampal sclerosis, quantitative measures of both the abnormal morphology (volume) and abnormal signal (T_2 relaxation measurement) have allowed this diagnosis to be made

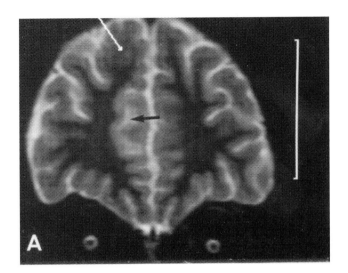

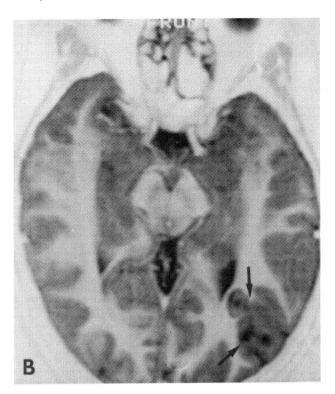

FIGURE 5-2. A. Malformations of cortical development (dysplasias) can be subtle and have either increased T$_2$-weighted signal (*black arrow*) or signal similar to gray matter (*white arrow*). This lesion was not apparent on x-ray CT. B. On heavily T$_1$-weighted images, these abnormalities can show dark signal (*arrows*). This patient had temporal lobe epilepsy. C and D. Lesions can appear similar to gray matter in signal characteristics (*arrows*).

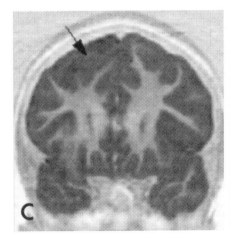

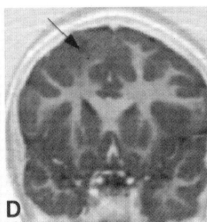

objectively (see Chapter 6). However, visual analysis (in expert hands) is just as powerful and in some cases reveals subtleties of interpretation that are not detectable with quantitative means, because of the limited focus of quantitative methods.

The new MR techniques allow many aspects of brain structure, function, and biochemistry to be investigated in the clinical setting, and this has revolutionized the ability to detect brain abnormalities underlying epilepsy. In some surgical programs for the treatment of epilepsy, MR has become at least as important as electroencephalography (EEG). The information from MR is also having a major impact on the classification and understanding of epilepsy syndromes and is shifting the emphasis from the electro-clinical syndrome diagnosis of these conditions to the brain substrates, or the structural abnormalities, from which the electrical and clinical features of an epilepsy syndrome originate (Table 5-1). Currently, it is unclear how far this trend will progress, how frequently substrates can be identified in patients with epilepsy, what the relationships of these structural abnormalities are to the site of seizure origin, and what role they have in the pathogenesis and expression of epilepsy. Also, it is not known whether all the important structural abnormalities that may exist in the

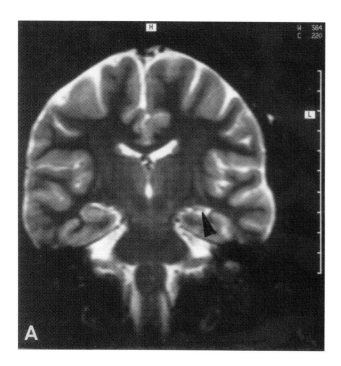

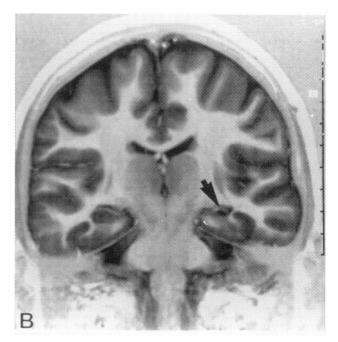

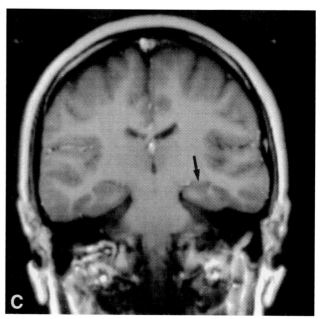

FIGURE 5-3. The classic features of hippocampal sclerosis. A. A 5-mm-thick T_2-weighted image through the body of the hippocampus. The hippocampus is small, and its most prominent feature is the increased signal from the gray matter (*arrowhead*). B. In a 5-mm-thick heavily T_1-weighted inversion recovery sequence, hippocampal anatomy can be seen. The hippocampus is small and easily distinguished from the alveus (*thin white line between the hippocampus and CSF*) and on the abnormal left side has a dark signal within it (*arrow*). By comparison, the normal internal microarchitecture of the hippocampus is seen on the right side. C. In a minimally T_1-weighted image, the hippocampus (*arrow*) is small, but the abnormal signal is not seen within it. The inversion recovery sequence in this orientation is the easiest for the diagnosis of hippocampal sclerosis because the structure is easily identified and the signal abnormality and internal features assist in the diagnosis of abnormality. (A and B. From Jackson et al.[44] By permission of the American Society of Neuroradiology.)

brains of these patients are being detected or whether only the most apparent lesions are seen.

MAGNETIC RESONANCE IN EPILEPSY

In epilepsy, as in other disorders, the information obtained from an MR examination depends on several factors. Important among these are the following:

1. Planning the investigation before the imaging study. How long will the study be, and what abnormalities must be either demonstrated or excluded by the study?

2. The choice of the sequence, for example, T_1-weighted for anatomy, T_2-weighted for abnormal signal, proton-density-weighted, or other sequences such as T_2^* or diffusion-weighted. Special sequences such as T_2 mapping or volume acquisition.

3. The imaging axis used in acquiring or displaying the images. This can be critical in interpreting subtle abnormalities of the temporal lobe, such as in the hippocampus.

4. The skill of the reporting specialist, including the threshold for defining abnormality (sensi-

TABLE 5-1. Classification of Temporal Lobe Epilepsy by Substrate and Electroclinical Syndrome

Surgically remedial epilepsy substrates based on MRI findings
Mesial temporal sclerosis
Hippocampal sclerosis
Hippocampal sclerosis and other temporal lobe abnormalities
Hippocampal sclerosis and extratemporal abnormalities (dual pathology)
Mass lesions
Tumor
Vascular malformation
Cortical developmental malformations
for example, focal dysplasia
Acquired lesions
for example, focal gliosis
Electroclinical syndromes of temporal lobe epilepsy—subtype by site of onset*
Hippocampal-amygdalar (temporobasal)
Temporal polar or amygdalar-polar
Lateral temporal neocortical
Opercular-insular
Frontobasal-cingulate

*Wieser (1988).[46]

tivity) and the knowledge of normal and pathologic anatomy of the disease or structure to be imaged (specificity). In epilepsy, it is essential that the reporting specialist has a specific interest in the problem of epilepsy, because often a different approach is required, different structures need to be carefully examined, and specific hypotheses about the epileptic condition have to be confirmed or excluded.

5. The criteria used to make a diagnosis of abnormality. For example, the diagnosis of hippocampal sclerosis will be reported differently if only atrophy is assessed or if signal change or architecture of the hippocampus is also considered. This also depends on the imaging sequences and orientation that are available.

6. What abnormalities the study is designed to diagnose. A standard protocol, even if extensive, cannot detect all abnormalities. If it does, then often nothing further is required,

but if it does not, then additional MR investigations need to be "hypothesis driven." If a short standard screening study has been performed, it does not mean that the "MR is normal" if no abnormality is identified. The principle is that if a lesion or abnormality is not seen on the MR study, this does not mean that a lesion cannot be seen using MR techniques. It is critical to decide how many pulse sequences and how much imaging time should be used and what new techniques should be applied in the search for an abnormality in a patient.

Although it should be apparent from this list, it needs to be emphasized that the MR investigation of a patient with epilepsy must involve close interactions between clinicians and imaging specialists if all the relevant structural information important to the treating physician is to be obtained.

LEVELS OF MAGNETIC RESONANCE INVESTIGATION

The way in which MR should be used can be considered to be analogous to EEG[47] (Table 5-2). After an initial routine interictal surface EEG (stage 1), no one would think that all the information that could be gained from EEG had been acquired. In some cases, the diagnosis of epileptic discharges and their location and character could be obtained from this most basic study. In most medical centers, the routine study would consist of a simple interictal recording and some different montages, including provocation procedures such as photic stimulation and hyperventilation (stage 2). This increases the yield of relevant information. If this provides all the required diagnostic information, additional EEG studies may not be needed. However, in cases in which the diagnosis is still unclear, additional investigations can be considered. This step involves much greater interaction between the neurologist and neurophysiologist. For example, sleep studies may be considered or an ictal recording under conditions in which videomonitoring is available may be required (stage 3). The final step in the EEG investigation might be further consultation among neurosurgeons, neuropsychologists, neurophysiologists, and neurologists. Also, invasive depth electrodes may be implanted so that a recording can be made from the surface of the brain or from deep within its substance. This step is expensive, time-consuming, and involves morbidity; therefore, it must be pursued with a specific hypothesis in mind. It is largely this invasive step that noninvasive investigations such as MR can replace.

Similarly, MR can be performed at different levels that involve differing levels of consultation, time com-

TABLE 5-2. Protocol for Magnetic Resonance Studies in Epilepsy

---

Level 1. Routine imaging in epilepsy patients (recommendation): major sequences

Sequence 1: 3D T_1-weighted

Heavily T_1-weighted 3D sequence with default reconstruction parasagittally (for example, MPRAGE)

The parasagittal images are then used as scout views for accurate placement of the imaging plane for the coronal imaging and the T_2 relaxation mapping. The coronal plane is placed at right angles to the hippocampus (or halfway between the two hippocampi if these are at different angles).

Hippocampal angulation is noted. The central slice is placed at the anterior border of the brain stem. The T_2 map is placed so that the anterior limit is immediately posterior to the hippocampal head.

Images are reconstructed in the tilted coronal plane (both 5-mm thick for visual analysis and 1.8-mm thick for volumetric analysis) and in the axial plane (5-mm thick with a slice gap so that slices are centered on the parahippocampal gyrus, hippocampus, amygdala, and basal ganglia).

Sequence 2: coronal T_2-weighted

Coronal (oriented as above) heavily T_2-weighted sequence covering the whole brain

Sequence 3: coronal inversion recovery

Coronal (oriented as above) inversion recovery sequence. TE26,TI300,TR3000, 5-mm thick, covering the temporal lobe. In some medical centers, this may be considered a level 2 study, but the additional basic information provided about the hippocampus and temporal white matter justifies it as an important component of a level 1 study.

Sequence 4: coronal T_2 map

Coronal T_2 map (single slice) 8-mm thick, oriented and positioned from the 3D sequence (sequence 1 above); 16 echoes from TE 24 ms–TE 264 ms. This sequence may also be considered a level 2 study, but in an epilepsy center, we find the information about severity and bilaterality as well as the quantitative check on the visual findings justify using this in a level 1 study.

Level 2. Additional studies in patients with partial epilepsy and negative findings on MR

Depending on the clinical question, these sequences may be used to provide additional information. Sequence 3 and 4 above may be considered in this category if only basic screening is required, but in this case, not all hippocampal abnormalities will be detected. Similarly, volume measurement may be considered a level 1 study in some epilepsy centers.

Measurement of hippocampal volume and side-to-side asymmetry

FLAIR sequence, either coronal or axial, to demonstrate the hippocampus, parahippocampal gyrus, entorhinal area, or amygdala

Amygdala T_2 mapping

Image reconstruction in special planes from the 3D study

Additional inversion recovery studies oriented to examine a particular region of suspicion

Level 3. Other investigations that may provide additional data in patients with partial epilepsy and negative findings on MR— usually involve additional time or expertise

MR spectroscopy of the temporal lobes

Surface rendering to demonstrate the gyral pattern

Cortical ribbon analysis with special sequences or with post-processing analysis (for example, fractal analysis of cortical pattern or quantitative measurement of cortical complexity)

---

mitment, and effort and that, in turn, give different and additional information. In the first stage, a routine MRI study is performed. It is designed for whole-brain coverage in minimal time, without special sequences optimized for epilepsy. In some specialist epilepsy centers, extra sequences or special imaging orientations may be performed at this initial stage (stage 2, a recommended protocol for epilepsy is discussed below). This may be sufficient if the imaging study defines structural abnormalities that can be understood in the context of the electroclinical information. In some cases, the results of the imaging study are equivocal or negative and additional studies should be undertaken. This third stage may involve additional investigations (MR spectroscopy, T_2 imaging, volume imaging, or other sequences such as inversion recovery [IR], or fast low-angle inversion recovery [FLAIR], if not already performed) or it might involve additional analysis (volumetrics, reconstructions in particular planes, and inspection of the images on the console). In the future, functional MRI (fMRI) may also be used for special purposes. The general rule is that MR investigations should aim to exclude the existence of abnormality as well as to detect abnormality if it happens to be seen. If a pathologic abnormality is present but is not seen on a "routine" MR study, this does not mean that the abnormality cannot be seen with optimal use of MR techniques.

IMAGING BEFORE MAGNETIC RESONANCE

Many radiologic features have been proposed for the diagnosis of hippocampal sclerosis. However, until MRI techniques were optimized, the noninvasive diagnosis of hippocampal sclerosis was not reliable. For example, the isolated dilatation of the temporal horn of the lateral ventricle was generally found with CT or pneumoencephalography on the side of seizure origin, but it was not a reliable indicator of hippocampal abnormality because occasionally the dilatation was seen on the side contralateral to that proven to have hippocampal sclerosis.[21,48-62] Since MR studies have been available, it is clear that temporal horn dilatation usually occurs on the side of hippocampal sclerosis; however, it is not uncommon to find the dilatation on the opposite side. Therefore, dilatation of the temporal horn should not be used in deciding which temporal lobe may be abnormal and, particularly, which hippocampus may have underlying damage. However, dilatation of the temporal horn may be a guide to the presence of other lesions in the adjacent hippocampus or temporal lobe, but this has not been established.[36,63,64] Other CT orientations were developed to improve visualization of the mesial temporal regions, but for the detection of hippocampal sclerosis, these are not reliable.[63] Although CT has developed since these early studies, it still does not reliably detect lesions in the temporal lobe unless they are larger than 2 cm or calcified.

EARLY MAGNETIC RESONANCE STUDIES IN EPILEPSY

The detection of hippocampal sclerosis on MRI was initially a matter of controversy. In most reports, hippocampal sclerosis was not recognized at all.[65,66] In isolated case reports, the description of T_2-weighted mesial temporal signal increase was not supported by pathologic confirmation.[55,67] Confusion existed about what criteria were needed for the diagnosis of hippocampal sclerosis, and in many cases, vaguely localized signal change in the mesial temporal region was labeled as hippocampal sclerosis. This led to confusion with arti-

facts in the region (field inhomogeneity, pulsation from local arteries, and partial volume from the regional CSF) and also to confusion between hippocampal sclerosis and other lesions. It was suggested that increased signal in the mesial temporal region reflected underlying sclerosis.[33,68] This was not initially a sensitive correlation, because it was present in only a portion (65%) of the cases in which hippocampal sclerosis was pathologically proven.[33] In these cases, signal abnormality was more commonly detected when severe abnormalities existed in the hippocampus.[33,59,69,70] The difficulties in diagnosis can be understood if one realizes that these early studies were often at low field strength and demonstrated poor signal-to-noise ratio (SNR) and field inhomogeneity. Coupled with suboptimal image orientation, diagnostic features were difficult to appreciate. An example of early studies is shown in Figure 5-4.

The recognition that optimal imaging of the hippocampus requires coronal images, with images oriented in a plane perpendicular to the long axis of the hippocampus, meant that the diagnosis of hippocampal sclerosis could be made with high sensitivity and specificity.[3,71] Using this imaging plane, both the side-to-side symmetry of the hippocampal gray matter (reflecting lateralized atrophy and best shown on inversion recovery or other heavily T_1-weighted sequences) as well as altered signal (increased hippocampal signal on T_2-weighted sequences and decreased signal on heavily T_1-weighted or inversion recovery sequences that reflect changes in the free water content of the hippocampus) are necessary for the reliable detection of hippocampal sclerosis. In our initial series of 81 patients undergoing temporal lobectomy, reported in 1990,[3] a sensitivity of 93% and specificity of 86% percent was found. This series relied on the presence of asymmetry and signal change. Since then, MR imaging of the hippocampus has been optimized with advances in image sequences and improvements in the specificity of interpretation, including sequences that allow internal features of the hippocampus to be defined.[44] The sensitivity and specificity of visual assessment of the MR images has now been confirmed by several authors.[8,12,24-26,42,72] The important principle is that diagnosis based on a single feature is not as sensitive or as specific as assessment of all features. Even in optimized series, not all features are present in all cases that can be diagnosed to have hippocampal sclerosis.

METHODS OF DETECTING LESIONS WITH MAGNETIC RESONANCE: PRINCIPLES

In principle, an MR study can detect abnormality in the brain either (1) by demonstrating signal contrast between normal and abnormal tissue or (2) by allowing the abnormal structure of the brain to be detected.

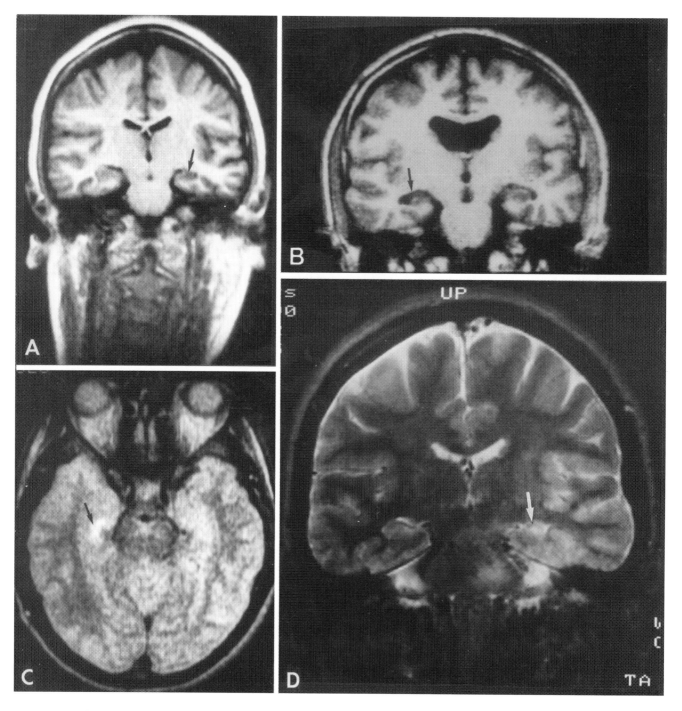

FIGURE 5-4. The diagnostic features of hippocampal sclerosis can be detected even at 0.3 T, and this enabled the diagnosis of hippocampal sclerosis with high sensitivity and specificity on early CT studies. A and B. Atrophy and signal change are seen on these T_1-weighted inversion recovery images. C and D. Signal change localized to the hippocampus could also be detected in early studies. In many early studies, artifacts were a problem and undermined the confidence of diagnosis in many cases. In the early T_2-weighted study (D), there is field inhomogeneity; this image is severely affected by artifact. These artifacts are uncommon in modern imaging systems. However, even in this early case, the hippocampus (*arrow*) can be seen to be small, and the signal is abnormal relative to the surrounding gray matter. With detailed knowledge of the anatomy of this region, the diagnosis of hippocampal sclerosis could still be made. The confident and reliable diagnosis of hippocampal sclerosis depends on the acquisition of optimized imaging and on optimized interpretation of these images, which requires a detailed appreciation of the anatomy of the mesial temporal lobe as well as a clear understanding of which abnormalities can be due to MR artifacts and which ones cannot be.

1. *The generation of contrast between normal and abnormal tissue* so that tissue characteristics that reflect abnormality can be identified by alterations in signal intensity or by measuring T_1 or T_2 relaxation times. Signal contrast depends on differing MR properties between the structures that are to be distinguished and that can be detected as alterations in signal. This signal can be acquired in such a way that it can emphasize several different properties of the tissue (for example, proton density, T_1-weighted and T_2-weighted for routine imaging, diffusion weighted, T_2^* weighted, magnetization transfer contrast, and others for special problems).

In the case of T_1- and T_2-weighted images, the major component of contrast is dependent on the free water content of the tissue as well as on the mobility of the protons and the presence of large molecules (microviscosity). Some sequences can make the MR image more sensitive to signal contrast which might not be apparent on routine images (for example, inversion recovery provides good contrast between gliosis, white matter, and gray matter, which is not necessarily the case in proton density or other T_1-weighted images). The use of special imaging sequences can even generate contrast that is dependent on other MR properties, such as diffusion of water, or on the state of oxygenation of the blood, but these are not used for routine MR studies and are not considered further in this chapter. Hence, if an abnormality is not seen on one type of MR study, this does not mean that it cannot be seen on an MR study performed using a different imaging technique.

2. *Detailed morphological analysis of a structure* can demonstrate changes in size or appearance that correlate with an underlying pathologic process. Careful volumetric measurements of a given structure compared with normal values or with serial measurements or side-to-side asymmetries may demonstrate variations in volume that correlate with pathologic processes.

All these methods have been applied to the problem of detecting the lesion of mesial temporal sclerosis.

VISUAL ANALYSIS

Definition

The term "visual analysis" refers to the whole process of analysis of the images acquired from an imaging study. This is in distinction to quantitative, or number-based analysis, of regions or structures such as the hippocampus. It represents the information that a properly trained and experienced observer should be able to extract from the study. There are two main aspects to this. One, has the study resolved, either anatomically or by detection of contrast with normal tissue, the abnormality so that it is capable of being detected? Two, has the abnormality actually been diagnosed with sensitivity and specificity by the observer? Both these elements are important, and

clearly, the better the base images are at distinguishing the relevant abnormality, the greater the chance of detecting it. However, even marked MR findings can potentially be dismissed as artifact or as insufficient to make a definite diagnosis. Therefore, visual analysis depends both on the imaging technique and the observer's skill.

Protocols for Magnetic Resonance Imaging and Assessment in Intractable Epilepsy: Principles

Before listing a protocol, the factors and principles on which this protocol are based are discussed, because specific imaging sequences may alter, and it is important to be able to choose an approach that balances imaging time and information acquired. Cost versus benefit is important in all imaging studies and is related mostly to imaging time. All elements of an imaging protocol have to be justified. The type of information that is gained from different sequences and why these sequences are used must be understood.

The final protocol depends on what clinical information is sought and what hypotheses about underlying brain abnormality must be excluded. In general, the aim of the MR study should be to reveal the substrate of the epileptic condition in all conditions in which brain abnormalities exist. In the case of epilepsy surgery, the MR detection of a surgically remedial substrate of the epilepsy is so important that any effort to reveal it is justified. Our suggested protocol (see Table 5-2) and the principles on which it is based are discussed below. Such protocols require collaboration among physicists, radiologists, and physicians so that all relevant information is acquired in the most cost-effective way.

Discussion of image acquisition inevitably requires a discussion of what features we wish to detect. Although any proposed imaging strategy must include all the brain, the special problem of intractable epilepsy dictates that the hippocampus must always be assessed carefully and hippocampal sclerosis must be excluded. To miss identifying this lesion can have significant clinical consequences. Our epilepsy protocol, and all the illustrative images, are acquired according to the following principles.

Image Orientation

The most important factor in any protocol for imaging the temporal lobe is the orientation of the imaging plane. This must be in the temporal axis (Figure 5-5). Using this plane has a great many advantages. The anatomical boundaries of the temporal lobe are easier to define, and the partial volume effects of the edges of a tubular structure such as the hippocampus are reduced when the imaging axis is at right angles to it[3,71,73] (see Figure 5-3). Also, the internal features of the hippocampus can be seen because they are oriented along this hippocampal

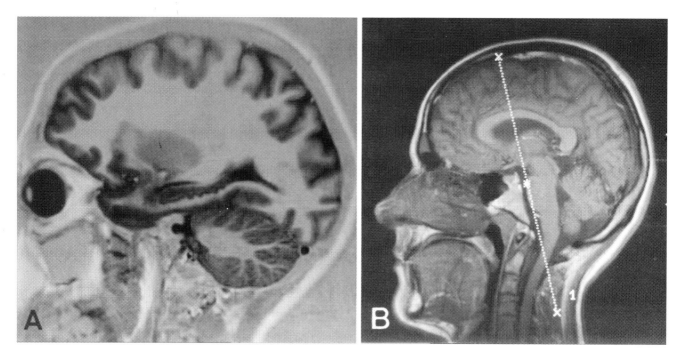

FIGURE 5-5. Orientation of the imaging plane is of utmost importance in optimization of the imaging of the hippocampus. A. The aim is to have a plane at right angles to the hippocampal body. This can be done by taking parasagittal scout images through the hippocampus (this can be taken from the three-dimensional imaging sequence). B. The alternative plane (*dotted line*) that can be used is along the angle of the anterior border of the brain stem, with the central slice located in the anterior part of the brain stem. It is important to standardize imaging, so that the imaging plane, central slice position, and other variables are reproduced between patients and over time (see Figure 5-18).

axis (it is usually not apparent when the imaging axis is not carefully oriented [see below]).[44] Imaging at right angles to the hippocampus in the coronal plane is essential in epilepsy. If an axial sequence is acquired, it should be oriented along the long axis of the hippocampus. Although it can be difficult to make the diagnosis of hippocampal sclerosis exclusively on the axial images, there are some advantages of the axial plane. This axial plane allows (1) the anterior-posterior distribution of the mesial temporal abnormality to be defined visually, (2) the white matter core of the temporal lobe to be assessed, and (3) the posterior temporal regions to be well visualized (Figure 5-6).

It is also important that this imaging plane be standardized by reference to orienting landmarks visible in the brain itself (rather than some standard based on head position). This standardized plane and position of the central slice are needed to properly compare the hippocampi of different persons and for sequential studies. The internal landmark that we find the easiest to use is the anterior border of the brain stem cutting across the pons (see Figure 5-5).[44] This approximates a right angle to the hippocampus.

Also, the hippocampus itself can be used if parasagittal scout images are acquired; the image plane is then oriented at right angles to the hippocampus itself. There are two things to be aware of if this latter orientation is used. The first thing to be aware of is that the left and right hippocampi often are not aligned in exactly the same plane, sometimes differing by 20° or more, particularly in epileptic patients. This can produce an artifactual side-to-side asymmetry from partial volume effects if one of the hippocampi is always used to orient the imaging plane (the hippocampus used for the image orientation will always seem slightly smaller). Very thin slices will avoid this to some extent, particularly for volume measurements. Another solution may be to use an axis oriented at right angles to a plane passing midway between the long axis of the two hippocampi. We choose to use the brain stem as our standardized reference and to note the orientation of the hippocampi relative to this, but this is a matter of preference as long as the orientation of the hippocampi is noted at the time of imaging. For most cases, this is not a particular problem because the hippocampal changes that are due to a pathologic process are greater than those due to artifacts of this kind, but for

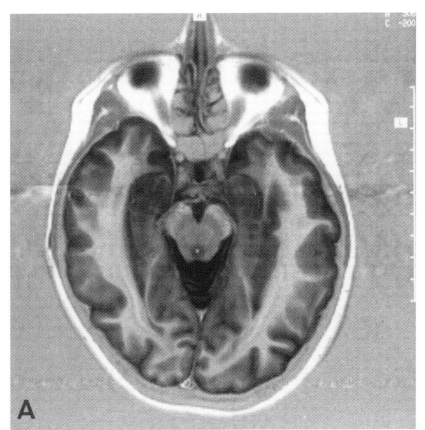

FIGURE 5-6. The axial images provide information that can be considered adjunct to the specific diagnosis of hippocampal sclerosis, which is based on optimally oriented coronal images. A. Normal hippocampus in a 5-mm-thick slice. B. The right hippocampus is atrophic throughout its length (*arrowheads*), but in (C) the posterior hippocampus appears to be normal size, with marked signal change in the hippocampal head and amygdala (*arrowheads*). This orientation is useful for assessing the white matter core of the temporal lobe for signal abnormalities and for determining the posterior extent of the hippocampal abnormality. Images in this orientation (5-mm-thick, 2.5-mm slice gap, centered on the hippocampus and then the amygdala; see Figure 5-12) can be reconstructed from the 3D sequence and can provide valuable information for visual analysis without increasing imaging time. (From Jackson et al.[44] By permission of the American Society of Neuroradiology.)

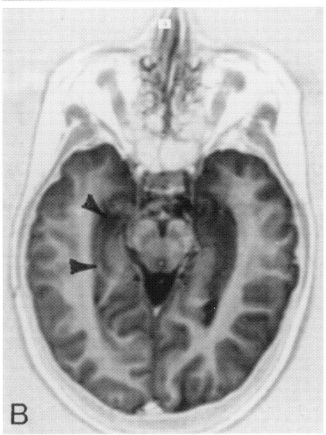

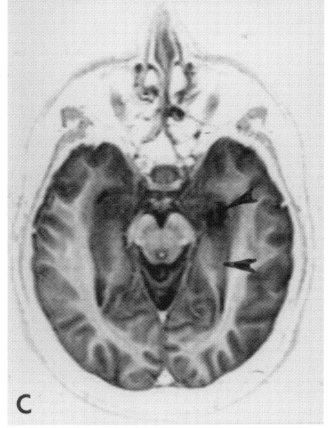

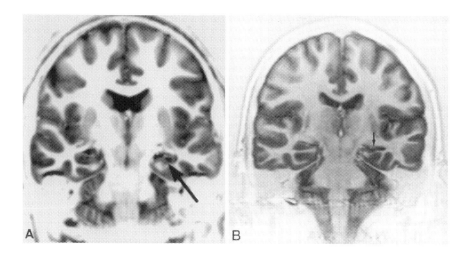

Figure 5-7. A and B. Heavily T$_1$-weighted inversion recovery images showing hippocampal atrophy and signal change (*arrows*). (*Continued*)

proper interpretation of less severe cases in which the findings are more subtle, these details can be essential.

The second thing to be aware of is that slices need to be acquired in the same anterior-posterior position. For visual analysis, it is easier to inspect images from a standardized position so that the features in each particular slice can be become familiar—and, thus, easier to interpret—and comparisons over time can be determined. The important lesions in epilepsy are often considered to be subtle, and all factors that assist the interpretation of images are important.

Slice Thickness

Optimal slice thickness is a controversial issue because the assumption is often made that thinner is better. In some aspects, this is true theoretically and intuitively compelling, but for reasons discussed below, this does not always translate into improved diagnostic accuracy and, in some cases, can lead to errors of diagnosis.

Thin slices need to be acquired and assessed, but for visual analysis, a large number of images (up to 64 for the temporal lobe at 1-mm slice thickness) can overwhelm the ability to assess them. Minor anatomical variations can sometimes lead to errors of interpretation because of the difficulties in assessing small asymmetries and determining whether the slice is taken from the same part of the hippocampus on each side. Normal subjects from control series can appear to have asymmetries in some slices, although this is rarely the case when thicker slices are assessed. When minor asymmetries can be due to factors other than the existence of a lesion, either errors are made or sensitivity is sacrificed in less severe cases. Therefore, although the information that thin slices contain is important, their use in visual analysis can sometimes lead to overinterpretation or unnecessary caution in making the diagnosis of asymmetry between the two hippocampi.

Visual analysis is not necessarily easier with thin slices, because side-to-side asymmetry is usually the only feature that can be assessed (internal structure is often not visible, and signal contrast is often poor because of the thin slices and pulse sequences used to acquire these images [fast T$_1$-weighted three-dimensional volume sequences]). The coexistence of signal change and asymmetry is the most reliable indicator of hippocampal sclerosis (see below).

Thick slices can introduce partial volume effects or miss minor and very focal abnormalities. Somewhat paradoxically, thicker slices can average out these small variations and make visual comparisons easier. It might be possible to establish the optimal balance between useful visual information and artifacts in this situation (both partial volume artifacts and the problem of inappropriate comparison of different parts of the hippocampus), but we have found empirically that it is most useful to examine the thicker (5-mm thick) slices first for the overall impression and for details of signal and internal structure. Next, thin slices are assessed to confirm the impression gained from thick slices and to resolve in finer detail the reason for hippocampal asymmetry (note that asymmetry does not always mean atrophy). For initial assessment of the hippocampus, 5-mm-thick slices in the coronal plane acquired in a standardized position are appropriate. For optimal diagnosis, thick slices with good contrast and SNR and thin slices oriented at right angles to the hippocampus are useful.

Pulse Sequences

1. The inversion recovery sequence using 5-mm slices with a 2.5-mm slice gap in the angled coronal plane (with the central slice oriented on the anterior brain stem [see Figure 5-5]) is an indispensible sequence if optimal visual diagnosis of hippocampal abnormalities is to be achieved. This provides good definition of the hippocampus and temporal lobe with excellent contrast, allowing all the features of hippocampal sclerosis to be detected in one image (Figure 5-7). This sequence allows

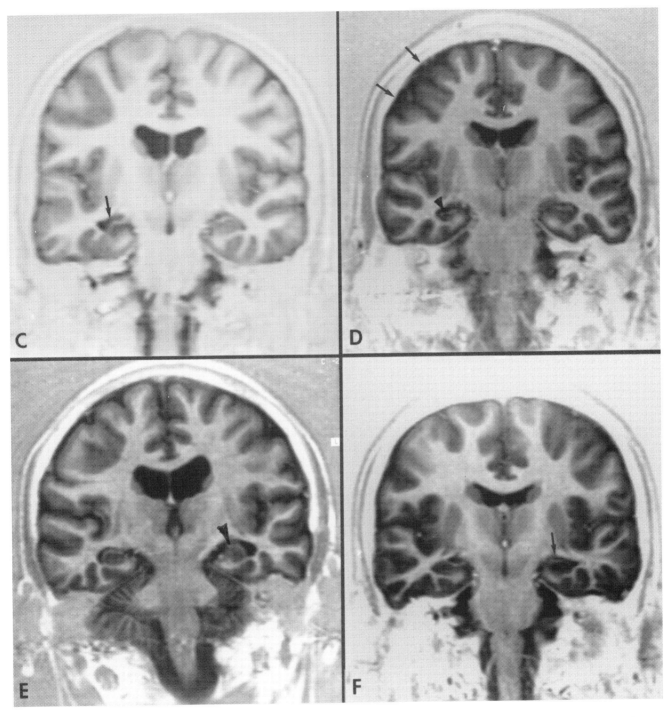

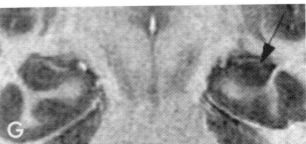

FIGURE 5-7. (*continued*) C. The signal change (*arrow*) is more obvious than the asymmetry. D. Cortical abnormality in ipsilateral frontal lobe (*arrow*). In other T_1-weighted images, signal change may not be seen, and atrophy alone must be relied on. E. There is little signal change or atrophy, but the microarchitecture is disturbed and mild atrophy (*arrowhead*) is seen in the whole hemisphere. F. No atrophy, but the signal change and disturbed microarchitecture allow the correct diagnosis of hippocampal sclerosis (*arrow*). G. Findings similar to those in F can be seen on high-resolution images (*arrow*).

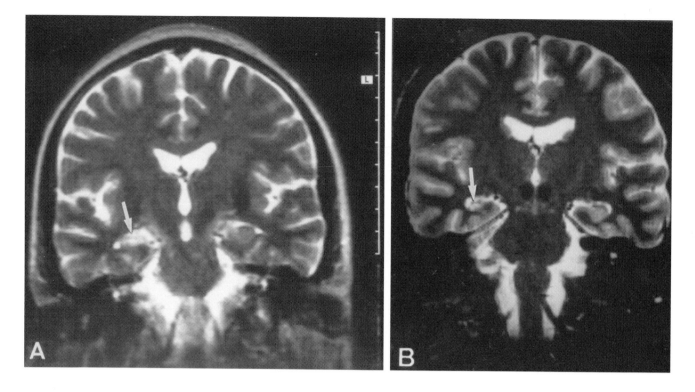

Figure 5-8. A–D. Examples of hippocampal sclerosis (*arrows*) as seen on 5-mm-thick T_2-weighted images. Note the signal change and the atrophy. E and F. Examples in which this signal change, although definite, is less marked. G. This signal change is shown in a T_2 relaxation map in which longer T_2 relaxation times are seen as higher signal. H and I. The T_2 relaxation time measured in a region of interest placed within the hippocampus (H) is described (I). Normal T_2 is 108 ms or greater. Therefore, there are bilateral abnormalities in the case shown in I.

atrophy to be assessed, demonstrates the internal architecture of the hippocampus, and provides good signal contrast among gray matter, white matter, and gliosis. We have not found that thinner inversion recovery slices (3 mm at the cost of a worse SNR) improve the detection of abnormality. To decrease imaging time, we use an asymetrical field of view (135×256), which makes acquisition time 8 minutes long. This is the sequence most likely to be dispensed with in epilepsy protocols because of the time required for the sequence, the inherent difficulties in providing whole-brain coverage or contiguous slices, and the fact that it is not implemented on some imaging systems. However, there often is signal change in the hippocampus and the temporal white matter that is clinically significant and that is not seen on other sequences. This sequence should be added to protocols if the visual detection rate of hippocampal sclerosis does not approach 100% in surgical series of patients with temporal lobe epilepsy. Other heavily T_1-weighted sequences may be developed that provide the same information, but currently, none have the same contrast sensitivity. In some cases, better contrast is more important than increased signal or spatial resolution. In our imaging laboratory, diagnostic accuracy is increased in cases with

subtle asymmetry using this sequence. This sequence cannot be the only sequence used because it does not cover all of the brain.

2. A T_2-weighted sequence covering the whole brain in the tilted coronal (temporal) plane with 5-mm-slice thickness is always acquired (Figure 5-8). A double echo STIR sequence is useful as the T_2-weighted sequence in younger children and whenever there are issues of delayed myelination. This sequence provides a clear distinction between gray and white matter despite the state of myelination. In older children and adults, any heavily T_2-weighted sequence appears to be appropriate. More heavily T_2-weighted sequences (80–120 ms) have been suggested to detect more signal change, although it is not uncommon to find cases in which the signal change is more apparent in the short TE sequence or even in the proton density image. Fast T_2 sequences appear to be as good as more conventional images.

3. A T_1-weighted three-dimensional (3D) sequence covering the whole head is now virtually mandatory and is probably the one sequence that cannot be dispensed with. We acquire a magnetization prepared rapid gradient echo (MPRAGE-Siemens) sequence covering the whole brain with a $256 \times 256 \times 128$ 3D matrix, with the

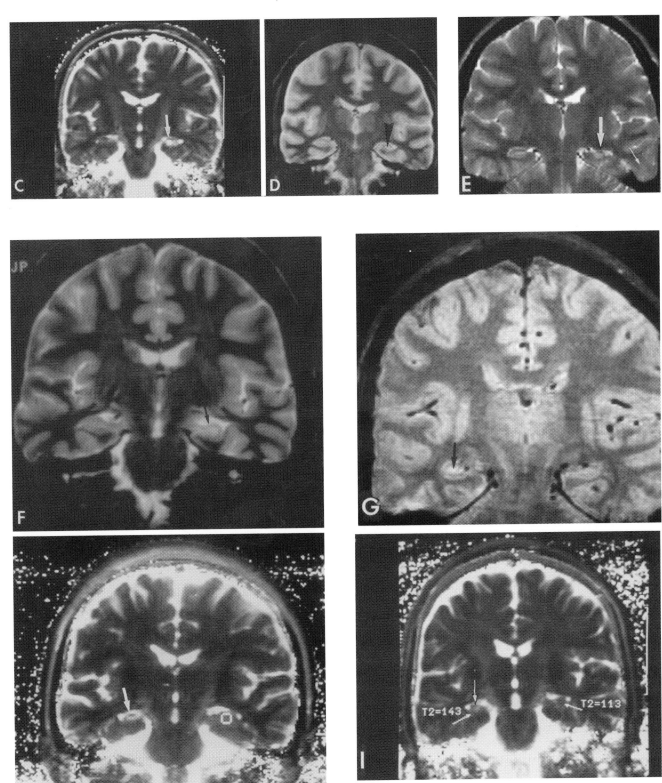

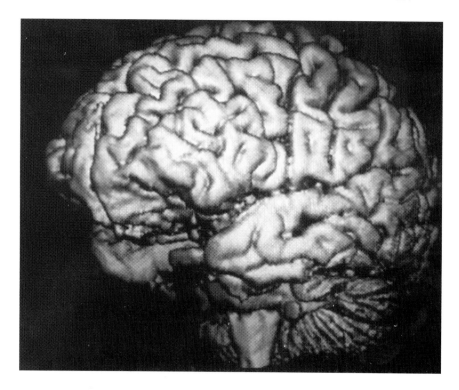

FIGURE 5-9. After a 3D data set is acquired, it is possible to reconstruct various surfaces, including the surface of the brain. This may be of value for the visual diagnosis of subtle abnormalities of gyral organization. (Figure courtesy of Dr. Ruben Kuzniecky, Alabama.)

128 partitions across the thinnest dimension of the head (in the sagittal direction, making each voxel 0.98 × 0.98 × 1.2 mm). Orientation in this manner gives the greatest resolution in the reconstructed images for this particular sequence. Default reconstruction in the sagittal plane also allows these images to be used as scout images for orientation of the other sequences from the parasagittal slice that includes the body of the hippocampus.

This is a true 3D data set (as opposed to a multislice sequence) and is the most heavily T_1-weighted 3D sequence available (the equivalent, although less heavily T_1-weighted sequence, is a spoiled gradient sequence [SPGR] on the GE system). The aim of this sequence is to enable high resolution in all three dimensions, allowing images to be reconstructed in any plane with any thickness at any time after the data set is acquired (down to the size of the individual voxels). This is a fast sequence that provides a great deal of data and processing options and, among other attributes, is ideal for hippocampal volume measurements.

For visual analysis, we reformat this 3D data set in different ways: first, as 1.5-mm slices in the tilted coronal plane covering the whole brain and, second, as 5-mm-thick tilted axial images centered on the hippocampus. This provides appropriately oriented axial images without additional imaging time for the axial sequence. Additional reorientation can be performed to examine regions of questionable cortical morphology suggestive of focal dysplasia.

The 3D imaging acquisition allows imaging of the whole brain in a relatively brief time (less than 10 minutes), and thin slices can be viewed in several orientations. This can help resolve the issue of partial volume artifacts.

These reconstructed images can be used for qualitative and morphometric analysis, and accurate estimates of hippocampal volume can be made from them. These sequences are also useful for the assessment of abnormalities of the neocortex. Because of the large amount of data these sequences generate, they often are best used to evaluate further an area that has been identified as possibly abnormal. The ability to reformat images in secondary planes is often essential for a specific diagnosis of minor cortical abnormalities. This same data set can also be used to generate 3D surface reconstructions of the brain (Figure 5-9), and it has been suggested that this can improve the diagnosis of abnormalities of gyral patterns. After a 3D data set such as this has been acquired, post acquisition manipulation, such as surface rendering and volume measurement, is relatively easy.

4. A T_2 relaxation time sequence is acquired to quantitate the signal change in the hippocampus and to confirm the visual impression of hippocampal sclerosis (particularly in cases in which the visual diagnosis is borderline). It is acquired particularly because of the issue of bilateral abnormalities (see Chapter 6).

Conclusion About Imaging Protocols

Full assessment of the hippocampus and temporal lobe relies on assessing different features in different image sets. Reliance on a single feature or a single imaging sequence is not optimal because the main features of a pathologic process are not always expressed in a single dimension (this would be equivalent to assessing all lesions by examining hematoxylin-eosin stained sections and expecting to detect all the abnormalities). Approximate imaging and analysis times are listed in Table 5-3.

General Findings

Detailed analysis of MR images reveals a high percentage of abnormalities that can be detected in the brains of patients with intractable partial epilepsy. As MR techniques improve, it is becoming clear that most patients with intractable epilepsy have detectable imaging abnormalities. Table 5-4 shows the range of abnormalities detected in a combined series of patients from several epilepsy centers.[74] Although previously no cause could be identified for many cases of intractable partial epilepsy, it is becoming clear that most adults and children with this condition have defined brain abnormalities that can be visualized with appropriately optimized imaging.[3,14,15,21,23,30,44,75–79]

Specific Findings

Optimized imaging of the hippocampus and temporal lobe structures depends on image orientation and image sequences optimized to display the anatomy and signal abnormality of hippocampal sclerosis and temporal lobe lesions.[80] MRI allows the visualization of brain anatomy with remarkable detail. This places new, and rather severe, demands on the neuroanatomical knowledge of many imaging specialists who previously have had no reason to know such fine details of normal structure of gray matter and its variations. The diagnosis of hippocampal sclerosis is a clear example in which this new level of detail is needed, because the MRI features of hippocampal abnormality are more subtle than those that

TABLE 5-3. Imaging of Hippocampal Sclerosis: Time Commitment for the Protocol

Recommended basic imaging and visual analysis
   Image acquisition (machine time), ~ 20 min
      3D T_1-weighted sequence, 8.5 min
      Coronal fast T_2, 4 min
      Coronal inversion recovery, asymmetric field of view 135 × 256, 8 min
   Image analysis
      Reformat of 3D data in axial and coronal orientation (radiographer), ~ 10 min
      Visual analysis (radiologist), ~ 5 min
Volume calculation of hippocampal size and asymmetry
   Image acquisition
      No additional time, 3D sequence routinely acquired
   Image analysis
      Image reconstruction (from the 3D data set), ~ 5–10 min
      Measurement of volume (expert-trained person), ~ 15–45 min (average, 30 min per patient)
T_2 relaxation maps
   Image acquisition
      16 image multi-echo sequence, 4–9 min (9 min for standard two-phase Siemens sequence)
   Image analysis
      Calculation of T_2 map (radiographer), ~ 2 min
      Placement of regions of interest (radiologist), ~ 1 min

TABLE 5-4. Findings in Patients with Intractable Epilepsy*

MRI diagnosis	Number (location) n = 340	%
Hippocampal sclerosis	194	57.0
Foreign tissue lesion (glioma, astrocytoma, or dysembryoplastic tumor)	46 (36 temporal, 10 extratemporal)	13.5
Cortical developmental malformation	35 (12 temporal, 23 extratemporal)	10.5
Vascular malformations (12 cavernous hemangiomas, 2 high-flow lesions)	14 (6 temporal, 8 extratemporal)	4.0
Cystic lesions	5 (4 temporal, 1 extratemporal)	1.5
Miscellaneous	17 (5 trauma, 1 tuberous sclerosis, 2 epidermoid, 4 extensive white matter lesions, 1 cerebellar atrophy, 4 uncertain)	5.0
No lesion demonstrated	29	8.5

*From a combined series of patients from the Austin Hospital (Melbourne, Australia; courtesy of Dr. Berkovic), Institute of Neurology (London, England; courtesy of Dr. Cook), and Great Ormond Street Hospital and NHS Trust (London).

TABLE 5-5. MRI Features of Hippocampal Sclerosis

MRI feature	Suggested histopathologic correlate	Found visually, % of cases
Unilateral atrophy (R cf. L)	Hippocampal atrophy (mostly CA1)	83–90
Loss of internal morphological structure on inversion recovery images	Loss of neurons in CA1, CA2, and CA4 and replacement gliosis	89
Increased signal on T_2-weighted images	Gliosis	77–85
Decreased signal on T_1-weighted images (inversion recovery)	Gliosis	83

Modified from Jackson et al.[44] By permission of the American Society of Neuroradiology.

previously were identified as pathologic. Without detailed knowedge of both the normal and pathologic anatomy of the hippocampus,[10,11,80-82] these features could easily be dismissed as normal variation, head tilt in the scanner, or occult partial volume effects. Training to achieve this new level of information requires the involvement of specialist epilepsy centers that frequently deal with these problems and use the clinical and imaging resources in a cooperative endeavor.

TUMORS

Approximately 20% of all patients with intractable epilepsy have a relatively large (that is, macroscopic) and localized lesion (tumor) that is the cause of their epilepsy. Before the advent of MRI, about only 50% of these lesions located in the temporal lobes were detected preoperatively (with CT).[3,61,69,83,84] Because patients with these lesions generally have an excellent outcome after surgical resection of the tumor, it is essential to identify them.[69,85-87] Many series have now established that MRI detects virtually all tumors, including dysembryoplastic lesions, hamartomas, and gliomas. Specific and important issues still exist, particularly in the ability to noninvasively distinguish between specific pathologic processes and to diagnose specific entities, such as dysembryoplastic neuroepithelial tumors.[31,88-90]

MESIAL TEMPORAL SCLEROSIS

Mesial temporal sclerosis refers to neuronal loss and gliosis that affect mesial structures, including the hippocampus, amygdala, entorhinal cortex, subiculum, and parahippocampal gyrus. We use the term "hippocampal sclerosis" in cases in which only the hippocampus has specifically been examined.

Hippocampal sclerosis is one of the most common lesions found in the brains of patients with intractable epilepsy.[91-93] Hippocampal sclerosis is a highly epileptogenic lesion. The side of the brain with the more affected hippocampus is almost always the side from which most temporal lobe seizures originate.[46,94] The detection

of hippocampal sclerosis with MRI may obviate invasive EEG monitoring with its attendant morbidity in patients being considered for surgical treatment. Until new MR techniques became available, hippocampal sclerosis was considered nonlesional epilepsy. The reliable detection of hippocampal sclerosis has changed the clinical perspective with regard to these patients.

Until after 1990, reports of the MR detection of hippocampal sclerosis were confusing. Although encouraging results were reported in some small studies, sclerosis was confused with artifacts in other studies, and there was inadequate pathologic verification in many studies. Since that time, optimized imaging at 1.5 T has shown that four main features visible on MRI are, in combination at least, specific for hippocampal sclerosis (Table 5-5).[44]

The criteria for assessing these optimized images include both morphological and signal intensity changes. The morphological features are atrophy and disruption of internal hippocampal structure. Abnormal signal in the hippocampus can be seen on both inversion recovery (T_1) and T_2-weighted imaging. The imaging of the fine anatomical structure of the hippocampus to a level of detail previously possible only with microscopic examination (Figure 5-10 shows details of this) may become an even more important method for detecting hippocampal sclerosis with improvements in imaging resolution (see Figure 5-10).

FIGURE 5-10. ▶ Internal structure of the hippocampus. A and B. The internal microarchitecture can be seen on routine inversion recovery images (5-mm thick). C and D. These features are shown in pathologic specimens. Note the absence of neurons (*arrow and arrowheads*) in the specimen showing hippocampal sclerosis, as compared with the normal case. E and F. Atrophy, loss of neurons, and diffuse gliosis are apparent on high-resolution inversion recovery images. These changes are shown diagrammatically in G and H. (Pathologic specimens courtesy of Dr. W. Van Paesschen, London.) (A, B, G, and H, from Jackson et al.[44] By permission of the American Society of Neuroradiology. E and F, courtesy of Dr. A. Connelly, London.)

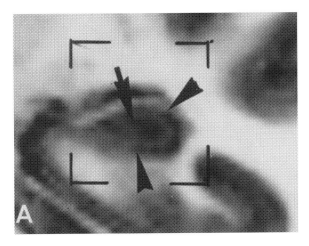

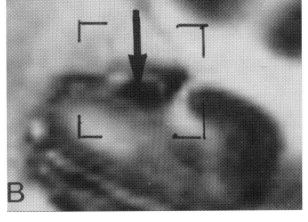

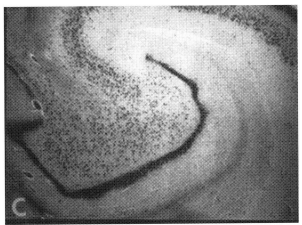

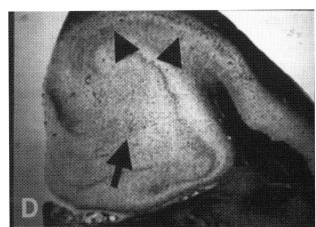

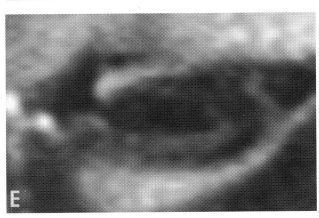

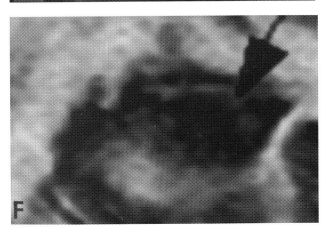

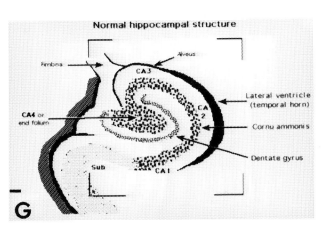

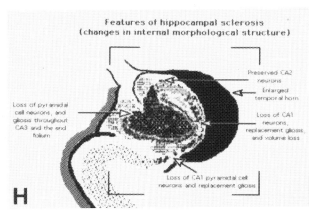

The visual diagnosis of hippocampal sclerosis can be highly subjective, and even experienced neuroradiologists may have difficulty detecting this subtle lesion. It must be emphasized that not all features are seen in all cases. Unequivocal signal change (as long as the hippocampus is not enlarged) or atrophy may be accepted as diagnostic of hippocampal sclerosis, with increased certainty if both are present. Added to this, the loss of internal structure can be helpful if the abnormality is subtle. In my experience, no single feature (such as atrophy) on its own is sensitive enough for reliable routine visual diagnosis, although in medical centers specializing in surgical epilepsy cases, an accurate diagnosis may be achieved in about 80% of cases.[13,28] After MR examination, it is important that the hippocampi can be assessed as being normal if abnormality does not exist.

Abnormal T_2-Weighted Signal

Visual analysis of T_2-weighted changes was the first method that demonstrated a correlation between a hippocampal abnormality and an MR detectable signal abnormality.[3,33,59,95-98] In a retrospective study correlating pathologic findings with T_2-weighted images, MRI abnormalities were detected in 65% of patients with mesial temporal sclerosis.[33] Among 14 patients with severe neuronal loss and gliosis, 11 (79%) had abnormal signal changes corresponding to the epileptogenic focus. Involvement of the hippocampus, amygdala, or parahippocampal gyrus (or some combination) was noted in 10 of these 11 patients. Other studies conducted during the same period demonstrated variability with respect to the number of studies with abnormal results.[33,65,76,99,100] Most of these early studies used the axial plane, and if done on the coronal view, they were performed without slice angulation. Slice thickness varied from 6 mm to 1.7 cm, and there was little standardization or optimization of pulse sequences. With these uncertainties, the sensitivity of MRI for the diagnosis of hippocampal sclerosis ranged from 0% to 80%.[2,3,7,20,21,30,33,36,37,39,65,67,70,76,99,101-109]

It was not until 1990 that the importance of the anatomical localization of this increased T_2 signal was established in a large clinical series of 81 patients undergoing temporal lobectomy with subsequent pathologic correlation. It became clear that the potential sensitivity and specificity of MRI using visual analysis were high. The diagnosis of hippocampal sclerosis was made with 93% sensitivity and 87% specificity using 0.3 T images.[3] It was emphasized in that study that the experience of the observers was an important factor in the detection of this lesion. In two series of patients, the correlation between observers was greater in the later series, and the diagnosis was made by both observers with greater sensitivity. Observer experience remains an important factor in this diagnosis, even in optimized images.

An early problem concerned the specificity of T_2-weighted signal changes. The presence of abnormal high signal from the mesial temporal region could have been related to an underlying foreign tissue lesion or even a vascular process, and, indeed, these were sometimes confused. It is important to recognize common artifacts in this region, in particular pulsation artifacts from blood vessels and from field inhomogeneity. With improving MR technology, these artifacts are less commonly present, but distinction of artifact from anatomical signal change is still important.

The possibility of mistaking the high-intensity signal from CSF in the temporal horn with abnormal hippocampal signal was another problem. This, too, depends on detailed anatomical knowledge and optimally oriented images. CSF and hippocampal tissue can be distinguished, and hippocampal signal can be assessed in virtually all situations if optimized images are obtained. In cases of real dilemma, a fluid-attenuated inversion recovery sequence can be performed in which the CSF is null (black) but the signal characteristics in the hippocampus and other tissues are preserved.[9]

Using optimized T_2-weighted sequences (orientation and sequence), the presence of increased signal from the hippocampal body can easily be detected (Figure 5-8), and this can clearly be distinguished from artifact and CSF. In the first echo, usually with echo times of 30 to 40 ms, the signal arising from the hippocampal formation may sometimes be subtle. Often, the abnormal signal is appreciated best in more heavily weighted T_2 sequences (echo times, 80–120 ms). Surprisingly, clear signal change sometimes is seen on the shorter T_2 echo, and this may even be more obvious at low (0.3–0.5 T) as compared with high (1.5 T) field strength. We recommend acquiring the second echo with echo times longer than 80 ms, although these occasional cases in which the proton density image demonstrates the abnormality most clearly are not yet fully understood. If inversion recovery sequences are acquired, signal change is usually seen on those images. Slight improvement in sensitivity by increasing the echo time to about 100 to 120 ms has been suggested, but this is not necessary if optimized images are used.

In normal subjects, the T_2- (and T_1-) weighted signal is usually isointense with gray matter, and this can be used as a comparison when judging signal change. Small changes of signal intensity are important in the context of temporal lobe epilepsy. The high signal is localized to the hippocampal gray matter and usually can be seen in the middle of the structure if the corresponding T_1-weighted image is used for definition of anatomical detail.[3,33,36,44,71,110] Careful attention to the location of this signal change within the hippocampus (in the coronal views) enables the diagnosis of hippocampal sclerosis to be made (see Figures 5-3, 5-7, 5-8, and 5-10). The process of creating hard copies of the images for visual reporting is also important. It is essential that appropriate "windowing" is established so that small changes in T_2-weighted signal are not obscured.

Orientation of the imaging slice perpendicular to the long axis of the hippocampus also avoids significant partial volume effects in most cases. After it is appreciated that one can have confidence in abnormal signal if it is localized anatomically to the hippocampal gray matter, the features of hippocampal sclerosis are easily appreciated, and one might wonder (as the authors of a recent publication did[111]) why there ever had been any problem with this.

Although the abnormal T_2 signal is a reliable finding for hippocampal sclerosis, several issues need to be considered. An uncommon problem may arise from the presence of normal dilatation of the hippocampal fissure. This may be diagnosed incorrectly as a high signal from the hippocampus, but it is rare and unlikely to be mistaken for hippocampal sclerosis if one is aware of it. Bilateral hippocampal T_2 signal abnormalities may be present and create difficulties because of the lack of a control side for comparison. The quantification of T_2 relaxation times has confirmed that T_2 signal abnormality is almost invariably associated with hippocampal sclerosis, even when it cannot be seen by visual analysis.[112]

In summary, increased T_2-weighted signal localized imprecisely to the mesial temporal region may be due to foreign tissue (such as a glioma or hamartoma), gliotic tissue in the hippocampus, increased CSF in the atrophied region, flow artifacts, and, occasionally, a developmental cyst in the hippocampal head stemming from failure of closure of the lateral aspect of the hippocampal fissure. Careful determination of the exact location of this signal change by detailed examination of the anatomical features allows the correct diagnosis. It is important to have sufficient knowledge of both the hippocampal anatomy and the easily recognizable artifacts that can occur in this region so that artifacts are not confused with significant signal abnormalities in the hippocampal gray matter.

Hippocampal Atrophy

The anatomy of the hippocampus and the adjacent limbic structures is complex; the appropriate imaging planes should be used to correctly visualize these structures. It must be remembered that the hippocampus, as fits the Latin derivation of its name, indeed has the shape of a sea horse, curving around itself with a superior rostrocaudal angulation of approximately 30° to 35°. Using MRI, the assessment of the cross-sectional size of the hippocampus must be made in images obtained in the modified coronal axis that transects the hippocampus at right angles (see Figure 5-5). This angulation avoids partial volume effects.

Initially, the visual assessment of hippocampal atrophy was questioned because of its subtle nature, often

being attributed to normal variation and head tilt in the scanner. It now is certain that visual assessment of optimally oriented images enables this feature to be recognized reliably,[3,33,36,44,68,71,113] and volumetry confirms the presence of this atrophy[19,28,82,114–118] (see Figure 5-7). In experienced hands, the visual assessment appears to be almost, but not quite, as good as volume estimation of hippocampal size in detecting hippocampal atrophy (it detects all cases in which the asymmetry is 85% or greater and some in which the asymmetry is less.[42]) Atrophy will be found in about 83% to 90% of cases by using optimized images and visual inspection alone (see Table 5-5). This is consistent with the experience in most epilepsy centers; however, in some, the detection rate appears to be about 50%. This may reflect the absence of optimized image acquisition, the use of only the criteria of hippocampal volume loss, ignoring signal and structural changes, inexperience in examining these structures, or an inappropriately high threshold for diagnosing abnormality. Whenever we discuss visual analysis, it must be remembered that we are not limited to a single feature, and other features can be used to help make the final diagnosis. The final detection rate of hippocampal sclerosis should not be confined to its success in detecting atrophy as compared with volumetric evaluation. It is the presence of more than one feature that enables sensitivity and specificity with visual assessment. In some cases, signal change may be detected more easily than atrophy or morphological abnormality, and in other cases, the reverse may hold true.

A word of caution needs to be added. Thin slices (1-2 mm) are not always the best for visual analysis, because side-to-side asymmetry may be more confusing with such a large number of images and minor irregularities may be more difficult to interpret. Conversely, thin slices may improve the diagnosis of atrophy in some patients, because changes may be localized to specific hippocampal sections. For detecting atrophy, a combination of thin (1.5 to 3 mm) and thicker high-contrast (5-mm inversion recovery) images is recommended for the detection of all abnormalities in the temporal lobes of patients with intractable epilepsy. The normal hippocampi are symmetrical when viewed in this way (Figure 5-11).

The use of qualitative comparisons between the right and left hippocampi demonstrates unilateral atrophy in most patients with mesial temporal sclerosis. We compare the cross-sectional circumference of each hippocampus in the coronal plane (see Figures 5-3, 5-7, and 5-8). Occasionally, the axial or sagittal reconstruction can help (see Figure 5-6), but the coronal plane is the one in which the diagnosis of hippocampal sclerosis is made most reliably. At the most anterior level, it may be difficult to distinguish the hippocampus from the amygdala, thus making an appropriate evaluation of atrophy difficult. At the level of the head of the hippocampus, atrophy may be

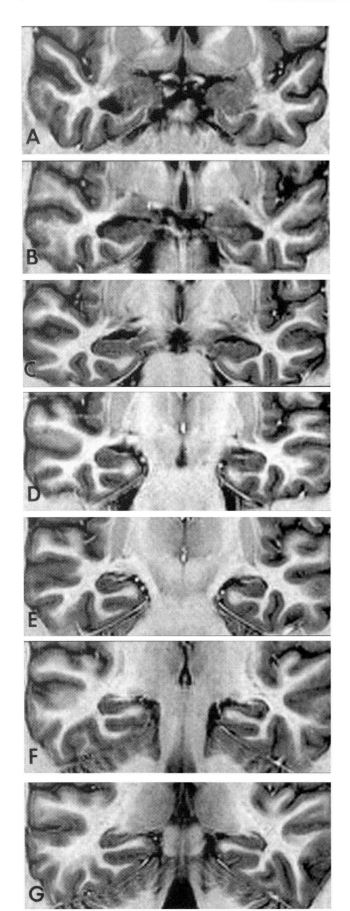

of a different degree when compared with the atrophy seen at the level of the hippocampal body. Conversely, abnormalities can sometimes be more prominent in the hippocampal head, and the region of the hippocampal head where it abuts the amygdala must be assessed carefully for atrophy and signal change (Figure 5-12). This may be due, in part, to the difficulty of distinguishing the hippocampal head from the amygdala. In those cases in which this is an issue, spending time unravelling the anatomy can often lead to a confident diagnosis that may not have been appreciated initially. Differing patterns of atrophy have also been described with quantitative and qualitative cross-sectional analysis of the hippocampus.[19,35]

The use of 3D acquisitions permits reconstruction in all planes. In addition to allowing thin slices to be obtained in the tilted coronal orientation, it permits reconstructions in the axial and sagittal planes. These additional planes may be useful in some cases and for specific purposes. In the axial plane, atrophy can be visualized and the posterior limit of the abnormality can sometimes be detected more easily (see Figure 5-6). For assessment of the cortex, additional planes may be useful in determining whether slight abnormalities in the appearance and pattern of the gyri are due to artifact or a pathologic process.

In summary, the assessment of the cross-sectional size of the hippocampus must be made in images obtained in the modified (tilted) coronal axis that transects the hippocampus at right angles. In this plane, a hippocampus assessed to be smaller by either qualitative or quantitative methods reliably predicts the side of the epileptogenic focus in cases of temporal lobe epilepsy, but absolute measures of hippocampal size must be interpreted with caution unless considerable effort is made to ensure standardization of the measurement process.[27] Quantitation of only the atrophy (hippocampal volume measurement) is slightly more sensitive than visual assessment of hippocampal size. However, with the addi-

◀ FIGURE 5-11. The normal hippocampus and amygdala are shown in this series of seven contiguous 5-mm-thick T_1-weighted images oriented in the tilted coronal plane. A. The amygdalae are symmetrical, but a normal asymmetry is seen in the temporal horns of the lateral ventricle. B. The hippocampal head can be distinguished from the amygdala. Note that the hippocampal head can appear asymmetrical in size at this level, even though there is no angulation of the image orientation. This can be even more apparent on thin slices. From the hippocampal head (C) and posteriorly (D–G) there is symmetry between the left and right hippocampi, and this region appears symmetrical in most normal subjects. No signal abnormalities are seen in any normal subjects, and the combination of asymmetry and signal change provides the most accurate means for diagnosing hippocampal sclerosis. T_2 maps are acquired from the region of images D and E.

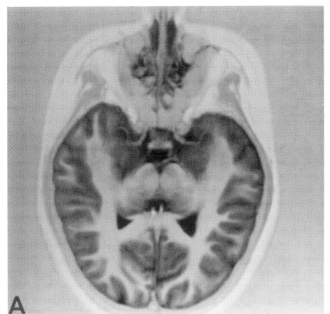

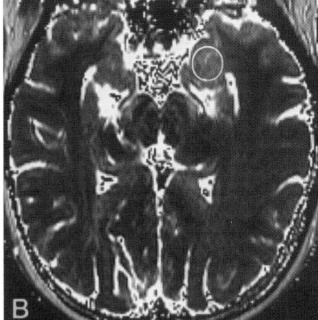

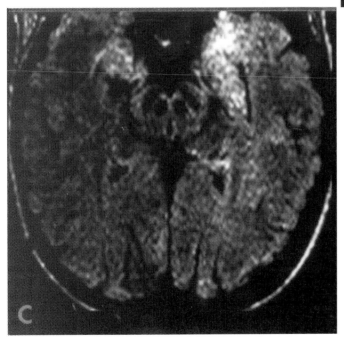

FIGURE 5-12. A. The normal amygdala in an axial T_1-weighted image oriented along the long axis of the hippocampal body. In some patients, with normal imaging using the basic protocols, additional imaging can reveal structural abnormalities that are the basis of temporal lobe seizures. B and C. In this patient, imaging results were normal, but an amygdala T_2 map (B) showed long T_2 relaxation times in the left amygdala (*circle*). This was visualized with a FLAIR sequence, which revealed signal increase in the amygdala and entorhinal region. (Images B and C courtesy of Dr. W. Van Paesschen, London.)

tion of signal abnormalities and architectural change in the hippocampus, visual assessment is as sensitive as quantitative methods in the population of patients being considered for temporal lobectomy (and for whom pathologic confirmation is available).

Loss of the Internal Structural Features (Microarchitecture) of the Hippocampus

The normal internal structure of the hippocampus is formed by the alveus, the molecular cell layer of the dentate gyrus, the pyramidal cell layer of the cornu ammonis, the internal medullary lamina, and white matter tracts. This structure can be seen on optimized coronal MR images (see Figure 5-10). This is clearly seen in histologic sections. Special surface coils placed on the temporal lobe to increase the SNR, thereby increasing spatial resolution, have also shown these abnormalities and correlated them with pathologic findings, showing a high degree of correlation.[119] Whereas the SNR is increased by these surface coils, their use requires considerable additional time (to place the coils, to replace the patient in the scanner, and to reset the MR). Also, these coils can create additional

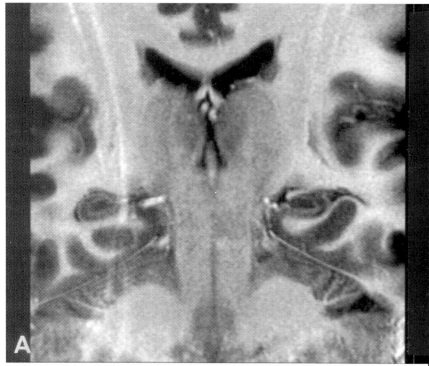

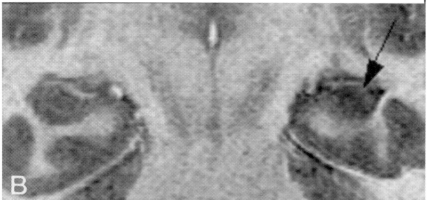

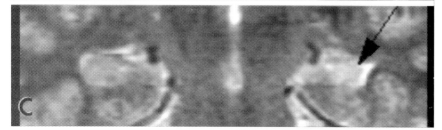

FIGURE 5-13. High-resolution imaging of the hippocampus depends on a good SNR and good contrast in the imaging sequence. This can be achieved at high field strength, with special coils, or with developments of current imaging systems. A. High-resolution inversion recovery image (9 min) using conventional imaging. The internal microarchitecture is clearly seen. B. A patient with left hippocampal sclerosis (pathologically confirmed after temporal lobectomy): note the loss of internal features (*arrow*). This is associated with signal abnormality (darker, long T_1). The internal structure of the contralateral hippocampus is clearly seen, and atrophy is not a prominent feature. C. T_2-weighted signal change (*arrow*) is present. (Figures B and C courtesy of Dr. A. Connelly, London.) (A from Kuzniecky and Jackson.[47] By permission of Raven Press.)

difficulties in eliminating head movement, because it is more difficult to immobilize the head. Improved techniques using conventional equipment may provide an alternative approach (Figure 5-13).

The loss of the internal microarchitecture in hippocampal sclerosis is a consequence of neuronal cell loss and replacement of normal anatomical layers with gliotic tissue (see Figure 5-10). It is difficult to describe this feature precisely, but after it is recognized, it is important for confidence of diagnosis in cases in which other fea-

tures are only mildly abnormal. Inversion recovery images are important because they produce stronger contrast within the normal anatomical layers of the hippocampus and also between normal tissue and gliosis. Important advances in this area can be anticipated in the near future, with attention being paid to high-resolution images (see Figure 5-13).

High-spatial resolution and good contrast are the two requirements for visualizing the internal structure of the hippocampus. By increasing the number of pixels covering the region and by lengthening the time of image acquisition, high-resolution images of the hippocampus can be generated. An alternative is to increase the signal by using temporal surface coils. Another alternative is to use an imaging sequence that allows the visualization of contrast between the various structures of the hippocampus. In some cases, increased contrast can be as useful as increased resolution. We have found that the use of inversion recovery images in 5-mm-thick slices oriented perpendicularly to the long axis of the hippocampus is an excellent routine sequence for identifying these features.[44] The increased contrast that this sequence provides between abnormal tissue (gliosis) and the normal structures of the hippocampus assists in diagnosing the disruption of this normal internal architecture that occurs in hippocampal sclerosis (see Figures 5-3, 5-7, and 5-10). The presence of a normal microarchitecture of the hippocampus without signal change should be taken as evidence that hippocampal sclerosis is not present, even when a significant asymmetry exists with the other side (this usually means that the bigger hippocampus is the abnormal one; this is a situation that occasionally is seen and that can create clinical confusion unless recognized). This is a case in which visual analysis can prevent an incorrect interpretation of the results of a volumetric quantitation study.

Careful evaluation of hippocampal microarchitecture increases the confidence with which the diagnosis of hippocampal sclerosis can be made in cases in which other features, for example, T_2 signal change and atrophy, are less prominent. It is not always possible to detect clearly the internal structure of the hippocampus or to determine whether it is normal or abnormal. However, one can detect the hippocampal microarchitecture in a large number of cases, and after this feature has been appreciated properly, it is of great help. With improvements in techniques and spatial resolution, it is likely that this feature will become one of the most important for the diagnosis of hippocampal abnormality. Neuronal loss in the CA1 region of the cornu ammonis in conjunction with gliosis is the pathologic hallmark of hippocampal sclerosis; thus, direct visualization of these features should provide accuracy about pathologic processes in a given hippocampus.

In summary, the normal internal morphological structure of the hippocampus is formed by the alveus, the molecular cell layer of the dentate gyrus, the pyramidal cell layer of the cornu ammonis, the internal medullary lamina, and the white matter tracts. It can be visualized on optimized coronal MR images (see Figures 5-3, 5-7, 5-10, and 5-13). In hippocampal sclerosis, the loss of this normal internal structure is a consequence of neuronal cell loss and the replacement of the normal anatomical layers with gliotic tissue (see Figure 5-10). This feature of hippocampal sclerosis potentially is important, because with increasing spatial resolution, thinning of the CA1 region of the cornu ammonis may prove to be a sensitive and specific means of diagnosing hippocampal sclerosis.

Signal Hypointensity on T_1-Weighted Inverse Recovery Images

The use of the inversion recovery sequence is valuable for the study of hippocampal sclerosis and other pathologic processes. It is used as part of our epilepsy protocol because it provides information not seen on our 3D or other T_1-weighted sequence. This is because of the high contrast between gray matter, white matter, and gliosis that is provided by the inversion recovery sequence. The main disadvantage is the time the sequence takes. With an asymmetrical field of view (128 x 256 matrix), it requires 7 to 9 minutes. With improved contrast in the hippocampus itself, it may be possible to define some structures such as the fimbria and cerebral vessels. In T_1-weighted spin-echo sequences and fast 3D T_1-weighted images (gradient echo), gliosis can be difficult to distinguish from gray matter signal intensity, but the inversion recovery sequence allows white matter, gray matter, and gliosis to be distinguished from one another more accurately.

For example, at 1.5 T, using a TR of 3,500 and a T_1 of 300 ms, a sclerotic hippocampus appears dark and small and the internal features are obscured (see Figures 5-3, 5-7, 5-10, and 5-11). The atrophic hippocampus demonstrates decreased signal, with a dark appearance. The signal hypointensity can be striking, and at times, the hippocampus is so severely atrophic that it resembles a cystic cavity (see Figures 5-3 and 5-10), although it is clear that this is not a cavity but a solid area of gliosis.[44] Proton density images show that this signal is not due to fluid but arises in solid tissue with proton density (and less heavily T_1-weighted) signal characteristics similar to those of gray matter. It is likely that this hypointensity (if the images are processed so that the CSF appears black) is due to a similar process that gives rise to the hyperintense signal in the T_2-weighted images. This signal change is due to increased T_1 relaxation time in the tissue. It must reflect predominantly a change in the content or situation of the protons in the tissue of interest. Because the etiology of this process is assumed to be the same as for T_2 signal abnormalities, it might be assumed that T_1 hypointensity would always be found in the same cases as T_2 hyperintensity. Whereas this is largely true, there appears to be differences among individuals. In some, no signal abnormality was detected on the T_2-weighted images, but clear T_1-weighted signal abnormalities were present.[44]

We find that analysis of these heavily T_1-weighted images is essential for detecting all cases of hippocampal abnormality. The inversion recovery sequence may be the only abnormal finding in some cases of hippocampal sclerosis, in particular, cases with minimal atrophy.[72] Therefore, for the optimized visual diagnosis of hippocampal sclerosis, these or equivalent images that provide these signal characteristics are essential. It is likely that fast sequences will be developed that will provide both the spatial resolution and contrast of this inverse recovery sequence. New techniques will need to be judged against this current standard.

In summary, it is the presence of the three features—asymmetry implying atrophy, signal change, and loss of normal microarchitecture—in a single coronal (inversion recovery) image that assists in the visual diagnosis of hippocampal sclerosis. This makes it possible to detect mild degrees of abnormality with greater sensitivity and specificity. The presence of signal change in this sequence, which also provides excellent anatomical information, has remained essential for confident visual analysis of the hippocampus in our center. The use of reconstructed slices from a 3D data set allows atrophy to be assessed, but it usually does not provide as much information about internal structure or signal change.

Summary of Hippocampal Sclerosis: Visual Diagnosis

An abnormal signal on T_1- or T_2-weighted images arising from an atrophic hippocampus nearly always represents hippocampal sclerosis. An abnormal signal arising from an apparently enlarged hippocampus may represent a hamartoma or glioma. If one relies on only a single feature such as atrophy, then, occasional cases in which the larger hippocampus is the abnormal one would be incorrectly lateralized. In many cases, hippocampal sclerosis is obvious and is the likely cause of epilepsy. In such cases, it can be diagnosed on the basis of a single feature, such as atrophy or T_2-weighted signal change. However, for cases in which hippocampal atrophy is less obvious, other features such as signal change or loss of normal microarchitecture are needed to make the diagnosis.

Epilepsy surgery requires a definitive diagnosis of hippocampal sclerosis if other investigations are to be replaced. This means that the occasional exceptional cases that cannot be diagnosed correctly with the assessment of a single feature (such as asymmetry) must be routinely detected. This requires routine assessment of signal abnormalities and abnormal microarchitecture.

ROLE OF GADOLINIUM IN HIPPOCAMPAL SCLEROSIS

Gadolinium has an important role in the study of mass lesions or vascular malformations in patients with pathologic features in the central nervous system associated with epilepsy.[120-122] However, contrast agents are not necessary for the diagnosis of hippocampal sclerosis.[123] Its use is unwarranted for the following reasons: (1) hippocampal sclerosis is not associated with significant structural vascular changes or disruption of the blood-brain barrier that warrant the use of contrast agents, (2) no enhancement occurs with MRI-based contrast agents in hippocampal sclerosis, (3) the use of contrast agents may be associated with side effects, and (4) gadolinium increases the cost and imaging time and more information can be obtained by performing an additional sequence (as discussed above) than by using contrast agents.

CURRENT EXPECTATIONS OF IMAGING IN INTRACTABLE EPILEPSY

An MRI study is undertaken in many cases to exclude the presence of a tumor or other structural lesion. In imaging centers in which an interest is taken in epilepsy, the question asked of imaging must include whether hippocampal sclerosis or cortical dysplasia is present.

Volumetric measurement of the hippocampus has been relied upon in many cases because the features of hippocampal sclerosis were considered too subtle for visual detection (in "routine" images). Reliance on quantifying the feature of hippocampal side-to-side asymmetry (volumetric assessment) is remarkably successful in detecting hippocampal sclerosis in patients with intractable temporal lobe epilepsy,[7,19,26,124–126] but as discussed above, reliance on a single feature may lead to errors in a minority of cases, whether because of variations in the pathologic process or occasional errors in calculation. Optimized visual analysis is important in providing a check on numerically derived measures of abnormality.[72] To date, the presence of asymmetry (attributed to hippocampal atrophy on the smaller side) has concentrated on whether hippocampal sclerosis is present and which side is affected (and, thus, likely to be the origin of the seizures).

Several other questions may be important in the assessment of patients with epilepsy, even in those with demonstrable hippocampal sclerosis:

1. Is the hippocampal sclerosis strictly unilateral or is the contralateral hippocampus or temporal lobe affected to some degree?
2. Is the pathologic abnormality confined to the hippocampus or does it involve the amygdala, entorhinal cortex, anterior temporal lobe, or other structures in the ipsilateral hemisphere?
3. Is hippocampal sclerosis the only lesion that may cause the epilepsy?
4. Are we able to demonstrate progression of hippocampal disease? Should efforts be addressed at preventing hippocampal damage at the onset of the epileptic condition?

Now that tools are available for the detection of hippocampal disease, it is important that some of these questions be answered and that the clinical significance of such findings be established. For example, the importance of bilateral disease can now be assessed with quantitative T_2 and evolving measurement techniques, both in a person and in populations. Early data suggest that the presence of contralateral hippocampal sclerosis is not a predictor of poor outcome after an operation on the anterior temporal lobe but that it may be important for cognitive outcome.[127]

TEMPORAL LOBE ABNORMALITIES OTHER THAN IN THE HIPPOCAMPUS

Mesial temporal sclerosis involves structures outside the boundaries of the hippocampus, and regional abnormalities are commonly present in these patients (Figure 5-14). These include the amygdala, uncus, subiculum, and parahippocampal gyrus. Abnormalities may extend into the other temporal gyri or even involve the entire ipsilateral hemisphere. In about half of these cases, the contralateral side may also be involved.[91,128] The principles discussed above in regard to the hippocampus apply also to these other structures, that is, abnormality is detected by signal change (contrast) or by atrophy or changes in architecture (morphology). In general, temporal lobe abnormalities more extensive than the hippocampus are common. There is an impression that in patients being investigated for possible surgical treatment (thus, a group with intractable epilepsy) isolated hippocampal sclerosis is uncommon if these other areas are examined carefully. This appears to be true more in pediatric than in adult patients, but this may reflect selection bias. The focus given to the hippocampus by quantitative methods of analysis causes a degree of tunnel vision. Because only the hippocampus is assessed with these methods, visual analysis is needed to ensure that the hippocampal abnormalities are evaluated in their proper context. When only the hippocampus is assessed, we should talk about "hippocampal sclerosis," which may be either isolated or exist in the context of more widespread abnormalities. "Mesial temporal sclerosis" should be reserved for discussion of all the structures listed above.

The Amygdala: Sclerosis and Other Abnormalities

Although much attention has been given to the hippocampus, the amygdala is also involved in the pathologic process in mesial temporal sclerosis,[86,128–130] and amygdalar lesions can be a cause of temporal lobe epilepsy independently of the hippocampus (see Figure 5-12). Anatomical study of the amygdala with MRI can be difficult. The amygdala is the superior relation of the head of the hippocampus at the level of the anterior commissure, and without heavy T_1-weighting in optimally oriented images, it can be difficult to separate the hippocampal head from the lateral amygdaloid nucleus at this level.[80] As pointed out by Jack et al.,[82,131] disarticulating the uncus, amygdala, and hippocampus anteriorly sometimes requires arbitrary judgment unless these optimized images are obtained. Cendes et al.[17] and Watson et al.[132] performed volumetric studies on the amygdala and hippocampus in selected patients and reported a statistically significant difference between controls and left-right temporal lobe seizures. Atrophy of the amygdala permitted lateralization in 20 of 30

(67%) patients, whereas hippocampal atrophy revealed lateralization in 26 of 30 (87%). However, atrophy of the amygdala was not reported in any patient without concomitant hippocampal atrophy. Nonetheless, when taken together, amygdaloid and hippocampal atrophy increased correct lateralization by 6%, from 87% to 93% of patients. Despite these data and the fact that clinical and pathologic studies have suggested a role for the amygdala in temporal lobe seizures, the study of this structure remains difficult.

Temporal Neocortex Abnormalities

Signal change in the cortical gray matter ("cortical ribbon") is often hard to detect because of the proximity of the CSF in the subarachnoid space. Partial volume effects are also more difficult to avoid in the cortex. Except in unusual cases, such changes can be unequivocally distinguished only rarely. Change in signal in the white matter core of the temporal lobe is easier to detect. This is characterized by the white matter becoming similar in intensity to the gray matter (see Figure 5-14); it gives the impression that the white matter in the region has been filled in (loss of contrast between gray matter and white matter). In addition, the white matter core may seem smaller on the side ipsilateral to hippocampal sclerosis. This is likely to represent gliosis or ectopic neurons in the white matter of the temporal lobe. Anecdotes of the loss of gray matter and white matter definition have been reported.[133] This suggestion is supported by finding regional abnormalities on MR spectroscopy.[134] The clinical importance of these regional abnormalities has not been established. It seems likely that hippocampal sclerosis in this context may have consequences different from hippocampal sclerosis alone.

Temporal neocortical atrophy may be seen in patients with temporal lobe epilepsy.[36,121,135,136] Few studies have systematically evaluated the presence of MRI-detected neocortical atrophy in these patients, although it appears to be a frequent finding when looked for carefully. It is usually associated with hippocampal changes and, when appropriate imaging is performed, with signal changes in the temporal white matter. Often, it is associated with varying degrees of minor atrophy of the ipsilateral hemisphere.

Neocortical atrophy or signal change can occur in isolation (that is, without hippocampal sclerosis). There may be atrophy of the neocortex without associated changes in the mesial temporal structures. However, neocortical atrophy usually occurs in association with hippocampal sclerosis. The degree of atrophy varies but is often quite marked (see Figure 5-14). Atrophy of selected temporal gyri may also occur, and the superior temporal gyrus, particularly where it forms the temporal pole, commonly appears to be abnormal. In this case, these findings can easily be interpreted as partial volume

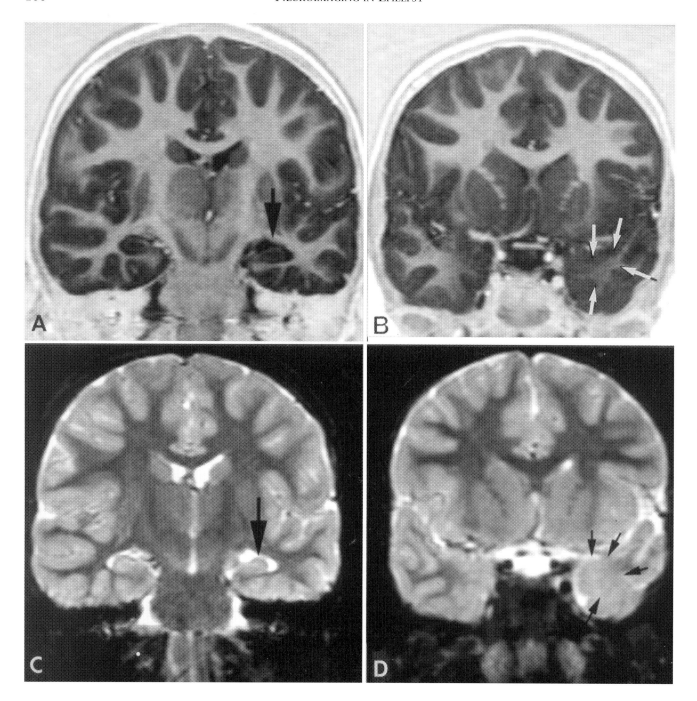

Figure 5-14. Patients with hippocampal sclerosis often have more extensive abnormalities of the ipsilateral temporal lobe, which are detected most easily as signal change on the heavily T_1-weighted (inversion recovery) images or on the T_2-weighted images. The white matter of the temporal core is distinct when images are acquired in the coronal plane. Partial volume is not an explanation of the loss of gray-white matter contrast. A–C. Images from a 9-year-old girl who had a prolonged febrile convulsion at age 2 and development of intractable temporal lobe epilepsy with nonfebrile seizures at age 5. A and C. Based on visual assessment and quantitative analysis, she has left hippocampal sclerosis (*arrows*). B. In addition there is marked signal change in the white matter core of the left temporal lobe (*area indicated by arrows*), and (D) in the same slice in the T_2-weighted image, the white matter core cannot be seen, and there is the appearance of a solid lesion (*area indicated by arrows*). Other abnormalities may be present in these images which can be detected only with visual analysis. Note the atrophy of the left thalamus and left basal ganglia. The girl had no focal neurologic findings. This is an obvious example, and it is difficult to determine whether the signal change in the temporal white matter is due to ectopic neurons (developmental malformation) or gliosis. Signal change of the type shown in B is commonly seen on inversion recovery images (not on other T_1-weighted images) in patients with hippocampal sclerosis.

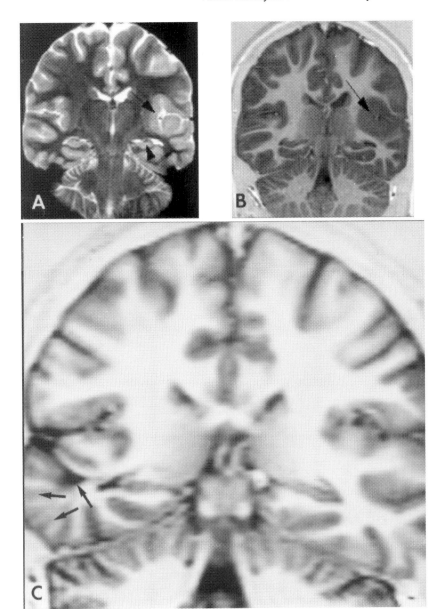

FIGURE 5-15. Hippocampal sclerosis can occur in association with other significant and possibly epileptogenic lesions. A–C. It appears that cortical developmental malformations (dysplasia) (*arrow*) are commonly associated with hippocampal sclerosis (*arrowhead*). A and B. Unilateral perisylvian dysplasia and ipsilateral hippocampal sclerosis. C. Schizencephaly (*vertical arrow*) with polymicrogyria involving the superior and middle temporal gyri (*two horizontal arrows*) of the right temporal lobe. This is associated with ipsilateral hippocampal sclerosis. Focal tumors can also be associated with hippocampal sclerosis. (*Continued.*)

effects at the temporal pole. Quantitative neocortical measurements have proved to be unreliable.[82,131]

Parahippocampal Gyrus Abnormalities

Another indirect feature of mesial temporal sclerosis commonly seen in patients with intractable temporal lobe epilepsy is atrophy or signal change in the parahippocampal gyrus. These changes can easily be overlooked, but with optimized images, the presence of thinning of the underlying white matter and blurring of the gray matter–white matter pattern can be evaluated. Similarly, thinning of the white matter located between the hippocampus and collateral sulcus is seen occasionally and may be a part of more generalized pathologic changes[135] (see Figure 5-14). The role of these structures in the epileptic process is not well known, and so they have received much less atten-

tion than the hippocampus. Gloor[137] has pointed out that the hippocampus may not be the only important structure in the genesis of seizures of mesial temporal lobe origin.

DUAL PATHOLOGY

Dual pathology means hippocampal sclerosis as well as a defined extrahippocampal structural abnormality. This usually means a tumor or focal dysplasia (Figure 5-15). As suggested above, hippocampal sclerosis alone may be an uncommon finding, but features that suggest atrophy or signal change in a more regional distribution cannot be considered dual pathology; currently, such a finding must be interpreted as part of the same abnormality that includes hippocampal sclerosis.

Dual pathology has been found in 7.5% to 30% of patients in pathologic and MR series.[128,138–140] It has

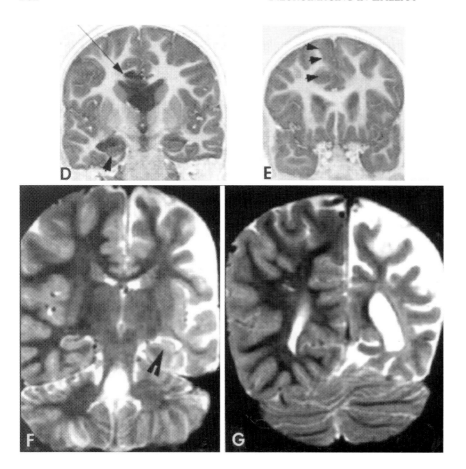

FIGURE 5-15 (*continued*). D and E. Images from a patient with a focal lesion involving the genu of the corpus callosum (*arrow*). On pathologic examination, this tumor had the histologic characteristics of an astrocytoma, but it was associated with adjacent cortical thickening and periventricular heterotopia (*arrowheads*). Most likely, it was a dysembryoplastic neuroepithelial lesion in a patient with cortical developmental malformation. F and G. Hippocampal sclerosis (*arrowhead*) can also be associated with diffuse abnormalities of the whole hemisphere, producing the syndrome of hippocampal sclerosis, hemiatrophy, and hemiplegia.

been suggested that the severity of the hippocampal changes interpreted as hippocampal sclerosis is less in cases of dual pathology than in cases of an "isolated" lesion and that the severity may depend on the type of pathologic process associated with hippocampal sclerosis.[140] It is tempting to speculate that the mild form of hippocampal sclerosis might be due to a mechanism such as kindling and that, in this context at least, hippocampal sclerosis may have originated secondary to seizures that initially arose from this other lesion.[141–143]

BILATERAL ABNORMALITIES

Bilateral abnormalities can be detected by visual analysis in some cases in which there are severe abnormalities. In general, visual assessment is not sensitive for detecting bilateral abnormalities. For routine detection of bilateral disease, quantitation with reference to a range of normal values is necessary. For this purpose T_2 relaxometry and MR spectroscopy are useful because there is a clear distinction between normal and abnormal, with little overlap.[127] Absolute volume measurements may also be helpful, although there may be greater overlap between normal and abnormal values, without unambiguous distinction between these normal and abnormal values in individual cases. For these reasons, quantita-

tion of the hippocampal asymmetry, absolute hippocampal volume, and T_2 relaxation time may be of clinical and research value.

VISUAL ANALYSIS COMPARED WITH QUANTITATIVE ANALYSIS OF VOLUME AND T_2 RELAXATION TIME

Studies have been performed in cases in which the hippocampal damage may be considered severe (as in surgical series). From experienced imaging and epilepsy centers with emphasis on optimization of visual reporting, a consensus is emerging that visual analysis detects virtually all the hippocampal lesions that can be detected with quantitative methods. This should be the aim of implementing an imaging protocol and clear criteria for visual assessment. Bronen et al.[12] recently reported that atrophy was found in 93% of cases assessed visually and signal abnormalities in 86%. All cases of hippocampal sclerosis were detected visually, with two having signal change without atrophy and five having atrophy without signal change. These results are remarkably similar to those of ours,[44] of Jack,[25,26] and of Kuzniecky et al.[35,77]

We recently compared optimized visual analysis with quantitative volume and T_2 relaxation time measurements[42] (Figure 5-16). Overall, in 50 cases exam-

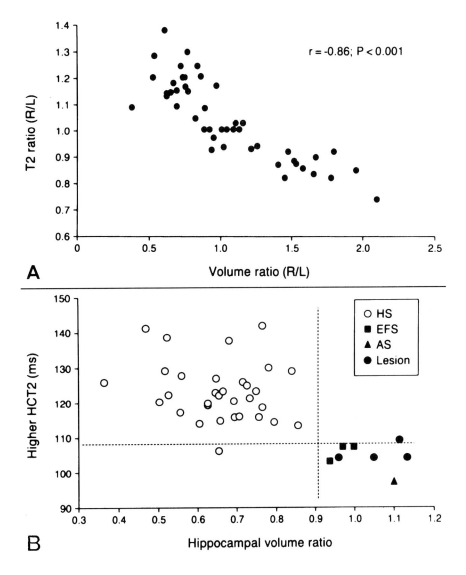

FIGURE 5-16. The relationship between the features of signal change and volume. A. The ratio of T$_2$ relaxation time (right to left) and hippocampal volume (right to left) are strongly correlated. B. The absolute hippocampal T$_2$ relaxation time compared with the hippocampal volume ratio as a function of the pathologic process identified after temporal lobectomy. *Dashed lines*, limit of normal (>0.92 ms and <108 ms). This shows that both features are usually present, but measurement of the severity of hippocampal damage depends on having an absolute measurement of hippocampal damage (a ratio of right to left ignores bilateral damage that occurs in up to 50% of cases[91]). (AS) amygdala sclerosis, (EFS) end folium sclerosis, (HS) hippocampal sclerosis. (B. From Van Paesschen et al.[42] By permission of American Academy of Neurology.)

ined, there was no case in which visual analysis differed from quantitative analysis in terms of making the definite diagnosis of hippocampal sclerosis. There was a definite cut-off point for complete concordance of the two observers in the analysis of both signal change and atrophy. Signal change was detected by both observers when the T$_2$ relaxation time was ≥ 114 ms (normal ≤ 106 ms). Lateralized atrophy was detected by both observers in all cases in which the asymmetry was greater than 15%. In many of the other cases, one or the other observer detected abnormality, but this was not unanimous. In all cases, the abnormalities detected visually were always on the side of quantitative abnormality and the side of eventual temporal lobe resection. Occasionally, there was an exception. For example, one case had a clear, visually apparent signal change but no T$_2$ relaxation time abnormality on the side subsequently proved to have hippocampal sclerosis. This study investigated a surgical series in which the pathologic abnormality was often at the severe end of the spectrum. It is not known whether these conclusions apply to cases with less severe lesions.

The ratio of T$_2$ relaxation time measurements (left to right) correlated very highly with the ratio (left to right) of volume measurements (see Figure 5-16). The use of absolute T$_2$ relaxation times enabled bilateral abnormalities to be detected in 20% to 25% of cases.

CLINICAL ISSUES

With the advent of information about substrates that can be identified in the brains of patients with epilepsy and that may be the cause of epileptic seizures, the classification of epilepsy is being revised. Epilepsy syndromes are based on electrical (EEG) and clinical information that place emphasis on the ictal events. Anatomical and pathologic information (which is present both ictally and interictally) is not usually included in the classification of an epilepsy syndrome. Now that the diagnosis of hippocampal sclerosis can be made noninvasively with MRI, it has been suggested that the syndrome of mesial temporal sclerosis should be defined.[47] The features of this syndrome are listed in Table 5-6. Even in patients who fulfill these criteria, a heterogeneity of abnormalities can be identified in the temporal lobes of these patients. Occasionally, virtually identical abnormalities seen on MR do not have the same electroclinical features. It has not been determined whether this structural information can usefully be applied to the concept of epilepsy syndromes or whether it must be considered separately.

THE FUTURE OF VISUAL ANALYSIS

I expect that the greatest sensitivity will come from detailed analysis of the internal architecture of the hippocampus in high-resolution images, which have not yet been fully explored in clinical series. It seems likely that direct visualization of the information that is used by pathologists to make the diagnosis of hippocampal sclerosis will be more sensitive and specific than current visual analysis or, indeed, than quantitative methods of analysis. This expectation will depend on the development of high-resolution images with good contrast. It is likely that in the next 5 years such sequences will become routinely available, either through the availability of high field systems or the availability of new sequences or hardware.

PREDICTION OF OUTCOME

Because surgical treatment can provide such a good outcome in selected cases of intractable epilepsy, it is clinically important to know how the different types of abnormalities affect surgical prognosis. Because this MR information has been available preoperatively for only a few years, long-term outcome is only beginning to emerge. It is known from pathologic studies that the presence of hippocampal sclerosis is a good factor for prognosis after anterior temporal lobectomy with resection of the mesial structures. Berkovic et al.[8] recently reported on a series of 123 patients followed for up to 5 years. This included a cohort with visual diagnosis of hippocampal sclerosis and showed, using actuarial methods, that the preoperative MR findings were a major predictor of surgical outcome (Figure 5-17). When a foreign tissue lesion was present, eventual seizure-free outcome was greater than 80%, and when hippocampal sclerosis was visually diagnosed (cohort from reference 3), an eventual 2-year seizure-free period was achieved in 63%. The interesting finding in this group was that, unlike in other groups, even after 6 years an occasional patient with MR-diagnosed hippocampal sclerosis who had been seizure-free had seizures. This may be a clinically important finding for postoperative advice and management. When no abnormality was seen on the MR study, only 38% of the patients became seizure-free. This study used

TABLE 5-6. Features of the Syndrome of Mesial Temporal Sclerosis

Clinical

    Increased familial incidence of febrile convulsions in childhood

    Silent period (~ 3–30 yr) followed by development of complex partial seizures

    Intractable seizures

    Epigastric aura, oroalimentary automatisms

    Postictal confusion

EEG

    Anterior temporal interictal sharp and slow waves in interictal period

    Ictal lateralization, often theta rhythm

Imaging

    Hippocampal sclerosis with or without regional abnormalities in anterior and mesial temporal lobe

Treatment

    Frequently unresponsive to medications

    Excellent outcome with surgical treatment

actuarial methods and defined outcome as no seizure of any sort for a 2-year period.

Less strict definitions of good outcome (seizure-free, auras only, or occasional seizures) suggest that hippocampal sclerosis is associated with a good outcome with regard to seizure frequency in 70% to 80% of patients.[28]

RESEARCH

The consensus is that quantitative analysis will be important for research analysis and for answering detailed questions of severity and bilaterality. Expert visual analysis of optimized images is usually sufficient for answering the simple questions of "Is there hippocampal sclerosis?" and "On which side?" In clinical practice, perhaps quantitative analysis should be used only when equivocal results are reported on visual analysis or, in the short term, to confirm and establish appropriate thresholds for visual reporting. It must be emphasized that proper visual analysis of scans for the purpose of diagnosing hippocampal sclerosis with high sensitivity is a special problem that requires specific training. The proper interpretation of MR images in the context of epilepsy, and particularly if surgical treatment is being considered, requires this new level of training in this problem.

The origins of hippocampal sclerosis may be unravelled by the application of MR techniques to the new

FIGURE 5-17. The outcome of patients undergoing temporal lobectomy as a function of the preoperative MRI diagnosis. Patients were followed for 5 years postoperatively. This method of actuarial analysis is stricter than measurement of "good outcome" categories. A. The percentage of patients who never had a seizure postoperatively. After 5 years, approximately 70% of patients with tumor (foreign tissue lesion), 50% with hippocampal sclerosis, and only 20% with no imaging abnormality had never had a seizure postoperatively. B. The percentage of patients who eventually achieved 2 years without a seizure. This criterion is also stricter than those of "good outcome." Note that no patient can be 2 years seizure-free until 2 years have passed. The eventual outcome will be better than in A because this takes into account patients who may have had seizures in the "neighborhood" of the operation. Note that 80% of patients with a tumor (foreign tissue lesion), 63% with hippocampal sclerosis, and 38% with no imaging abnormality eventually became completely seizure-free. The results for "good outcome," which includes only occasional seizures, are better than this. (From Berkovic et al.[8] By permission of *Neurology*.)

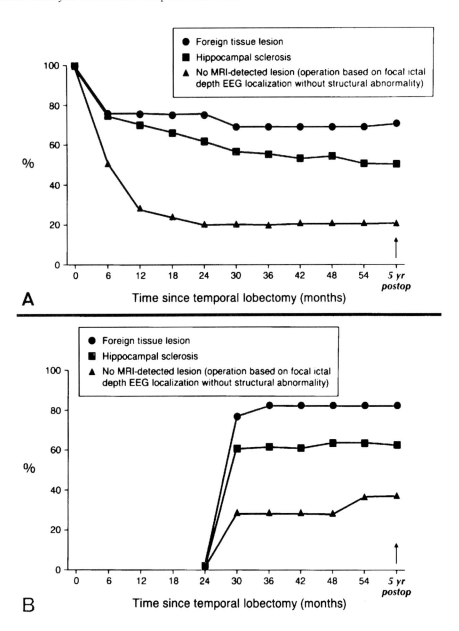

onset of seizures. For the first time, a technique is available that will allow the time course of these abnormalities to be determined. The long-running debate about whether hippocampal sclerosis pre-exists the onset of epilepsy (in particular, the febrile convulsion) or is caused by neurotoxic events associated with prolonged seizures may be addressed in a new way. Anecdotal reports that hippocampal sclerosis develops after prolonged status epilepticus in a child,[144] and even after prolonged seizures in an adult[145] (Figure 5-18), have been published.

CONCLUSION

The impact of MR and its application to clinical epilepsy is akin to the impact that EEG had in the 1940s. It allows abnormalities of the brain to be demonstrated noninvasively in many patients with epilepsy. This has clinical consequences, because the cause of the epilepsy can be defined in most patients with intractable partial epilepsy, and they can be considered for curative surgical procedures at an early stage of the disease.

The impact has been great in the field of epilepsy surgery in which patients who previously had required invasive depth electrode recordings are now often able to undergo a resective procedure based only on noninvasive studies, including noninvasive EEG, routine clinical evaluation, and new MR techniques. Even with this new level of information about the underlying abnormalities in patients with intractable epilepsy, it is important that epilepsy surgery be performed in medical centers dedicated to the problem. A comprehensive epilepsy program involves much more than the identification and removal

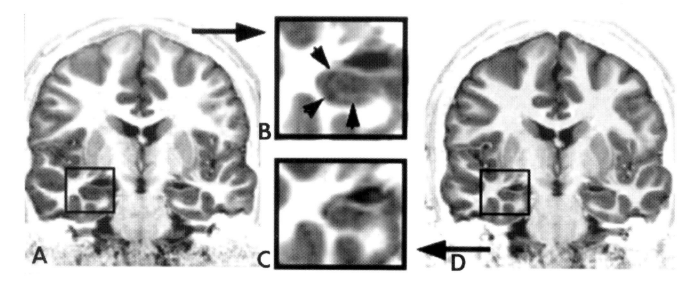

FIGURE 5-18. Severe seizures developed in a 23-year-old man who had had a single seizure at age 10 years. The initial imaging study (A and B) showed darkened internal features (*arrowheads in B*) in a normal, symmetrical hippocampus (inversion recovery image). The imaging study performed 6 months later (C and D) showed that the hippocampus was atrophic and had lost its normal internal microarchitecture. This demonstrates that hippocampal sclerosis can be acquired even in adulthood. Visual analysis can be important in determining these changes.

of the lesions that may cause the seizures, and in many cases, these needs are not reduced by the decreased use of invasive EEG studies.

In the broader field of clinical epilepsy, MR findings are having a large impact on our view of epilepsy and of the syndromes that can be defined. This will ultimately affect the classification of epilepsy, with new syndromes being defined, for example, temporal lobe epilepsy with hippocampal sclerosis. If it is economically and practically feasible, all patients with intractable epilepsy can benefit from optimized MR investigations, and visual analysis of the scans will continue to form the basis for all other MR investigations.

REFERENCES

1. Gerard G, Shabas D, Rossi D. MRI in epilepsy. Comput Radiol 1987;11:223–7.

2. Peretti P, Dravet CH, Raybaud CH, et al. Magnetic resonance imaging in partial epilepsies with an onset before 15 years. Epilepsia 1989;1:227–33.

3. Jackson GD, Berkovic SF, Tress BM, et al. Hippocampal sclerosis can be reliably detected by magnetic resonance imaging. Neurology 1990;40:1869–75.

4. Barkovich AJ, Chuang SH, Norman D. MR of neuronal migration anomalies. AJNR Am J Neuroradiol 1987;8:1009–17.

5. Barkovich AJ, Kjos BO. Gray matter heterotopias: MR characteristics and correlation with develop-mental and neurologic manifestations. Radiology 1992;182:493–9.

6. Baulac M, Granat O, Lehericy S, et al. MRI of developmental abnormalities of mesiotemporal lobe in adult patients with partial epilepsy. Epilepsia 1993;34 Suppl 6:130. (Abstr.)

7. Baulac M, Granat O, Gao X, et al. Hippocampal sclerosis and temporal lobe epilepsy: a MRI study. Epilepsia 1991;3:2–3.

8. Berkovic SF, McIntosh AM, Kalnins RM, et al. Preoperative MRI predicts outcome of temporal lobectomy: an actuarial analysis. Neurology 1995;45:1358–63.

9. Bergin PS, Fish DR, Shorvon SD, et al. FLAIR imaging in partial epilepsy: improving the yield of MRI. Epilepsia 1993;34 Suppl 6:121. (Abstr.)

10. Bronen RA, Cheung G. MRI of the normal hippocampus. Magn Reson Imaging 1991;9:497–500.

11. Bronen RA, Cheung G. MRI of the temporal lobe: normal variations, with special reference toward epilepsy. Magn Reson Imaging 1991;9:501–7.

12. Bronen RA, Fulbright R, Kim JH, et al. MR signal changes associated with pathology proven hippocampal sclerosis. Epilepsia 1994;35 Suppl 8:22. (Abstr.)

13. Cascino GD, Jack CR Jr, Hirschorn KA, et al. Identification of the epileptic focus: magnetic resonance imaging. Epilepsy Res Suppl 1992;5:95–100.

14. Cascino GD, Jack CR Jr, Parisi JE, et al. MRI in the presurgical evaluation of patients with frontal lobe epilepsy and children with temporal lobe epilepsy: patho-

logic correlation and prognostic importance. Epilepsy Res 1992;11:51–9.

15. Cascino GD, Jack CR Jr, Sharbrough FW, et al. MRI assessments of hippocampal pathology in extratemporal lesional epilepsy. Neurology 1993;43:2380–2.

16. Cendes F, Andermann F, Dubeau F, et al. Early childhood prolonged febrile convulsions, atrophy and sclerosis of mesial structures, and temporal lobe epilepsy: an MRI volumetric study. Neurology 1993;43:1083–7.

17. Cendes F, Andermann F, Gloor P, et al. MRI volumetric measurement of amygdala and hippocampus in temporal lobe epilepsy. Neurology 1993;43:719–25.

18. Cendes F, Andermann F, Preul MC, et al. Proton MR spectroscopic imaging in temporal lobe epilepsy (abstract). Neurology 1993;43 Suppl 2:A223.

19. Cook MJ, Fish DR, Shorvon SD, et al. Hippocampal volumetric and morphometric studies in frontal and temporal lobe epilepsy. Brain 1992;115:1001–15.

20. Dowd CF, Dillon WP, Barbaro NM, et al. Magnetic resonance imaging of intractable complex partial seizures: pathologic and electroencephalographic correlation. Epilepsia 1991;32:454–9.

21. Duncan R, Patterson J, Hadley DM, et al. CT, MR and SPECT imaging in temporal lobe epilepsy. J Neurol Neurosurg Psychiatry 1990;53:11–5.

22. Guerrini R, Dravet C, Raybaud C, et al. Epilepsy and focal gyral anomalies detected by MRI: electroclinico-morphological correlations and follow-up. Dev Med Child Neurol 1992;34:706–18.

23. Gulati P, Jena A, Tripathi RP, et al. Magnetic resonance imaging in childhood epilepsy. Indian Pediatr 1991;28:761–5.

24. Grünewald RA, Jackson GD, Connelly A, et al. MR detection of hippocampal disease in epilepsy: factors influencing T2 relaxation time. AJNR Am J Neuroradiol 1994;15:1149–56.

25. Jack CR Jr. MRI-based hippocampal volume measurements in epilepsy. Epilepsia 1994;35 Suppl 6:S21–9.

26. Jack CR Jr, Bentley MD, Twomey CK, et al. MR imaging-based volume measurements of the hippocampal formation and anterior temporal lobe: validation studies. Radiology 1990;176:205–9.

27. Jack CR Jr, Sharbrough FW, Twomey CK, et al. Temporal lobe seizures: lateralization with MR volume measurements of the hippocampal formation. Radiology 1990;175:423–9.

28. Jack CR Jr, Sharbrough FW, Cascino GD, et al. Magnetic resonance image-based hippocampal volumetry: correlation with outcome after temporal lobectomy. Ann Neurol 1992;31:138–46.

29. Jackson GD, Kuzniecky RI, Cascino GD. Normal hippocampal volumes in hippocampal sclerosis: MRI diagnosis based on other features (abstract). Epilepsia 1992;33 Suppl 3:71.

30. Kilpatrick CJ, Tress BM, O'Donnell C, et al. Magnetic resonance imaging and late-onset epilepsy. Epilepsia 1991;32:358–64.

31. Koeller KK, Dillon WP. Dysembryoplastic neuroepithelial tumors: MR appearance. AJNR Am J Neuroradiol 1992;13:1319–25.

32. Kuzniecky R, Berkovic S, Andermann F, et al. Focal cortical myoclonus and rolandic cortical dysplasia: clarification by magnetic resonance imaging. Ann Neurol 1988;23:317–25.

33. Kuzniecky R, de la Sayette V, Ethier R, et al. Magnetic resonance imaging in temporal lobe epilepsy: pathological correlations. Ann Neurol 1987;22:341–7.

34. Kuzniecky R, Garcia JH, Faught E, et al. Cortical dysplasia in temporal lobe epilepsy: magnetic resonance imaging correlations. Ann Neurol 1991;29:293–8.

35. Kuzniecky R, Faught E, Morawetz R, et al. MRI patterns of mesiotemporal atrophy in intractable temporal lobe epilepsy (abstract). Epilepsia 1993;34 Suppl:6:141.

36. Kuzniecky R, Suggs S, Gaudier J, et al. Lateralization of epileptic foci by MRI in temporal lobe epilepsy. J Neuroimaging 1991;1:163–7.

37. Lee AW, Cheng LO, Ng SH, et al. Magnetic resonance imaging in the clinical diagnosis of late temporal lobe necrosis following radiotherapy for nasopharyngeal carcinoma. Clin Radiol 1990;42:24–31.

38. Senzaki A, Okubo Y, Abe T, et al. Quantitative magnetic resonance imaging in patients with temporal lobe epilepsy. J Epilepsy 1993;6:243–9.

39. Swartz BE, Tomiyasu U, Delgado-Escueta AV, et al. Neuroimaging in temporal lobe epilepsy: test sensitivity and relationships to pathology and postoperative outcome. Epilepsia 1992;33:624–34.

40. Theodore WH. MRI, PET, SPECT: interrelations, technical limits, and unanswered questions. Epilepsy Res Suppl 1992;5:127–34.

41. Trenerry MR, Jack CR Jr, Ivnik RJ, et al. MRI hippocampal volumes and memory function before and after temporal lobectomy. Neurology 1993;43:1800–5.

42. Van Paesschen W, Sisodiya S, Connelly A, et al. Quantitative hippocampal MRI and intractable temporal lobe epilepsy. Neurology 1995;45:2233–40.

43. Watson C. Volumetric MRI in patients with extratemporal structural lesions (abstract). Epilepsia 1993;34 Suppl 6:128.

44. Jackson GD, Berkovic SF, Duncan JS, et al. Optimizing the diagnosis of hippocampal sclerosis using MR imaging. AJNR Am J Neuroradiol 1993;14:753–62.

45. Engel J Jr. Surgical treatment of the epilepsies. 2nd ed. New York: Raven Press, 1993.

46. Wieser HG. Human limbic seizures: EEG studies, origin, and patterns of spread. In: Meldrum BS, Ferrendelli JA, Wieser HG, eds. Anatomy of epileptogenesis. London: J Libbey, 1988:127–38.

47. Kuzniecky RI, Jackson GD. Magnetic resonance in epilepsy. New York: Raven Press, 1995.

48. Adams C, Hwang PA, Gilday DL, et al. Comparison of SPECT, EEG, CT, MRI, and pathology in partial epilepsy. Pediatr Neurol 1992;8:97–103.

49. Blom RJ, Vinuela F, Fox AJ, et al. Computed tomography in temporal lobe epilepsy. J Comput Assist Tomogr 1984;8:401–5.

50. Bogdanoff BM, Stafford CR, Green L, et al. Computerized transaxial tomography in the evaluation of patients with focal epilepsy. Neurology 1975;25:1013–7.

51. Broglin D, Vignal JP, Chodkiewicz JP, et al. Contribution of CT-scan and MRI to the pre-surgical evaluation of intractable partial epilepsies. Boll Lega Ital Epilessia 1988;63:39–44.

52. el Gammal T, Adams RJ, King DW, et al. Modified CT techniques in the evaluation of temporal lobe epilepsy prior to lobectomy. AJNR Am J Neuroradiol 1987;8:131–4.

53. Gastaut H, Gastaut JL. Computerized transverse axial tomography in epilepsy. Epilepsia 1976; 17:325–36.

54. Gaggero R, Donato A, De NM, et al. Magnetic resonance imaging (MRI) compared with computed tomography (CT) in child epilepsy. Boll Lega Ital Epilessia 1988;63:107–10.

55. Heinz ER, Heinz TR, Radtke R, et al. Efficacy of MR vs CT in epilepsy. AJR Am J Roentgenol 1989;152:347–52.

56. Jabbari B, Huott AD, DiChiro G, et al. Surgically correctable lesions detected by CT in 143 patients with chronic epilepsy. Surg Neurol 1978;10:319–22.

57. Jolles PR, Chapman PR, Alavi A. PET, CT, and MRI in the evaluation of neuropsychiatric disorders: current applications. J Nucl Med 1989;30:1589–606.

58. Price H, Danziger A. The role of computerised tomography in the diagnosis and management of intracranial abscess. Clin Radiol 1978;29:571–7.

59. Schörner W, Meencke HJ, Felix R. Temporal-lobe epilepsy: comparison of CT and MR imaging. AJR Am J Roentgenol 1987;149:1231–9.

60. Schörner W, Meencke HJ, Sander B, et al. Psychomotorische Epilepsie—Vergleich von CT und MR bei 100 Patienten. Rofo Fortschr Geb Rontgenstr Neuen Bildgeb Verfahr 1989;151:202–9.

61. Theodore WH, Katz D, Kufta C, et al. Pathology of temporal lobe foci: correlation with CT, MRI, and PET. Neurology 1990;40:797–803.

62. Oakley J, Ojemann GA, Ojemann LM, et al. Identifying epileptic foci on contrast-enhanced computerized tomographic scans. Arch Neurol 1979;36:669–71.

63. Wyler AR, Bolender NF. Preoperative CT diagnosis of mesial temporal sclerosis for surgical treatment of epilepsy. Ann Neurol 1983;13:59–64.

64. Adams CBT, Anslow P, Molyneus A, et al. Radiological detection of surgically treatable pathology. In Engel J, ed. Surgical treatment of the epilepsies. New York: Raven Press, 1987:213–33.

65. Sperling MR, Wilson G, Engel J Jr, et al. Magnetic resonance imaging in intractable partial epilepsy: correlative studies. Ann Neurol 1986;20:57–62.

66. Ormson MJ, Kispert DB, Sharbrough FW, et al. Cryptic structural lesions in refractory partial epilepsy: MR imaging and CT studies. Radiology 1986;160:215–9.

67. Maertens PM, Machen BC, Williams JP, et al. Magnetic resonance imaging of mesial temporal sclerosis: case reports. J Comput Tomogr 1987;11:136–9.

68. Berkovic SF, Ethier R, Robitaille Y, et al. Magnetic resonance imaging of the hippocampus: II. Mesial temporal sclerosis (abstract). Epilepsia 1986;27:612.

69. Heinz ER, Crain BJ, Radtke RA, et al. MR imaging in patients with temporal lobe seizures: correlation of results with pathologic findings. AJNR Am J Neuroradiol 1990;11:827–32.

70. Grant R, Hadley DM, Condon B, et al. Magnetic resonance imaging in the management of resistant focal epilepsy: pathological case report and experience of 12 cases. J Neurol Neurosurg Psychiatry 1987;50:1529–32.

71. Berkovic SF, Andermann F, Olivier A, et al. Hippocampal sclerosis in temporal lobe epilepsy demonstrated by magnetic resonance imaging. Ann Neurol 1991;29:175–82.

72. Jackson GD, Kuzniecky RI, Cascino GD. Hippocampal sclerosis without detectable hippocampal atrophy. Neurology 1994;44:42–6.

73. Press GA, Amaral DG, Squire LR. Hippocampal abnormalities in amnesic patients revealed by high-resolution magnetic resonance imaging. Nature 1989;341:54–7.

74. Jackson GD. New techniques in magnetic resonance and epilepsy. Epilepsia 1994;35 Suppl 6:S2–13.

75. Cross JH, Jackson GD, Neville BG, et al. Early detection of abnormalities in partial epilepsy using magnetic resonance. Arch Dis Child 1993;69:104–9.

76. Jabbari B, Gunderson CH, Wippold F, et al. Magnetic resonance imaging in partial complex epilepsy. Arch Neurol 1986;43:869–72.

77. Kuzniecky R, Murro A, King D, et al. Magnetic resonance imaging in childhood intractable partial epilepsies: pathologic correlations. Neurology 1993; 43:681–7.

78. Miura K, Kito M, Hayakawa F, et al. Neuroimaging in intractable partial epilepsy of children: comparison of MRI and SPECT. J Jpn Epilepsy Soc 1990;8:159–66.

79. Spencer SS. The relative contributions of MRI, SPECT, and PET imaging in epilepsy. Epilepsia 1994;35 Suppl 6:72–89.

80. Duvernoy HM. The human hippocampus: an atlas of applied anatomy. München: JF Bergmann Verlag, 1988.

81. Bronen RA, Cheung G. Relationship of hippocampus and amygdala to coronal MRI landmarks. Magn Reson Imaging 1991;9:449–57.

82. Jack CR Jr, Gehring DG, Sharbrough FW, et al. Temporal lobe volume measurement from MR images: accuracy and left-right asymmetry in normal persons. J Comput Assist Tomogr 1988;12:21–9.

83. Graux P, Frigard B, Merlier LB. Tumoral epilepsy. Rev Geriat 1983;8:213–4.

84. Kishikawa H, Ohmoto T, Nishimoto A. Brain tumor with seizures in children. Brain Develop Tokyo 1980;12:19–26.

85. Drake J, Hoffman HJ, Kobayashi J, et al. Surgical management of children with temporal lobe epilepsy and mass lesions. Neurosurgery 1987;21:792–7.

86. Hankey GJ, Davies L, Gubbay SS. Long term survival with early childhood intracerebral tumours. J Neurol Neurosurg Psychiatry 1989;52:778–81.

87. Rasmussen TB. Surgical treatment of complex partial seizures: results, lessons, and problems. Epilepsia 1983;24 Suppl 1:S65–76.

88. Daumas-Duport C. Dysembryoplastic neuroepithelial tumours. Brain Pathol 1993;3:283–95.

89. Prayson RA, Estes ML. Dysembryoplastic neuroepithelial tumor. Am J Clin Pathol 1992;97:398–401.

90. Daumas-Duport C, Scheithauer BW, Chodkiewicz JP, et al. Dysembryoplastic neuroepithelial tumor: a surgically curable tumor of young patients with intractable partial seizures. Report of thirty-nine cases. Neurosurgery 1988;23:545–56.

91. Margerison JH, Corsellis JA. Epilepsy and the temporal lobes. A clinical, electroencephalographic and neuropathological study of the brain in epilepsy, with particular reference to the temporal lobes. Brain 1966;89:499–530.

92. Falconer MA, Serafetinides EA, Corsellis JAN. Etiology and pathogenesis of temporal lobe epilepsy. Arch Neurol 1964;10:233–48.

93. Falconer MA. Mesial temporal (Ammon's horn) sclerosis as a common cause of epilepsy. Aetiology, treatment, and prevention. Lancet 1974;2:767–70.

94. Wieser H-G, Engel J Jr, Williamson PD, et al. Surgically remediable temporal lobe syndromes. In: Engel J Jr, ed. Surgical treatment of the epilepsies. 2nd ed. New York: Raven Press, 1993:49–63.

95. Sostman HD, Spencer DD, Gore JC, et al. Preliminary observations on magnetic resonance imaging in refractory epilepsy. Magn Reson Imaging 1984;2:301–6.

96. Rougier A, Biset JM, Kien P, et al. I.R.M. et chirurgie de l'epilepsie. Neurochirurgie 1988;34:188–93.

97. Laster DW, Penry JK, Moody DM, et al. Chronic seizure disorders: contribution of MR imaging when CT is normal. AJNR Am J Neuroradiol 1985;6:177–80.

98. Berkovic SF, Ethier R, Olivier A, et al. Magnetic resonance imaging of the hippocampus: I. Normal anatomy. Epilepsia 1986;27:611–2.

99. Lesser RP, Modic MT, Weinstein MA, et al. Magnetic resonance imaging (1.5 tesla) in patients with intractable focal seizures. Arch Neurol 1986;43:367–71.

100. Brooks BS, King DW, el Gammal T, et al. MR imaging in patients with intractable complex partial epileptic seizures. AJR Am J Roentgenol 1990;154:577–83.

101. Furune S, Negoro T, Maehara M, et al. Magnetic resonance imaging in complex partial seizures. Jpn J Psychiatry Neurol 1989;43:361–7.

102. Ryvlin P, Garcia-Larrea L, Philippon B, et al. High signal intensity on T2-weighted MRI correlates with hypoperfusion in temporal lobe epilepsy. Epilepsia 1992;33:28–35.

103. Kodama K. MRI in patients with temporal lobe epilepsy: correlation between MRI findings and clinical features. Seishin Shinkeigaku Zasshi 1992;94:26–57.

104. Convers P, Bierme T, Ryvlin P, et al. Apport de l'imagerie par resonance magnetique dans 100 cas d'epilepsie partielle rebelle a scanner X normal. Rev Neurol (Paris) 1990;146:330–7.

105. Stefan H, Pawlik G, Bocher-Schwarz HG, et al. Functional and morphological abnormalities in temporal lobe epilepsy: a comparison of interictal and ictal EEG, CT, MRI, SPECT and PET. J Neurol 1987;234:377–84.

106. Tamaki K, Okuno T, Ito M, et al. Magnetic resonance imaging in relation to EEG epileptic foci in tuberous sclerosis. Brain Dev 1990;12:316–20.

107. Guyot M, Duche B, Loiseau P, et al. Magnetic resonance imaging in partial epilepsies. Boll Lega Ital Epilessia 1988;63:111–2.

108. Theodore WH, Dorwart R, Holmes M, et al. Neuroimaging in refractory partial seizures: comparison of PET, CT, and MRI. Neurology 1986;36:750–9.

109. Froment JC, Mauguiere F, Fischer C, et al. Magnetic resonance imaging in refractory focal epilepsy with normal CT scans. J Neuroradiol 1989;16:285–91.

110. Ryvlin P, Cinotti L, Froment JC, et al. Metabolic patterns associated with non-specific magnetic resonance imaging abnormalities in temporal lobe epilepsy. Brain 1991;114:2363–83.

111. Williamson PD, French JA, Thadani VM, et al. Characteristics of medial temporal lobe epilepsy: II. Interictal and ictal scalp electroencephalography, neuropsychological testing, neuroimaging, surgical results, and pathology. Ann Neurol 1993;34:781–7.

112. Jackson GD, Connelly A, Duncan JS, et al. Detection of hippocampal pathology in intractable partial epilepsy: increased sensitivity with quantitative magnetic resonance T2 relaxometry. Neurology 1993;43:1793–9.

113. Jackson GD, Duncan JS, Connelly A, et al. Increased signal in the mesial temporal region on T2-weighted MRI: a quantitative study of hippocampal sclerosis. Neurology 1991;41 Suppl 1:170–1.

114. Cahan LD, Engel J Jr. Surgery for epilepsy: a review. Acta Neurol Scand 1986;73:551–60.

115. Cascino GD, Jack CR Jr, Parisi JE, et al. Magnetic resonance imaging-based volume studies in temporal lobe epilepsy: pathological correlations. Ann Neurol 1991;30:31–6.

116. Jack CR Jr, Sharbrough FW, Marsh WR. Use of MR imaging for quantitative evaluation of resection for temporal lobe epilepsy. Radiology 1988;169:463–8.

117. Lencz T, McCarthy G, Bronen RA, et al. Quantitative magnetic resonance imaging in temporal lobe epilepsy: relationship to neuropathology and neuropsychological function. Ann Neurol 1992;31:629–37.

118. Spencer SS, McCarthy G, Spencer DD. Diagnosis of medial temporal lobe seizure onset: relative specificity and sensitivity of quantitative MRI. Neurology 1993; 43:2117–24.

119. Ojemann LM, Tsuruda JS, Holmes MD, et al. Comparison of clinical features, histology and high resolution fast spin MRI using a phased array coil in patients undergoing surgery for temporal lobe epilepsy (abstract). Epilepsia 1993;34 Suppl 6:136.

120. Elster AD, Mirza W. MRI imaging in chronic partial epilepsy: role of contrast enhancement. AJNR Am J Neuroradiol 1991;12:165–70.

121. Kuzniecky RI, Cascino GD, Palmini A, et al. Structural neuroimaging. In: Engel J Jr, ed. Surgical treatment of the epilepsies. 2nd ed. New York: Raven Press, 1993:197–209.

122. Runge VM. Clinical magnetic resonance imaging. Philadelphia: JB Lippincott Company, 1990.

123. Cascino GD, Hirschorn KA, Jack CR, et al. Gadolinium-DTPA-enhanced magnetic resonance imaging in intractable partial epilepsy. Neurology 1989;39:1115–8.

124. Cendes F, Andermann F, Gloor P, et al. Atrophy of mesial structures in patients with temporal lobe epilepsy? cause or consequence of repeated seizures? Ann Neurol 1993;34:795–801.

125. Ashtari M, Barr WB, Schaul N, et al. Three-dimensional fast low-angle shot imaging and computerized volume measurement of the hippocampus in patients with chronic epilepsy of the temporal lobe. AJNR Am J Neuroradiol 1991;12:941–7.

126. Kuks JB, Cook MJ, Fish DR, et al. Hippocampal sclerosis in epilepsy and childhood febrile seizures. Lancet 1993;342:1391–4.

127. Incisa della Rocchetta A, Gadian DG, Connelly A, et al. Verbal memory impairment after right temporal lobe surgery: role of contralateral damage as revealed by 1H magnetic resonance spectroscopy and T2 relaxometry. Neurology 1995;45:797–802.

128. Bruton CJ. The neuropathology of temporal lobe epilepsy. Oxford: Oxford University Press, 1988.

129. Gloor P, Olivier A, Quesney LF, et al. The role of the limbic system in experimental phenomena of temporal lobe epilepsy. Ann Neurol 1982;12:129–44.

130. Hudson LP, Monuz DG, Miller L, et al. Amygdaloid sclerosis in temporal lobe epilepsy. Ann Neurol 1993;33:622–31.

131. Jack CR Jr, Twomey CK, Zinsmeister AR, et al. Anterior temporal lobes and hippocampal formations: normative volumetric measurements from MR images in young adults. Radiology 1989;172:549–54.

132. Watson C, Andermann F, Gloor P, et al. Anatomic basis of amygdaloid and hippocampal volume measurement by magnetic resonance imaging. Neurology 1992;42:1743–50.

133. Meiners LC, Valk J, Jansen GH, et al. Magnetic resonance of epilepsy: three observations. In: Shorvon SD, Fish DR, Andermann F, et al., eds. Magnetic resonance scanning and epilepsy. New York: Plenum Press, 1994:79–82.

134. Connelly A, Jackson GD, Duncan JS, et al. Magnetic resonance spectroscopy in temporal lobe epilepsy. Neurology 1994;44:1411–7.

135. Bronen RA, Cheung G, Charles JT, et al. Imaging findings in hippocampal sclerosis: correlation with pathology. AJNR Am J Neuroradiol 1991; 12:933–40.

136. Kuzniecky R, Burgard S, Faught E, et al. Predictive value of magnetic resonance imaging in temporal lobe epilepsy surgery. Arch Neurol 1993;50:65–9.

137. Gloor P. Cited by Engel J Jr. (45).

138. Babb TL, Brown WJ. Pathological findings in epilepsy. In: Engel J Jr., ed. Surgical treatment of the epilepsies. New York: Raven Press, 1987:511–40.

139. Babb TL, Pretorius JK. Pathologic substrates of epilepsy. In: Wyllie E, ed. The treatment of epilepsy: principles and practice. Philadelphia: Lea & Febiger, 1993:55–70.

140. Levesque MF, Nakasato N, Vinters HV, et al. Surgical treatment of limbic epilepsy associated with extrahippocampal lesions: the problem of dual pathology. J Neurosurg 1991;75:364–70.

141. Adamec RE. Does kindling model anything clinically relevant? Biol Psychiatry 1990;27:249–79.

142. Wada JA, Mizoguchi T, Komai S. Kindling epileptogenesis in orbital and mesial frontal cortical areas of subhuman primates. Epilepsia 1985;26:472–9.

143. Delgado-Escueta AV, Ward AA Jr, Woodbury DM, et al. New wave of research in the epilepsies. Adv Neurol 1986;44:3–55.

144. Nohria V, Lee N, Tien RD, et al. Magnetic resonance imaging evidence of hippocampal sclerosis in progression: a case report. Epilepsia 1994;35: 1332–6.

145. Jackson GD, Fitt GJ, Mitchell LA, et al. Hippocampal sclerosis developing in adults: progression of hippocampal MR findings (abstract). Epilepsia 1995;36 Suppl 3:S249.

Mesial Temporal Sclerosis: Magnetic Resonance– Based Hippocampal Volume Measurements

Clifford R. Jack, Jr.

The two most obvious microscopic changes that occur in mesial temporal sclerosis are gliosis and cell loss.[1-3] The respective magnetic resonance (MR) imaging correlates are prolonged T_1 and T_2 tissue relaxation (due to a relative increase in unbound tissue water) and atrophy. As mentioned in Chapter 5, simple visual inspection of properly acquired images from a modern MR imager can reveal the presence of mesial temporal sclerosis with around 90% accuracy.[4-10] Therefore, it is reasonable to ask whether it is necessary to perform formal hippocampal volume measurements to identify mesial temporal sclerosis for clinical purposes. If not, why measure hippocampal volumes at all? On the basis of our experience, the role for formal hippocampal volume measurements in daily clinical practice is small. However, measurements are essential in conducting statistically based research relating hippocampal size to relevant clinical variables in epilepsy. The rationale for performing MR-based hippocampal volume measurements in epilepsy research is not merely to identify the atrophy associated with mesial temporal sclerosis but, more importantly, to quantify its severity. In the study of brain morphometry, it is accepted that a fundamental relationship exists between brain structure and function, both normal and abnormal. Perhaps the most useful descriptor of morphometric structure that currently can be derived from a set of medical images is volume. Formal volume measurements introduce a level of precision in the estimation of hippocampal size that is not available with only visual inspection of a set of MR images. Precise quantitation of hippocampal volume provides ordinal data that can be correlated with quantitative pathologic, clinical, epidemiologic, or cognitive measures, thus enabling statistically based testing of hypotheses that relate brain structure to function. Therefore, formal volumetric measurement of brain structures, such as the hippocampus, should remain a useful research tool in epilepsy and other conditions in which global or local brain atrophy has a prominent role.

To produce accurate hippocampal volume measurements with MR imaging, attention must be directed to the two major components of the operation as a whole: MR image acquisition and image processing (that is, extracting a volume).[5,11,12] Optimization of *both* of these aspects of hippocampal volume measurement is essential to obtaining a useful result. No image processing scheme can extract meaningful volumetric data from an MR imaging data set that was improperly acquired. Likewise, an optimally acquired MR study will yield useless quantitative information if the image processing steps are carried out in a haphazard fashion.

MAGNETIC RESONANCE IMAGE ACQUISITION

An optimized pulse sequence for in vivo quantitation should cover the anatomical area of interest, in this case the hippocampi, in a reasonable amount of time, while maximizing spatial resolution and contrast to noise. In selecting a set of MR imaging variables (also known as a pulse sequence) appropriate for hippocampal volume measurement, two major principles must be observed.

1. The ability to spatially resolve brain structure is a function of the inherent spatial resolution of the images. Given the fact that the hippocampus is small, MR images used to measure its volume must be of high resolution. The higher the resolution of the images, the more accurate and precise the volume measurements will be. Attention to this is most critical in the slice select dimension, because this dimension of a voxel is typically greater than the dimensions in the plane of the imaging slice.

2. The MR images must have gray scale contrast properties that clearly demarcate the boundary of the hippocampus from adjacent white matter and cerebrospinal fluid (CSF).

From a historical perspective, the MR pulse sequence that provided the best possible set of images for hippocampal volume measurement has changed with the technical progress made in MR imaging. At the Mayo Clinic, we have changed MR acquisition techniques with each new technical development. For example, in 1986, state-of-the-art MR imaging permitted, at best, interleaved contiguous 5-mm-thick spin echo slices.[11] In 1989, 4-mm-thick spin echo images and, in 1990–1991, 3-mm-thick spin echo images became commercially available. In 1990–1991, the major MR vendors introduced three-dimensional gradient echo sequences, and these have been used with a slice thickness less than 2 mm by several groups to measure hippocampal volume. Currently, the pulse sequence we use is a three-dimensional *oblique* coronal volumetric radiofrequency (RF) spoil gradient echo (SPGR) with the following: 124 partitions or slices, 256×192 matrix, 1 signal average, 45° flip angle, minimum TR and TE, and 22-cm $\times$ 16.5-cm field of view. Spatial resolution is 0.859 mm $\times$ 0.859 mm in plane and 1.6 mm in the "slice" select direction, producing a voxel volume of 1.1816 mm.[3] This takes less than 7 minutes to acquire.

IMAGE PROCESSING

The image processing operations required to extract a precise hippocampal volume measurement from a set of MR images can be summarized as follows:

1. Manipulation of the input images to achieve proper orientation and display of the hippocampi. The long axis of the hippocampi are angled with respect to the sagittal imaging plane; the degree of this angulation varies from subject to subject (Figure 6-1).

Ideally, MR images used for volume measurement are acquired perpendicular to the hippocampal long axis (that is, in an oblique coronal plane).[12] If this is not possible, then the images may be reformatted, provided that the original MR images have been acquired in a three-

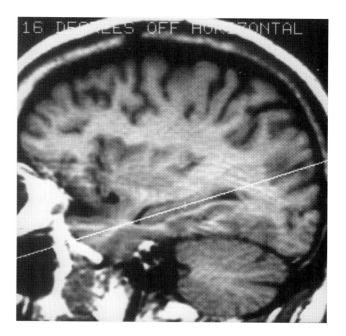

FIGURE 6-1. Hippocampal angulation. Parasagittal image through the hippocampus of a normal subject. The long axis of the hippocampus is angled obliquely with respect to orthogonal magnet axes. The degree of angulation can vary significantly from individual to individual.

dimensional mode with voxel thickness not exceeding about 2 mm (Figure 6-2). Such a data set should first be interpolated to produce cubic voxels. At our institution, we "subvolume" the resulting data set so that the voxels outside of the temporal lobes are discarded. Excluding these nonessential regions speeds up subsequent steps and also reduces the memory space required to store the

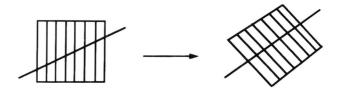

FIGURE 6-2. Reformatting. The diagonal line indicates the hypothetical orientation of the long axis of the hippocampus with respect to orthogonal magnet axes. The rectangular box with vertical lines, represents the orientation of a series of slices in a three-dimensional volumetric MR data set. The figure on the left indicates the oblique manner in which an unreformatted coronal data set might intersect the long axis of the hippocampus. The figure on the right illustrates the result of reformatting. After reformatting, each image is oriented perpendicular to the true long axis of the hippocampus.

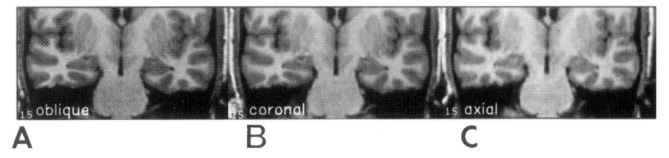

FIGURE 6-3. Effect of reformatting. Three different three-dimensional volumetric pulse sequences identical except for the plane of acquisition were acquired in the same subject. A. Image acquired in an *oblique* plane (acquired directly perpendicular to the principle axis of the left hippocampal formation), (B) in the *coronal* plane, and (C) in the *axial* plane. The coronal and axial acquisitions were then reformatted so that the slices were oriented perpendicular to the principal axis of the left hippocampal formation (Figure 6-2). The borders of the hippocampus are defined most clearly by the images acquired directly perpendicular to the principal axis of the hippocampus, that is, the oblique image in A, in which no reformatting was necessary. The borders of the hippocampus are least sharp in C, the image acquired axially. This figure illustrates that when nonisotropic MRI data are reformatted, the reformatted images become increasingly blurry as the angle between the original plane of acquisition and the reformatted plane increases. (From Jack et al.[14] By permission of Elsevier Science.)

processed images. The subvolumed data are then interpolated again in plane to the equivalent of a 512×512 matrix and magnified by a factor of 2. These steps have recently been described in detail.[13]

We have found that a direct coronal acquisition tailored to the anatomy of the subject results in sharper hippocampal boundaries than do orthogonal coronal three-dimensional SPGR images, which have been secondarily reformatted to be perpendicular to the hippocampus[14] (Figure 6-3).

2. The borders of the hippocampi are traced by hand sequentially on each imaging slice from posterior to anterior (Figure 6-4). This step is known as "segmentation." Several automated or semiautomated techniques have been described for whole brain volume measurement from MRI. However, because no gray scale differences separate the hippocampus from adjacent tissue along its inferomedial border, the hippocampi must be segmented manually.

3. The number of voxels within the traced outlines of the right and left hippocampi are counted by the computer and multiplied by voxel size to give volume in cubic millimeters.

ANATOMIC BOUNDARIES

Anatomic boundaries of the hippocampus must be defined both in the plane of the imaging slices, "in-plane boundaries" (oblique coronal), and in the anteroposterior direction, "anteroposterior boundaries."

In-Plane Boundaries

The structures to be included are the hippocampus proper (Ammon's horn), the dentate gyrus, and the subiculum. Laterally, the boundary of the hippocampus is

determined by CSF in the temporal horn, superiorly by the CSF in the choroidal fissure, medially by CSF in the uncal and ambien cistern, and inferiorly by the gray-white matter junction between the subiculum and the white matter in the parahippocampal gyrus. The gray matter of the subiculum is continuous with that of the parahippocampal gyrus, and it is necessary to trace a boundary through the gray matter at this location. This portion of the hippocampal boundary is the most subjective and produces most of the intrasubject and intersubject variability in boundary tracing. If the MR images are of high resolution and are acquired or reformatted perpendicular to the long axis of the hippocampal formation, then determining the in-plane boundaries of the hippocampal head (pes hippocampus) is straightforward. The hippocampal head must be disarticulated from the overlying amygdala. The uncal recess of the temporal horn provides a convenient superior landmark for the head of the hippocampus. When the hippocampal digitations are fused to the amygdala, the thin line formed by the alveus serves as a useful landmark (Figure 6-4). We include the intralimbic gyrus within the boundaries of the hippocampus. The choroid plexus is excluded.

Anteroposterior Boundaries

We include the entire hippocampal head in the measurement, and this serves as the anterior boundary of the hippocampus. Previously, we defined the posterior boundary of the hippocampus as the oblique coronal slice that intersected the posterior commissure when cross-referenced to the midline sagittal slice.[5,12] With this technique, only the head and body of the hippocampus are measured; the tail is excluded. More recently, Watson et al.[15] have identified an intrinsic landmark to define the posterior boundary of

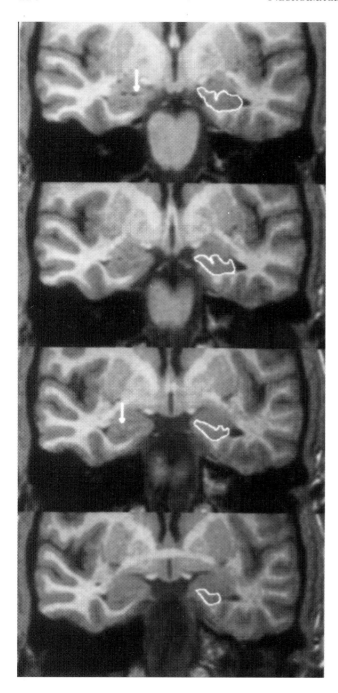

FIGURE 6-4. Tracing in-plane hippocampal boundaries. In this four-panel collage, traces (*in white*) of the outline of the head of the left hippocampus appear as they would on the workstation screen. The boundaries of the right hippocampal head appear as they would prior to tracing. The *arrow* in the top panel indicates the patent uncal recess of the temporal horn, which demarcates the boundary between the amygdala and the hippocampal head. The *arrow* in the next to bottom panel indicates the thin white line formed by the alveus, which indicates the boundary between the hippocampal head and amygdala in the more anterior portions of the hippocampal head.

the hippocampus, namely, the coronal section in which the crus of the fornix is seen in full profile (Figure 6-5). We have adopted this approach, because it has several advantages: (1) the total volume of hippocampal tissue is increased, (2) shifts in hemispheric anatomy after temporal lobectomy do not corrupt postoperative volume measurements, and (3) rotation of the head of the patient with respect to the coronal plane at the time of MR image acquisition becomes less of a technical problem. However, we do correct for head rotation by realigning the image data in the coronal plane when necessary.

ACCURACY AND REPRODUCIBILITY

Before applying the technique of hippocampal volume measurements to patients, studies of the validity of these measurements had to be assessed. Measurements that are neither accurate nor reproducible would defeat the purpose of volumetric quantitation. Several groups have performed such validation studies.[11,16-18] Not surprisingly, the reported accuracy and reproducibility of brain volume measurements have improved since the initial studies were published in 1988[11] because of the significant technical progress made in MR imaging. The most recently published validation studies cited a 1.2% intraobserver variability and a 3.4% interobserver variability.[17] Accuracy with respect to phantoms of known volume has been estimated at about 5%.[16,18]

NORMAL VALUES

To apply the technique of hippocampal volume measurements to the study of pathologic conditions, the range of values found in normal subjects in the general population must be known. Hippocampal volume measurements in normal subjects have been studied by several investigators,[12,15,18-22] who generally agree on the following:

1. *Body Habitus.* Larger people tend to have larger heads, brains, and hippocampi. In normal persons, hippocampal volume increases linearly with total intracranial volume. Therefore, in comparing absolute hippocampal volumes among different groups, the hippocampal volume values should be scaled by this measure of head size.

2. *Sex.* Hippocampal volumes of men, on average, are larger than those of women. However, this is accounted for by the difference in head size. When normalized by total intracranial volume, the difference in hippocampal volume between men and women is not significant.

3. *Age.* Hippocampal volumes appear to be stable during young adulthood, ages 20 to 40 years. However, at some as yet undetermined point, perhaps age 60, hippocampal volumes decline linearly with age, consistent with age-related generalized cerebral atrophy.

However, published studies of normal hippocampal volume in young adults are in sharp disagreement on two

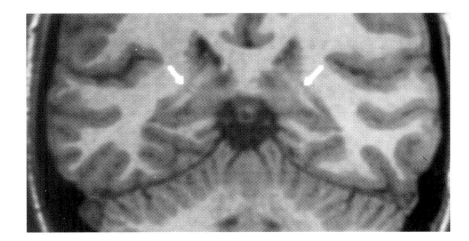

FIGURE 6-5. Posterior hippocampal boundary. This slice through the hippocampal tail shows the forniceal crura (*arrows*) in full profile as they lift away from the tail of the hippocampus. This appearance demarcates the posterior boundary of the hippocampus. (From Jack et al.[14] By permission of Elsevier Science.)

TABLE 6-1. Reported Values of Normal Hippocampal Volume (Unnormalized)

Hippocampus	Jack et al.[12]	Ashtari et al.[20]	Cook et al.[18]	Watson et al.[15]	Cendes et al.[17]	Bhatia et al.[22]
Right	2.8 cm^3	2,598 mm^3	3,185 mm^3	5,265 mm^3	4,711 mm^3	3.77 cm^3
Left	2.5 cm^3	2,727 mm^3	3,229 mm^3	4,903 mm^3	4,591 mm^3	3.78 cm^3

From Jack et al.[14] By permission of Elsevier Science.

issues. First, is there normal *relative* or side-to-side hippocampal volumetric asymmetry, and if so, which side is larger? In the original publication on normative hippocampal volume measures, we reported that the right hippocampus was slightly larger than the left (2.8 cm^3 vs 2.5 cm^3) in a sample of 52 normal young adult volunteers (these measurements excluded the hippocampal tail).[12] Weis et al.[23] analyzed stereologic measurements of the entire hippocampus from 29 preserved brain specimens and also reported that the right hippocampus was slightly larger than the left, 3.69 cm^3 versus 3.44 cm^3. In subsequent MR studies, some authors found a small right-left discrepancy in relative hippocampal volume in normal subjects, but others did not.[15,18–22] Second, what is "the" normal *absolute* volume of the right and left hippocampi? Table 6-1 summarizes results from different studies in which absolute right and left hippocampal volumes were measured.

Several explanations may be proposed for the disagreement among these different studies regarding relative hippocampal volume (right vs left) and absolute hippocampal volume. One explanation is related to differences in defining the anterior and posterior boundaries of the hippocampus. Ashtari et al.[20] and Spencer et al.[24] measured the tail and body but excluded the hippocampal head. We[12] measured the entire hippocampal head and body, but excluded the tail. Four other research groups, Cook et al.,[18] Watson et al.,[15] Cendes et al.,[17] and Bhatia et al.,[22] measured the entire anteroposterior extent of the hippocampus. The posterior landmark used by these investigators was the coronal section in which the crura of the fornices lift away from the hippocampal tail.[15]

Another possible explanation for the discrepancy among values reported for normal absolute hippocampal volume is the method of pixel counting used by the volumetric software at different institutions. As indicated above, the boundaries of the hippocampus must be traced on serial planimetric imaging sections. After this tracing is completed, a region of interest (ROI) is defined. The volume of the hippocampus is then calculated by counting the number of pixels within the traced ROI on successive anatomical slices and multiplying the total number of imaging voxels by voxel volume. However, minor differences in the way the pixels of a traced ROI are counted can produce major differences in calculated volume, as indicated in Figure 6-6. This highly idealized scheme illustrates three possible options: the pixel counting software could count (1) the pixels inside the trace, (2) include the row of pixels under the trace in the ROI, or (3) include the row of pixels outside the trace in the ROI calculation. A priori, there is no right or wrong approach; however, the difference in numeric output is substantial. This simple matter of pixel counting is obviously known to the software programmers but may be unknown to the user. In fact, none of the published papers on hippocampal volumetrics have commented on this aspect of methodology. Different groups of investigators probably have different software, and this could account for a substantial portion of the variation in absolute hippocampal volume reported in normal subjects.

In addition to differences among institutions, volumetric data produced at the same institution may be incompatible if produced with different techniques. Although it is important to remain technically state-of-the-art in terms of MR acquisition and image processing, to do so presents

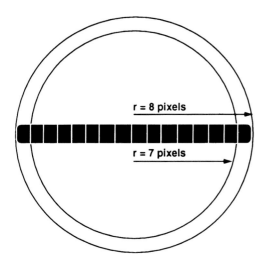

A) r = 7mm; area = 154mm²
B) r = 8mm; area = 201mm²
C) r = 9mm; area = 254mm²

31%
26%
65%

Figure 6-6. Pixel counting in a traced region of interest. Assume that the hippocampus is a perfectly cylindrical structure and that this image represents a single slice perpendicular to the principal axis of the hippocampus. The two concentric circles in this image represent the pixels on which the outer boundary of the hippocampus was manually traced. The area of this hippocampal slice could be calculated in three different ways. Option A: all those pixels inside the trace could be counted, giving an area of 154 mm². Option B: the pixels underneath the trace could also be included, giving an area of 201 mm². Option C: the row of pixels immediately outside the trace could also be counted, giving an area of 254 mm². These differences in counting pixels in relation to a traced region of interest, produce marked changes in the total calculated area (and, by extension, total volume) of the hippocampus. The difference in calculated area between methods A and B is 31%; between methods B and C, 26%; and between methods A and C, 65%. (From Jack et al.[14] By permission of Elsevier Science.)

significant problems with data consistency in a rapidly changing technical environment. Each change in MR acquisition technique or image processing technique (or both) has the potential to introduce a systematic change in the hippocampal volume measurements that are produced.

RESEARCH STUDIES IN EPILEPSY USING HIPPOCAMPAL VOLUMETRIC MEASUREMENTS

Initial studies of hippocampal volumetric measurements in epilepsy addressed the correlation between volumetrically defined hippocampal atrophy and electroclinical seizure lateralization in temporal lobe onset epilepsy.[5,20,21] These early MR-based hippocampal volumetric studies helped to establish the now widely accepted fact that mesial temporal sclerosis can be identified reliably with MR. These studies also helped to establish the concept that the syndrome of nonlesional temporal lobe epilepsy should be divided into two separate entities. The more common is a mesial temporal seizure onset syndrome with mesial temporal sclerosis as the histologic substrate of epileptogenesis. The less common is a neocortical onset syndrome with an uncertain neuropathologic basis.

During a measurement procedure, volumes of the right and left hippocampi are generated. To use this data to label one temporal lobe as abnormal, numeric criteria had to be established that segregate the paired right and left hippocampal volume measurements in a given patient into three domains: right hippocampal atrophy, indeterminate or nonlateralizing atrophy, and left hippocampal atrophy. Our approach has been to subtract the left from the right hippocampus.[5] In general, negative values indicate right hippocampal atrophy, positive values indicate left atrophy, and values around zero are nonlateralizing. Other medical centers have also used this right minus left approach (or a variant), a right-to-left ratio approach, or a discriminate analysis approach.[15,18–21,24] The sensitivity and specificity of volume measurements to seizure lateralization in nonlesional temporal lobe onset seizures that we reported initially were 76% specificity and 100% sensitivity.[5] Other groups have reported differing sensitivity and specificity values, ranging as high as 100% sensitivity and 100% specificity.[18] Again, interinstitutional variance in the reported accuracy of hippocampal volume measurements in seizure lateralization is expected. In any given epilepsy case series, the greater the percentage of nonlesional patients with mesial temporal sclerosis (as compared with neocortical onset seizures without mesial temporal sclerosis), the more accurate hippocampal volume measurements will be in lateralizing seizures for that group.[15,18–21,24] Also, it would be expected that early studies performed with less developed MRI technology would have lower reported accuracy than studies performed with more technically advanced MRI equipment.

Several authors have studied the relationship between hippocampal volume measurements and histologic analysis of subsequently resected temporal lobe specimens.[19,21,25] In every study, a strong correlation was found between MRI-defined volume loss and the histologic severity of mesial temporal sclerosis.

The central role of the hippocampal formation in declarative memory function is well established. Sass et al.[26] have shown a deficit in hippocampal-mediated memory function in patients with histologically proven mesial temporal sclerosis. The MR correlate of this relationship has been identified by several groups who have shown a significant relationship between the severity of hippocampal atrophy as determined with MRI volumetric measurements and standard tests of memory and learning (see Chapter 18).[21,27]

The relationship between mesial temporal sclerosis and several clinical variables has been a topic of considerable interest and controversy for decades. Several studies have convincingly demonstrated a significant relationship between MR-based hippocampal volume measurements and a history of febrile convulsions in early childhood.[28–30] In these studies, MRI-determined atrophy ipsilateral to the side of the seizure focus was significantly more common in persons with a history of early childhood prolonged febrile convulsions. Also, no significant relationship was identified between MRI-determined atrophy and either the estimated severity or the duration of the seizure disorder. These volumetric studies support the concept that a selective window of vulnerability exists in early childhood for the formation of mesial temporal sclerosis and that formation of the lesion (cell death mediated by excitotoxic neurotransmitters) is related to prolonged febrile convulsions that occur during this period of vulnerability. Conversely, these studies do not support the idea that mesial temporal sclerosis is a lesion that develops incrementally throughout life and worsens with each successive seizure.

The initial work in which a significant relationship was found between MRI-identified mesial temporal sclerosis and outcome after temporal lobectomy was performed with hippocampal volume measurements.[31] In this study, 97% of the patients in whom clinical EEG lateralization was concordant with volumetrically determined hippocampal atrophy had a favorable (seizure-free or near seizure-free) outcome. The percentage of patients with a favorable outcome decreases to 42% if the volume measurements were nonlateralizing, and if they were abnormal on the side opposite the lobectomy, the percentage of patients with a satisfactory outcome decreased to 33%. These general results have been replicated using visual criteria.[32,33]

Among epilepsy patients, the incidence of MRI-defined hippocampal volume loss is extremely low or nonexistent in those with documented extratemporal onset seizures.[17–19,34,35] In fact, if the hippocampus is atrophic in a patient with apparent extratemporal seizures, then reexamination of the electroclinical determination of extratemporal onset should be considered. The identification of hippocampal atrophy must be considered in the context of a patient's clinical presentation. Several well-known nonepileptic conditions are associated with hippocampal atrophy, including Alzheimer's dementia, certain amnestic syndromes, and schizophrenia.[36–41] However, in these conditions, the atrophy typically is bilaterally symmetrical. Although hippocampal atrophy is not specific for epilepsy, it seems to be quite specific for seizures of temporal lobe onset in patients with habitual seizures. This rule is not absolute; however, we have found rare cases in which the hippocampus in the nonepileptic temporal lobe is smaller than that in the temporal lobe of seizure onset.

In conclusion, formal volumetric measurements are of greatest utility in clinical research. Studying the relationship between hippocampal volume and other relevant variables has been a fruitful area of clinical research, and the precision of the technique will only improve with the inevitable advances in MR image acquisition and imaging processing technology.

REFERENCES

1. Babb TL, Brown WJ, Pretorius J, et al. Temporal lobe volumetric cell densities in temporal lobe epilepsy. Epilepsia 1984;25:729–40.

2. Dam AM. Epilepsy and neuron loss in the hippocampus. Epilepsia 1980;21:617–29.

3. Pringle CE, Blume WT, Munoz DG, et al. Pathogenesis of mesial temporal sclerosis. Can J Neurol Sci 1993;20:184–93.

4. Kuzniecky R, de la Sayette V, Ethier R, et al. Magnetic resonance imaging in temporal lobe epilepsy: pathological correlations. Ann Neurol 1987;22:341–7.

5. Jack CR Jr, Sharbrough FW, Twomey CK, et al. Temporal lobe seizures: lateralization with MR volume measurements of the hippocampal formation. Radiology 1990;175:423–9.

6. Jackson GD, Berkovic SF, Tress BM, et al. Hippocampal sclerosis can be reliably detected by magnetic resonance imaging. Neurology 1990;40:1869–75.

7. Berkovic SF, Andermann F, Olivier A, et al. Hippocampal sclerosis in temporal lobe epilepsy demonstrated by magnetic resonance imaging. Ann Neurol 1991;29:175–82.

8. Bronen RA, Cheung G, Charles JT, et al. Imaging findings in hippocampal sclerosis: correlation with pathology. AJNR Am J Neuroradiol 1991;12:933–40.

9. Jackson GD, Berkovic SF, Duncan JS, et al. Optimizing the diagnosis of hippocampal sclerosis using MR imaging. AJNR Am J Neuroradiol 1993;14:753–62.

10. Jack CR Jr, Mullan BP, Sharbrough FW, et al. Intractable nonlesional epilepsy of temporal lobe origin: lateralization by interictal SPECT versus MRI. Neurology 1994;44:829–36.

11. Jack CR Jr, Gehring DG, Sharbrough FW, et al. Temporal lobe volume measurement from MR images: accuracy and left-right asymmetry in normal persons. J Comput Assist Tomogr 1988;12:21–9.

12. Jack CR Jr, Twomey CK, Zinsmeister AR, et al. Anterior temporal lobes and hippocampal formations: normative volumetric measurements from MR images in young adults. Radiology 1989;172:549–54.

13. Jack CR Jr. MRI-based hippocampal volume measurements in epilepsy. Epilepsia 1994;35 Suppl 6:S21–9.

14. Jack CR Jr, Theodore WH, Cook M, et al. MRI-based hippocampal volumetrics: data acquisition,

normal ranges, and optimal protocol. Magn Reson Imaging 1995;13:1057–1064.

15. Watson C, Andermann F, Gloor P, et al. Anatomic basis of amygdaloid and hippocampal volume measurement by magnetic resonance imaging. Neurology 1992;42:1743–50.

16. Jack CR Jr, Bentley MD, Twomey CK, et al. MR imaging-based volume measurements of the hippocampal formation and anterior temporal lobe: validation studies. Radiology 1990;176:205–9.

17. Cendes F, Leproux F, Melanson D, et al. MRI of amygdala and hippocampus in temporal lobe epilepsy. J Comput Assist Tomogr 1993;17:206–10.

18. Cook MJ, Fish DR, Shorvon SD, et al. Hippocampal volumetric and morphometric studies in frontal and temporal lobe epilepsy. Brain 1992;115:1001–15.

19. Cendes F, Andermann F, Gloor P, et al. MRI volumetric measurement of amygdala and hippocampus in temporal lobe epilepsy. Neurology 1993; 43:719–25.

20. Ashtari M, Barr WB, Schaul N, et al. Three-dimensional fast low-angle shot imaging and computerized volume measurement of the hippocampus in patients with chronic epilepsy of the temporal lobe. AJNR Am J Neuroradiol 1991;12:941–7.

21. Lencz T, McCarthy G, Bronen RA, et al. Quantitative magnetic resonance imaging in temporal lobe epilepsy: relationship to neuropathology and neuropsychological function. Ann Neurol 1992;31:629–37.

22. Bhatia S, Bookheimer SY, Gaillard WD, et al. Measurement of whole temporal lobe and hippocampus for MR volumetry: normative data. Neurology 1993;43:2006–10.

23. Weis S, Haug H, Holoubek B, et al. The cerebral dominances: quantitative morphology of the human cerebral cortex. Int J Neurosci 1989;47:165–8.

24. Spencer SS, McCarthy G, Spencer DD. Diagnosis of medial temporal lobe seizure onset: relative specificity and sensitivity of quantitative MRI. Neurology 1993;43:2117–24.

25. Cascino GD, Jack CR Jr, Parisi JE, et al. Magnetic resonance imaging-based volume studies in temporal lobe epilepsy: pathological correlations. Ann Neurol 1991;30:31–6.

26. Sass KJ, Spencer DD, Kim JH, et al. Verbal memory impairment correlates with hippocampal pyramidal cell density. Neurology 1990;40:1694–7.

27. Trenerry MR, Jack CR Jr, Ivnik RJ, et al. MRI hippocampal volumes and memory function before and after temporal lobectomy. Neurology 1993;43:1800–5.

28. Trenerry MR, Jack CR Jr, Sharbrough FW, et al. Quantitative MRI hippocampal volumes: association with onset and duration of epilepsy, and febrile convulsions in temporal lobectomy patients. Epilepsy Res 1993;15:247–52.

29. Cendes F, Andermann F, Dubeau F, et al. Early childhood prolonged febrile convulsions, atrophy and sclerosis of mesial structures, and temporal lobe epilepsy: an MRI volumetric study. Neurology 1993;43:1083–7.

30. Cendes F, Andermann F, Gloor P, et al. Atrophy of mesial structures in patients with temporal lobe epilepsy: cause or consequence of repeated seizures? Ann Neurol 1993;34:795–801.

31. Jack CR Jr, Sharbrough FW, Cascino GD, et al. Magnetic resonance image-based hippocampal volumetry: correlation with outcome after temporal lobectomy. Ann Neurol 1992;31:138–46.

32. Kuzniecky R, Burgard S, Faught E, et al. Predictive value of magnetic resonance imaging in temporal lobe epilepsy surgery. Arch Neurol 1993;50:65–9.

33. Garcia PA, Laxer KD, Barbaro NM, et al. Prognostic value of qualitative magnetic resonance imaging hippocampal abnormalities in patients undergoing temporal lobectomy for medically refractory seizures. Epilepsia 1994;35:520–4.

34. Cascino GD, Jack CR Jr, Parisi JE, et al. MRI in the presurgical evaluation of patients with frontal lobe epilepsy and children with temporal lobe epilepsy: pathologic correlation and prognostic importance. Epilepsy Res 1992;11:51–9.

35. Cascino GD, Sharbrough FW, Jack CR Jr, et al. Acute depth electrode investigations in temporal lobe epilepsy: correlation with magnetic-resonance-imaging-based volume studies and pathology. J Epilepsy 1992;5:49–54.

36. Seab JP, Jagust WJ, Wong ST, et al. Quantitative NMR measurements of hippocampal atrophy in Alzheimer's disease. Magn Reson Med 1988;8:200–8.

37. Kesslak JP, Nalcioglu O, Cotman CW. Quantification of magnetic resonance scans for hippocampal and parahippocampal atrophy in Alzheimer's disease. Neurology 1991;41:51–4.

38. Jack CR Jr, Petersen RC, O'Brien PC, et al. MR-based hippocampal volumetry in the diagnosis of Alzheimer's disease. Neurology 1992;42:183–8.

39. Squire LR, Amaral DG, Press GA. Magnetic resonance imaging of the hippocampal formation and mammillary nuclei distinguish medial temporal lobe and diencephalic amnesia. J Neurosci 1990;10:3106–17.

40. Suddath RL, Christison GW, Torrey EF, et al. Anatomical abnormalities in the brains of monozygotic twins discordant for schizophrenia. N Engl J Med 1990;322:789–94.

41. Bogerts B, Lieberman JA, Ashtari M, et al. Hippocampus-amygdala volumes and psychopathology in chronic schizophrenia. Biol Psychiatry 1993;33:236–46.

Postoperative Imaging

*Neil D. Kitchen, Louis Lemieux,
and David R. Fish*

Neuroradiology, especially magnetic resonance imaging (MRI), is now widely recognized to be of paramount importance in the preoperative assessment of patients with medically intractable epilepsy, and in this sense, epilepsy surgery is becoming much more "image-guided." Until recently, little attention has been given to the use of postoperative imaging. Consequently, the anatomical results of surgical procedures guided in large part by imaging have not been assessed by imaging, resulting in a significant loss of information about the actual procedure performed. Precise delineation of the extent of the surgical resection is fundamental to the following issues:

1. Quality control of surgical practice through the comparison of planned and actual resections.[1]
2. The identification of structural reasons that may account for individual surgical failures.[2] The likelihood of a good outcome postoperatively depends mostly on the nature of the underlying abnormality and the extent of its removal.[2] Potential structural reasons for surgical failures are inadequate resection of the primary pathologic substrate (Figure 7-1), contralateral hippocampal sclerosis (bitemporal disease), hippocampal sclerosis associated with nonresected adjacent or distant foreign tissue lesions (Figure 7-2), and multiple foreign tissue lesions or postoperative gliosis (Figure 7-3). Cases with nonresectable abnormalities present difficult management issues[3] but are becoming increasingly recognized. For example, Raymond et al.[4] documented MRI-determined evidence of extrahippocampal cortical dysplasia in 15 of 100 patients with hippocampal sclerosis.

3. The prognostic significance of the extent of resection of the lesion and surrounding brain in relation to postoperative outcome. In temporal lobe resections, specific consideration can be given separately to different subcompartments (hippocampal formation, entorhinal cortex, parahippocampal gyrus, amygdala, lateral cortex), although nonresected cortex nevertheless may sometimes be functionally disconnected. In addition, hippocampal sclerosis is a heterogeneous condition. The extent of the atrophy varies according to the cause. Patients with a history of a prolonged childhood febrile seizure may have atrophy affecting the whole length of the hippocampus, whereas in other patients it may be focal, usually affecting the anterior segment.[5]

4. The prognostic significance of presurgical tests in relation to the actual operation performed rather than to the planned resection.

5. The precise anatomical substrate of changes in brain function, such as specific neuropsychometric deficits after limited resections. This is particularly important in assessing deficits after temporal lobe surgery when the volume of mesial resection may be quite variable.

6. The integration of research data from different surgical centers (currently limited by uncertainty about

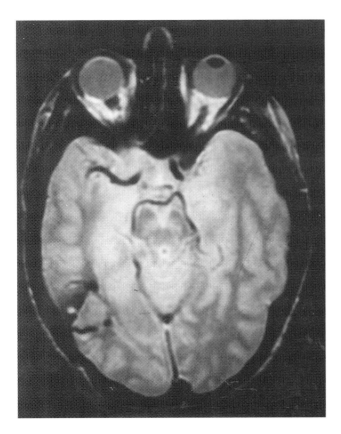

Figure 7-1. Postoperative volumetric magnetic resonance image showing only partial resection of a large vascular malformation, with remaining hemosiderin-stained surrounding gliosis.

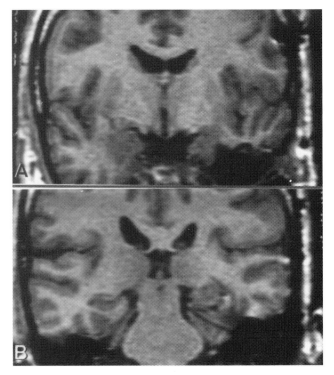

Figure 7-2. Postoperative volumetric magnetic resonance image. A. Anterior temporal coronal slice showing resection cavity (hippocampal sclerosis was confirmed histologically). B. Posterior temporal coronal slice showing an independent mesial lesion with features of a dysembryoplastic tumor.

the comparability of resections performed by different surgeons).

7. With the use of serial scans, the occurrence and effect of secondary degenerative changes can be studied, with particular reference to the "running down" phenomenon.

Traditionally, the extent of a neurosurgical procedure has been described by one or more of the following: the surgeon's visual assessment, intraoperative linear measurements, and postoperative photographs. These methods provide a very restricted view of the surgical field and relatively crude information. Also, they may be difficult to interpret because of problems of orientation. Nevertheless, broad statements may be possible. For example, Bengzon et al.[6] reported that complete rather than partial hippocampal resections were more often associated with postoperative seizure control. Alternative techniques have included the linear measurement or weight of the resected specimen.[7] These techniques do not include material removed by suction and do not provide information about different anatomical compartments. However, Smith et al.[8] reported a good correlation

between the linear measurement of the fresh hippocampal specimen and postoperative seizure control. This would be corroborated by the success of second operations involving extension of the mesial excision in patients whose seizures were not controlled by an initially limited temporal lobe resection.[9]

Recognizing the importance of the extent of resection in epilepsy surgery, Penfield and Jasper[10] and Rasmussen[11] both described the use of tantalum clips placed around the edges of cortical resections in conjunction with postoperative plain film radiography to supplement the operative record. Subsequently, postoperative computed tomography (CT) was used to demonstrate the operative cavity. However, this fails to provide the necessary anatomical detail for accurately delineating the extent of mesial temporal resections and is often influenced by artifact (Figure 7-4).

Several groups have used semiquantitative postoperative MRI techniques to estimate the extent of hippocampal or temporal neocortical resections.[12–17] Awad et al.[14] divided the temporal lobe into five coronal regions based on 1-cm-thick T_1-weighted images and subdivided each of these into quadrants, thus describing 20 compartments. Each compartment was scored as "0" (no resection), "1" (partial resection), or "2" (complete resection). They demonstrated that (1) the

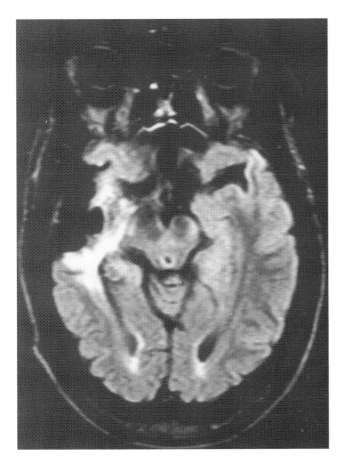

FIGURE 7-3. Postoperative fluid-attenuated inversion recovery (FLAIR) magnetic resonance image showing extensive signal change posterior to the margin of the resection.

volume of resection varied considerably among patients, even when a standard procedure was attempted; (2) the surgical record from visual inspection consistently overestimated the extent of the resection that had been performed; and (3) overall, the extent of inferolateral and basal resection correlated with the probability of a good outcome. Siegel et al.[17] used 3- to 5-mm-thick slices obtained in three planes through the operative site after selective amygdalohippocampal resections. They estimated the volume of hippocampal resection with "a best-fitting approximation model of a truncated cone." Again, larger resections were more likely to be associated with a good outcome, although more detailed analysis only revealed a significant effect for the proportion of the parahippocampal gyrus that was resected.

MRI methodology at the National Hospital for Neurology and Neurosurgery[18,19] has been developed to routinely obtain matched preoperative and postoperative volumetric MRI in epilepsy surgery cases using the following identical image variables: currently, a 1.5-Tesla Signa Unit (GE Medical Systems; Milwaukee, WI) is used with a 24-cm field of view. The volumetric sequence is performed in the coronal plane using a T_1-weighted spoiled echo gradient technique. Contiguous 1.5-mm-thin slices are thus obtained of the whole brain with a 35/5/1 (TR/TE/NEX) pulse sequence, flip angle 35°, and a matrix size of 256 × 128. These provide excellent anatomical detail, can be reformatted in any plane, and provide sufficient data to obtain reliable volumetric assessments of even partial hippocampal resections, according to the Cavilieri principle.[18]

FIGURE 7-4. Postoperative computed tomographic scan. Note failure of the scan to demonstrate adequately mesial temporal anatomy; also, note degradation by artifact. (*L*) left, (*R*) right.

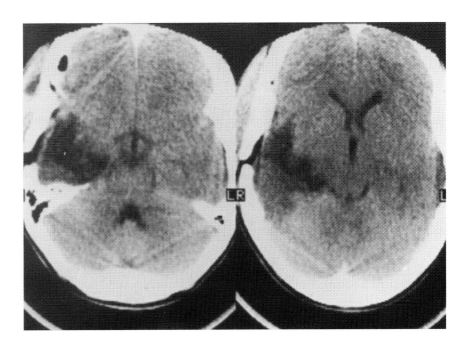

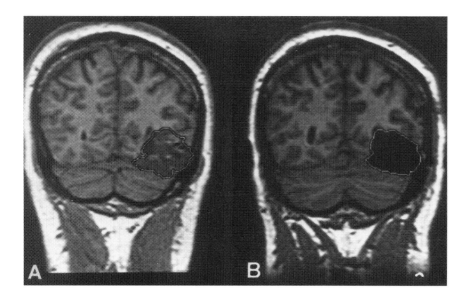

FIGURE 7-5. A. Preoperative magnetic resonance image showing a large tumor, histologically confirmed to be a dysembryoplastic neuroepithelial tumor, outlined by trackerball technique (calculated volume of lesion, 27,900 mm^3). B. Postoperative magnetic resonance image of same patient after planned total lesionectomy, with resection margin outlined by trackerball technique (volume of cavity, 28,600 mm^3).

Currently, preoperative volumetric information and surgical resection volumes are measured by manually outlining the regions of interest with a trackerball-driven cursor (Figure 7-5). Preoperatively, we apply these techniques to the hippocampi and structural lesions and postoperatively to the resection and any residual abnormality (that is, nonresected structural lesions or hippocampal remnant). Comparison of these data sets may provide quantitative information about the extent of resection. Qualitative three-dimensionally reconstructed views may help to display the site of resection (Figure 7-6), but quantitative measures are calculated from the two-dimensional images from the volumetric sequence.

There are three key aspects of validation:

1. Preoperative data set. Preoperative volumetric imaging has been well validated.[18] The main limitation is the difficulty in measuring structures such as the hippocampus which have a complex geometry and subtle borders, sometimes disrupted by the primary lesion. Therefore, considerable training and practice are often required to obtain reliable data.
2. Postoperative data set. In contrast to preoperative data, identification of the resection cavity is usually obvious because it is filled with cerebrospinal fluid density signal and is well demarcated from the surrounding brain (see Figure 7-5). It is relatively easy to follow the curvature of the brain at the superficial cortical margin, although artifact from underlying air cells or hemostatic clips may occasionally be a problem.
3. Correlation of the volume of the residual defect with the extent of the resection performed at the time of operation.

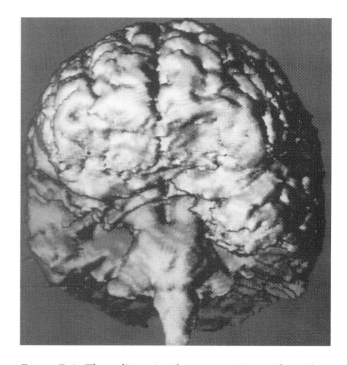

FIGURE 7-6. Three-dimensional reconstruction, performed on an Allegro workstation (ISG Technologies; Toronto, Ontario, Canada), of temporal lobe resection.

If the intracranial contents react to the surgical procedure by permanently swelling, contracting, or shifting, this correlation will be impaired. Such considerations are the main limitation in the interpretation of postoperative images. A priori, these exclude quantitative analysis in the following situations: extrinsic tumors such as meningiomas, high-grade intrinsic tumors, other lesions with mass effect or indistinct margins, and patients who have received radiotherapy. However, in epilepsy work, the common

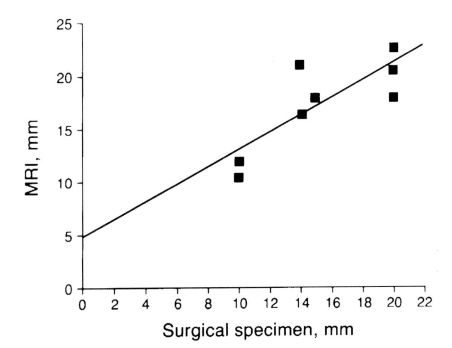

FIGURE 7-7. Correlation between hippocampal resection lengths determined from fresh (surgical) specimen and postoperative magnetic resonance imaging (MRI).

abnormalities are foreign tissue lesions that are static, often with distinct margins, such as cavernomas, hamartomas, or other indolent tumors as well as hippocampal sclerosis.

Imaging within the first 3 months postoperatively may be associated with acute residual changes. However, in the setting of an indolent lesion, subsequent serial volumetric assessments in 12 patients scanned up to 18 months postoperatively revealed stable MRI-defined resection volumes (within 10%). Major shifts of the intracranial contents are readily excluded by inspection and comparison of anatomical landmarks on preoperative and postoperative imaging. We have not found these shifts to be a significant problem with hippocampal resections and small indolent lesions.

Even with stability over time and corroboration by inspection of anatomical landmarks, verification of the MRI-derived measurements of resection magnitude is by no means trivial. Comparison with en bloc surgical specimens would be ideal, but resections often are piecemeal and some tissue is not available because of suction dissection. Validation of MRI-defined length of hippocampal resection has been obtained by comparison with the fresh surgical specimen in eight cases: these showed a good correlation (correlation coefficient, 0.81; $P < 0.01$), and in seven of the eight cases, these measurements were within 3 mm (Figure 7-7).[20] The MRI-determined length of hippocampal resection tends to be slightly greater than that of the fresh specimen, possibly reflecting the loss of some tissue by suction dissection. Surgically straightforward total lesionectomies in cases of indolent tumors with visually obvious lines of demarcation, in which no attempt was made to remove adjacent brain, allow indi-

rect corroboration. In such cases, the MRI-defined preoperative lesion volume and the postresection defect volume are often similar (Figure 7-5 and 7-8), suggesting little effect on the surrounding brain at 3 months. Further comparison with fresh en bloc lesions using volume displacement techniques will provide additional assessment of reliability in different clinical situations.

Methodological advances will include better coregistration in appropriate cases and further sequences to identify additional postoperative changes. Currently, such coregistration is performed manually by matching the coronal slices in each series as they relate to the posterior hippocampal limit (coronal slice in which the fornix is maximum), which is a common landmark in both series. However, registration of the preoperative and postoperative volume scans can be improved with the surface-matching module in ANALYZE 6.2 (Mayo Foundation; Rochester, MN). The two data sets can be registered automatically to within 2 mm on the basis of the surface of the skin or the surface of the cortex. The difference between the preoperative and postoperative images can then be calculated by subtracting these two volumetric data sets, although thresholding may be necessary to remove any artifact due to the imperfect registration. The presumed resection volume may then be calculated by voxel counting (Figure 7-9).

Postoperative gliosis around the surgical margin may be difficult to identify on T_2-weighted images due to artifact from the cerebrospinal fluid-filled resection cavity. This may be overcome by using a spin density (first echo) image or a fluid-attenuated inversion recovery (FLAIR) sequence[21,22] (see Figure 7-3).

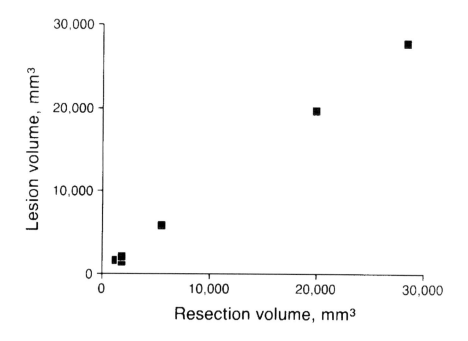

FIGURE 7-8. Correlation between magnetic resonance imaging–calculated preoperative lesion volumes and postoperative resection cavity volumes in patients with indolent, surgically accessible lesions undergoing planned total lesionectomies. Note that the correlation between the two measures is good. In all cases, the resection volume was slightly larger than the lesion volume; this could reflect suction dissection.

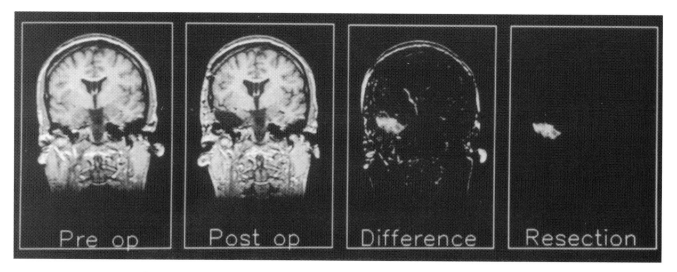

FIGURE 7-9. Preoperative (*Pre op*) and postoperative (*Post op*) volume-rendered magnetic resonance imaging scans coregistered with ANALYZE demonstrate the subtraction image (*Difference*) representing the resected tissue (*Resection*).

To date, we have obtained 125 postoperative volumetric MRI determinations on 103 patients after epilepsy surgery (54 cases of hippocampal sclerosis and 56 lesional cases, including 7 patients with both abnormalities) and have matched preoperative and postoperative MRI determinations for 58 of these subjects.

FINDINGS IN HIPPOCAMPAL SCLEROSIS

At the National Hospital for Neurology and Neurosurgery, several different operations are performed for temporal lobe epilepsy, ranging from selective stereotaxic amygdalohippocampectomy to standard or extended temporal lobectomy, according to the overall clinical, electroencephalographic, and neuroimaging findings. Consequently, the postoperative MRI-defined resection cavities have ranged from 2,600 mm³ (selective stereotaxic amygdalohippocampectomy) to 51,600 mm³ (extended temporal lobectomy). Cases with both preoperative and postoperative matched imaging allow a range of measures of the resections to be derived (Table 7-1; Figures 7-10 through 7-12).

Because of the differences in technique among surgeons and the different aims of the operation in a particular patient, the variability in volume of postoperative

TABLE 7-1.   Measurements Made with Magnetic Resonance Imaging in 10 Cases of Surgically Treated Temporal Lobe Epilepsy Due to Hippocampal Sclerosis

| | Hippocampal formation | | | | | | | Lateral resection | | | |
Case	Volume, mm³	Length, mm	Resection volume, mm³	%	Resection length, mm	%	Specimen length, mm	Volume, mm³	Length 1, * mm	Length 2, * mm	Total resection volume, mm³
1	1,735	25.5	1,665	96	22.5	88	20	22,025	44	53	23,690
2	2,000	31.5	1,280	64	16.5	52	14	12,465	19	29	13,745
3	1,790	30.0	680	38	10.5	35	10	10,030	25	27	10,710
4	2,030	34.5	1,440	71	20.5	59	ND	21,540	38	44	22,980
5	1,530	25.5	1,330	85	21.0	82	14	18,250	42	52	19,550
6	1,795	31.5	1,365	76	20.5	65	20	4,790	41	50	6,155
7	1,525	25.5	1,160	76	18.0	71	15	17,240	26	31	18,400
8	1,520	34.5	1,170	77	18.0	52	20	18,715	36	39	19,885
9	4,130	37.5	785	19	9.0	24	ND	4,955	21	21	5,740
10	2,475	30.0	1,430	58	12.0	40	10	10,450	26	38	11,880

ND, not determined.

*Linear measures 1 and 2 were taken from the console and are the distances from the lateral and medial margins, respectively, of the resection to the temporal pole.

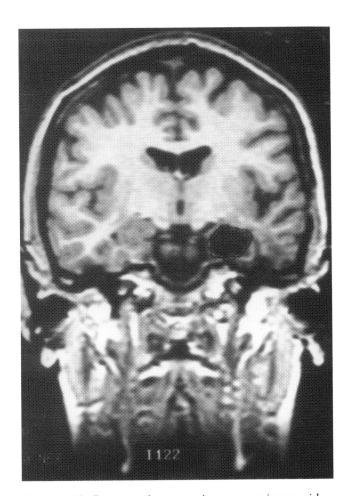

FIGURE 7-10. Postoperative magnetic resonance image with trackerball-driven delineation of the resection margin after hippocampal resection.

resection cavities is not surprising. This variability provides interesting data in terms of postoperative seizure control and psychometric changes (see below).

The follow-up period has been short (mean, 17 months), and 46 of 54 patients with temporal lobe epilepsy have become seizure-free. At this stage, we have identified some patients who are seizure-free despite incomplete resection of the atrophied hippocampus. However, firm conclusions about the optimum extent of resection will require a longer follow-up period and a larger number of failures: currently, most of our failures had other preoperatively identified poor prognostic features (for example, minimal or absent hippocampal volume loss, seizures of unknown cause, or dual pathology).

Findings in Lesional Epilepsy

In lesional epilepsy, both the pathologic nature of the surgical specimen and the completeness of resection as judged by postoperative MRI findings appear to be the key determinants of seizure outcome.[2,23] To date, we have studied 37 cases (mean follow-up period, 23.6 months). Lesion resections were categorized as "partial" or "complete," and outcome as either "seizure-free" or "persistent seizures." The lesions consisted of dysembryoplastic neuroepithelial tumors (12 cases), low-grade glioma (9 cases), cavernoma (10 cases), localized cortical dysgenesis (5 cases), and ganglioglioma (1 case). The percentage of patients in each group that became seizure-free were: dysembryoplastic neuroepithelial tumors, 75%; cavernoma, 70%; low-grade glioma, 40%; ganglioglioma, 100%; and localized cortical dysgenesis, 20%.

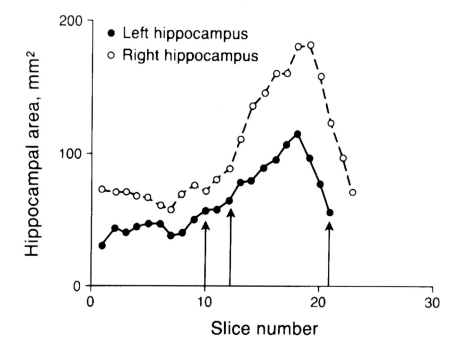

FIGURE 7-11. Preoperative volumetric analysis of case shown in Figure 7-10. The graph shows the hippocampal surface area in each 1.5-mm-thick slice from posterior (slice 1) to anterior (slice 30). The hippocampus on the left is diffusely smaller than the one on the right. *Arrows* at slices 10 and 21 indicate the extent of the resection as judged by postoperative magnetic resonance imaging (the postoperative coronal slice shown in Figure 7-10 corresponds to slice 12 [*middle arrow*]). The posterior atrophic hippocampus (slices 1 to 9) was not resected.

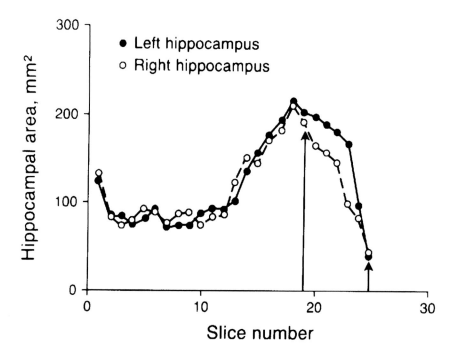

FIGURE 7-12. Preoperative volumetric magnetic resonance imaging showed focal hippocampal atrophy (slices 18 to 25) in a patient who underwent selective resection. The *arrows* delineate the extent of the hippocampal resection (that is, all the atrophic hippocampus removed, the symmetric posterior portion has been left in situ), as determined from postoperative imaging.

Of interest, in the dysembryoplastic neuroepithelial tumors and cavernoma groups, some patients (two and three, respectively) became seizure-free without complete resection. In contrast, in the low-grade glioma group, all the five patients with only partial resection had persistent seizures, whereas all four with complete resection were seizure-free. Completeness of resection may be crucially important for seizure control in patients with low-grade glioma but not always so in patients with cavernomas or dysembryoplastic neuroepithelial tumors. This may have implications for surgical practice.

More detailed studies have been possible in those cases with matched preoperative and postoperative MRI studies (Table 7-2; Figure 7-13). It may be possible to

TABLE 7-2.   Measurements Made with Magnetic Resonance Imaging After Lesional Surgery*†

| Case | Lesion volume | | | Total resection volume, mm³ | Brain resection volume, mm³ |
	Preoperative, mm³	Postoperative, mm³	% resected		
1	640	0	100	9,640	9,000
2	5,480	0	100	5,500	20
3	1,740	0	100	1,885	145
4	27,845	0	100	28,595	750
5	800	0	100	8,200	7,400
6‡	9,150	2,070	77	8,275	1,195
7	275	0	100	440	165
8‡	1,125	195	83	2,440	1,510
9	1,965	0	100	22,120	20,155
10	19,720	0	100	23,105	3,385
11	6,370	6,370	0	0	0
12‡	3,050	380	87	2,920	250
13	1,090	0	100	2,810	1,720

*The detailed information in the Table is possible only with the use of identical preoperative and postoperative volumetric magnetic resonance imaging scans.

†Various types of resective operations were used, except in case 11, in which nonresective Morrell's procedure was performed.

‡Lesion was removed only partially.

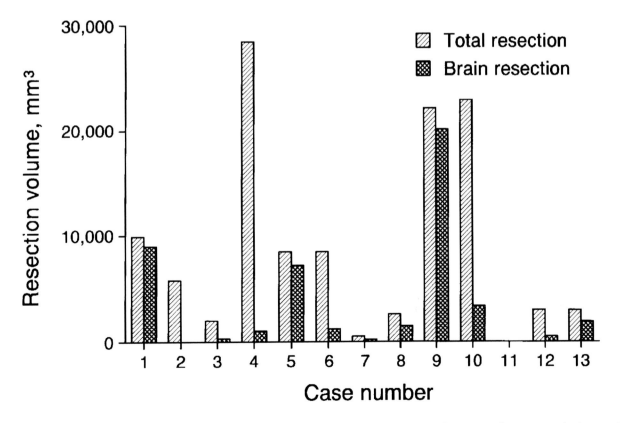

FIGURE 7-13.   The volume of surrounding brain tissue resected varies with the surgical technique used. For example, in case 4, a large, readily accessible lesion was resected with only minimal resection of surrounding brain.

make approximate estimations of the proportion of the lesion and the amount of surrounding brain that have been removed in certain static lesions.

PSYCHOMETRIC DATA

Postoperative MRI studies have enabled us to examine several issues relating to neuropsychologic outcome after epilepsy surgery.[24,25] Amygdalohippocampectomy, performed as a stereotaxic procedure, is reserved in our practice for those patients in whom there is concern about memory function postoperatively. We have studied six patients who have had this operation, with resection volumes ranging from 2,600 mm^3 to 7,500 mm^3. Even with such small resections, we found declines in test scores appropriate to the side of operation. We also found that there was not a marked protective effect on verbal memory, although this clearly was a highly selected group of patients. A larger group of 24 patients[24] who received surgical treatment for temporal lobe epilepsy due to various causes have also been studied in this context. All patients underwent preoperative and postoperative neuropsychometric testing. Postoperative MRI scans were used to estimate the extent of the resection and, in particular, to divide patients into those with solely neocortical resection (lesionectomy) and those with resection that included the mesiobasal structures. Preliminary findings indicate that completely sparing the mesiobasal structures could still be associated with significant psychometric deficits, that is, local lesionectomy procedures were not necessarily protective neuropsychologically and could result in changes comparable to those seen with anterior temporal lobectomies. However, the extent of resection, surgical pathologic findings, and side of operation all appeared to interact to give a more accurate prediction of the neuropsychologic outcome for individual patients.

CONCLUSIONS

The extent of resections is difficult to judge by visual inspection of the operative field and such estimates show considerable variation. Postoperative MRI study provides important data for individual patient management and research purposes. Matched preoperative and postoperative imaging techniques are essential, with volumetric data allowing the reconstruction of thin contiguous slices through the whole brain. In certain circumstances, quantitative data can be obtained about the extent of resection as well as about the identification of additional lesions or postoperative structural changes. Future work will concentrate on additional sequences to further characterize these changes and to delineate the range of abnormalities in which quantitative resection volumes can be investigated reliably with postoperative imaging.

REFERENCES

1. Kitchen ND, Cook MJ, Shorvon SD, et al. Image guided audit of surgery for temporal lobe epilepsy. J Neurol Neurosurg Psychiatry 1994;57:1221–7.

2. Cascino GD, Boon PAJM, Fish DR. Surgically remediable lesional syndromes. In: Engel J Jr, ed. Surgical treatment of the epilepsies. 2nd ed. New York: Raven Press, 1993:77–86.

3. Fish D, Andermann F, Olivier A. Complex partial seizures and small posterior temporal or extratemporal structural lesions: surgical management. Neurology 1991;41:1781–4.

4. Raymond AA, Sisodiya S, Cook M, et al. The frequency of cortical dysplasia in patients with hippocampal sclerosis. Neurology (in press).

5. Kuks JBM, Cook MJ, Fish DR, et al. Hippocampal sclerosis in epilepsy and childhood febrile seizures. Lancet 1993;342:1391–4.

6. Bengzon AR, Rasmussen T, Gloor P, et al. Prognostic factors in the surgical treatment of temporal lobe epileptics. Neurology 1968;18:717–31.

7. McMillan TM, Powell GE, Janota I, et al. Relationships between neuropathology and cognitive functioning in temporal lobectomy patients. J Neurol Neurosurg Psychiatry 1987;50:167–76.

8. Smith JR, King DW, Park Y, et al. Relationship of age and extent of hippocampal resection to the outcome of anterior temporal lobectomy. Epilepsia 1993;34 Suppl 6:28.

9. Tanaka T, Yonemasu Y, Olivier A, et al. Clinical analysis of reoperation in cases of complex partial seizures. No Shinkei Geka 1989;17:933–7.

10. Penfield W, Jasper H. Epilepsy and the functional anatomy of the human brain. Boston: Little, Brown and Company, 1954.

11. Rasmussen T. Cortical resection in the treatment of focal epilepsy. Adv Neurol 1975;8:139–54.

12. Jack CR Jr, Sharbrough FW, Marsh WR. Use of MR imaging for quantitative evaluation of resection for temporal lobe epilepsy. Radiology 1988; 169:463–8.

13. Katz A, Awad IA, Kong AK, et al. Extent of resection in temporal lobectomy for epilepsy. II. Memory changes and neurologic complications. Epilepsia 1989;30:763–71.

14. Awad IA, Katz A, Hahn JF, et al. Extent of resection in temporal lobectomy for epilepsy. I. Interobserver analysis and correlation with seizure outcome. Epilepsia 1989;30:756–62.

15. Awad IA, Rosenfeld J, Ahl J, et al. Intractable epilepsy and structural lesions of the brain: mapping, resection strategies, and seizure outcome. Epilepsia 1991;32:179–86.

16. Nayel MH, Awad IA, Luders H. Extent of mesiobasal resection determines outcome after temporal

lobectomy for intractable complex partial seizures. Neurosurgery 1991;29:55–60.

17. Siegel AM, Wieser HG, Wichmann W, et al. Relationships between MR-imaged total amount of tissue removed, resection scores of specific mediobasal limbic subcompartments and clinical outcome following selective amygdalohippocampectomy. Epilepsy Res 1990;6:56–65.

18. Cook MJ, Fish DR, Shorvon SD, et al. Hippocampal volumetric and morphometric studies in frontal and temporal lobe epilepsy. Brain 1992;115:1001–15.

19. Kitchen ND, Thomas DGT, Shorvon SD, et al. Volumetric analysis of epilepsy surgery resections using high resolution magnetic imaging—technical report. Br J Neurosurg 1993;7:651–6.

20. Kitchen ND, Thomas DGT, Fish DR, et al. Volumetric MRI to assess extent of resection in temporal lobe epilepsy. Epilepsia 1993;34 Suppl 6:105.

21. De Coene B, Hajnal JV, Gatehouse P, et al. MR of the brain using fluid-attentuated inversion recovery (FLAIR) pulse sequences. AJNR Am J Neuroradiol 1992;13:1555–64.

22. Bergin PS, Fish DR, Shorvon SD, et al. FLAIR imaging in partial epilepsy: improving the yield of MRI. Epilepsia 1993;34 Suppl 6:121.

23. Kitchen ND, Thomas DGT, Harkness W, et al. Influence of pathology on seizure outcome in lesional epilepsy surgery. Epilepsia 1993;34 Suppl 6:105.

24. Kitchen ND, Thompson PJ, Fish DR, et al. Neuropsychological sequelae after temporal neocortical lesionectomy: comparison with temporal lobectomy. Epilepsia 1993;34 Suppl 6:71.

25. Kitchen ND, Thomas DG, Thompson PJ, et al. Open stereotactic amygdalohippocampectomy—clinical, psychometric, and MRI follow-up. Acta Neurochir (Wien) 1993;123:33–8.

Proton Magnetic Resonance Spectroscopy in Epilepsy

Alan Connelly

The aim of this chapter is to provide an understanding of the role of proton magnetic resonance spectroscopy (^{1}H MRS) in the study of epilepsy. So that the strengths and limitations of this technique can be appreciated by those not familiar with spectroscopy, the initial section describes some of the principles underlying the acquisition of in vivo data and the type of biochemical information that may be derived from these data. Next, the information that has been obtained from the study of patients with epilepsy is discussed with regard to the neurobiology of the condition and the role of ^{1}H MRS in clinical investigation and management.

IN VIVO MAGNETIC RESONANCE SPECTROSCOPY: BASIC PRINCIPLES

Nuclear magnetic resonance (NMR) began as a spectroscopic technique, and in this form, it has been one of the most powerful analytical tools (particularly in chemistry) for several decades. In medicine, many people have become familiar with NMR through the more recent development of magnetic resonance imaging (MRI). The fundamental theory is the same for both techniques, because they each depend on the same nuclear properties and interactions. However, some important differences in practice arise from the fact that the primary aim of NMR is to obtain chemical information and that of

the MRI is to provide spatial information. The following discussion attempts to outline the basis for MRS and to describe the incorporation of imaging principles for the purpose of spatial localization.

Chemical Shift

In NMR, the resonance frequency of a nucleus is linearly proportional to the magnetic field strength experienced by that nucleus. In practice, this is dominated by the applied static magnetic field, which in most in vivo MRS studies in humans is 1.5 T or greater. The application of additional linear magnetic field gradients (that is, magnetic fields whose strength varies with spatial position) can be used to make the total magnetic field experienced by a collection of nuclei dependent on their position within such a field. This in turn means that their resonance frequencies are spatially dependent. In this manner, in imaging, frequency is used to provide spatial information.

In the absence of such externally applied gradient fields, similar nuclei do not necessarily experience the same field strength, even in a homogeneously applied field. This is because the nuclei are surrounded by electrons that also experience the applied magnetic field, causing them to circulate and, in turn, to produce a second magnetic field in the direction opposite to the applied field. Therefore, the magnetic field actually experienced by a nucleus is a combination of (1) the applied field and (2) the field produced by the surrounding electrons. As a result, the *effective* field at a nucleus (and, thus, the resonance frequency of that nucleus, because this is dependent on the field experienced by the nucleus) is different in different chemical environments. This effect is known as the "chemical shift," and the magnitude of the frequency shift is proportional to the applied field strength. Therefore, in spectroscopy, frequency is used to provide chemical information by means of this chemical shift.

For example, if we consider the NMR spectrum from a substance such as acetic acid, the hydrogen nuclei in the methyl group ($-CH_3$) give a separate NMR signal from the hydrogen of the carboxyl group (–COOH). The separation in this case would be about 10.5 parts per million. (Note that chemical shifts are conventionally quoted in terms of the dimensionless unit, parts per million [ppm], to allow direct comparison at different field strengths, because the separation in frequency terms is dependent on the applied field strength. For example, the resonance frequency of ^1H at 1.5 T is about 63 MHz, but at 1 T, it is about 42 MHz. A chemical shift difference between two hydrogen nuclei that was 63 Hz at 1.5 T would become 42 Hz at 1 T, but it would be 1 ppm in both cases.) The amplitude of the signal obtained from the nuclei at a particular site within a molecule is proportional to the number of equivalent nuclei at such a site. In the example given above, the signal obtained from the CH_3 group would be three times the intensity of that from the single ^1H in the COOH group. Such signals are usually displayed as a plot or graph of signal intensity against frequency in which the resonance signals appear as peaks against a flat baseline (see Figures 8-1 and 8-2 for examples of in vivo spectra).

The signal intensity of a spectral peak is indicated by the area under the peak (that is, the integral of the peak) rather than the height of the peak. The latter is dependent on the linewidth, which in turn is determined by the magnetic field homogeneity over the region from which signal is obtained and the T_2 relaxation time of the protons giving rise to the signal. The higher the field homogeneity, the narrower the linewidth (down to the limit referred to as the "natural linewidth" as determined by T_2).

The need frequently to distinguish between closely adjacent resonance lines in proton spectroscopy results in a major difference in the hardware specification for MRI and MRS. To decrease the overlap between resonances, it is essential that the MRS linewidths are minimized by having very high field homogeneity, necessitating a considerable improvement with respect to the requirements for MRI. A prerequisite for achieving such homogeneity is the facility to adjust the currents running in a set of coils known as the shim coils, which

lie on a cylindrical former inside the magnet bore, and which provide fine tuning of the field homogeneity. The process of optimization of these currents is referred to as "shimming" the magnet and must be carried out during each investigation on the particular local volume of interest to achieve good spectral quality. (Of particular relevance to this present work is that shimming is unusually difficult in the temporal lobe region because of large local variations in magnetic susceptibility.) By decreasing the linewidth, not only is the spectrum improved in terms of peak resolution but the peak height also increases (because the peak area is unaffected), allowing an improvement in the signal-to-noise ratio (SNR).

It is important to note that NMR is inherently an insensitive technique and, as a result, is limited frequently by SNR considerations. The amount of signal available is crucially dependent on the type of nucleus involved. Not all nuclei are NMR-active; for example, the most abundant isotopes of carbon and oxygen (^{12}C and ^{16}O) are NMR-inactive. Only those nuclei that have non-zero nuclear spin angular momentum give rise to an NMR signal, and these nuclei vary considerably in sensitivity. The nuclei that have been used in a biologic context include ^1H, ^{31}P, ^{13}C, ^{19}F, and ^{23}Na. For reasons given below, the most widely studied nuclei for in vivo spectroscopy are ^1H and ^{31}P.

The intensity of the NMR signal available from a particular type of nucleus depends primarily on the strength of the applied magnetic field (signal to noise is approximately linearly proportional to the field strength for in vivo MRS) and on a property of the nucleus known as the magnetogyric ratio. The larger this constant, the higher the signal from any individual nucleus. Each element (and, in fact, each isotope of a given element) has a different magnetogyric ratio associated with the nucleus. The hydrogen nucleus, which consists of a single proton (hence the term "proton NMR" commonly applied to the study of ^1H), has the highest magnetogyric ratio of all nuclei except for its own non-naturally occurring isotope, tritium. Therefore, the hydrogen nucleus is the most sensitive nucleus for NMR studies.

Another important factor that determines the strength of an NMR signal is the number of nuclei within the field of view of the receiver coil. If hardware considerations (including radiofrequency [RF] coils) are ignored, this is influenced primarily by three factors: (1) the concentration of the substance containing the nuclei concerned, (2) the size of the volume from which signal is acquired, and (3) the natural abundance of the NMR-active isotope of the element of interest.

In studies of chemical preparations, the dependence on factor 1 above frequently can be dealt with by increasing the concentration of the compound of interest. However, in human biologic studies, the concentrations of substances within the body are largely predefined, and, indeed, it most likely is this parameter that we

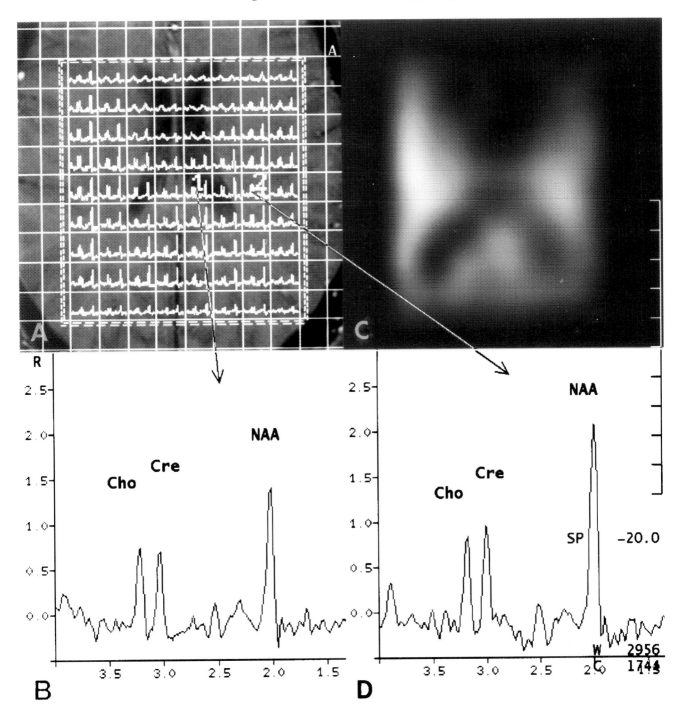

FIGURE 8-1. Example of an ¹H CSI data set showing (A) the large volume of interest (*dotted lines*) divided into smaller voxels (*solid lines*) by phase encoding; spectra obtained from individual voxels (B) (*from voxel labelled 1*) and (D) (*from voxel 2*). The three major peaks are indicated as choline-containing compounds (*Cho*), creatine + phosphocreatine (*Cre*), and N-acetylaspartate (*NAA*). C. The spatial distribution of an individual metabolite displayed as an image or "metabolite map" created by integrating the signal intensity over a particular frequency band within each spectrum (in this case, that around the NAA peak). (Figure courtesy of Dr. R. Sauter, Erlangen, Germany.)

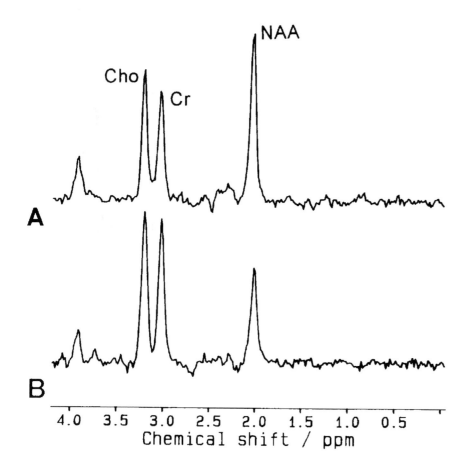

FIGURE 8-2. [1]H spectra obtained independently from $2 \times 2 \times 2$-cm single voxels in the (A) right and (B) left temporal lobes of a child with temporal lobe epilepsy. The spectrum from the left temporal lobe (ipsilateral to the seizure focus) shows a marked reduction in the N-acetyl-aspartate (*NAA*) signal intensity with respect to the right temporal lobe and to control data. (*Cho*) choline-containing compounds, (*Cr*) creatine + phosphocreatine.

would like to determine in disease states. As a consequence, nuclei such as fluorine (^{19}F), which give a relatively large signal per nucleus (fluorine sensitivity is 83% that of hydrogen) but which do not occur in high concentrations in the body, are not usually studied in vivo unless introduced as an external agent.

For a given concentration, the number of nuclei that potentially can contribute to the NMR signal is determined by the size of the volume from which signal is obtained (see below). Therefore, signal strength is linearly related to volume size for a homogeneously distributed substance (with the condition that any increase in the excited volume is within the field of view of the receiver coil).

Some elements that are potentially interesting biologically (and that are present in relatively high concentrations) do not give sufficient signal to be studied routinely in vivo because of the low natural abundance of the NMR-active isotope. For example, carbon is widely distributed throughout the body, but the main isotope of carbon (^{12}C) is NMR-inactive and the NMR-active nucleus (^{13}C) constitutes only 1.1% of natural carbon, resulting in very low sensitivity. As a result, carbon is better suited to the study of particular biochemical mechanisms and turnover rates using externally administered

[13]C-enriched agents than to the study of extensive patient populations. It is possible to obtain information regarding the destination of any ^{13}C labeling while observing ^{1}H signals (that is, with proton sensitivity) by the use of heteronuclear spectral editing techniques,[1,2] but a detailed discussion of such methods is not appropriate here.

Both ^{1}H and ^{31}P are of high natural abundance (99.98% and 100%, respectively), of relatively high sensitivity (although the sensitivity of phosphorus is only 1/15th that of hydrogen, it is still one of the more sensitive nuclei), and are present in sufficiently high concentrations in compounds that are of metabolic interest in vivo. They are also what is known as "spin-1/2 nuclei" (it is not appropriate to this text to discuss spin quantum numbers in detail), and, as a result, both nuclei are capable of generating narrow spectral lines. Together, these characteristics have resulted in the widespread use of these two nuclei for the study of in vivo metabolites. Because of initial technical difficulties with proton spectroscopy (mainly the need to suppress signals from water and lipids), most of the early in vivo MRS studies were performed with the phosphorus nucleus. However, in recent years, it has become possible to acquire high-quality ^{1}H spectra in vivo, which has led to an increase in the number of proton studies, taking advantage of the increased sensitivity available from this nucleus.

Signal-to-Noise Ratio

When an NMR signal is acquired, background RF noise is also acquired, even if all externally generated signals are excluded by housing the scanner in a RF-screened room. The dominant sources of noise in vivo are the RF coil and the patients themselves; the former is due to coil resistance and the latter to the fact that current flow in a conducting sample constitutes an additional resistance.

To detect NMR signals generated by metabolites, it is necessary to distinguish them from background noise. If the signal intensity is insufficient to allow identification of metabolite peaks, the SNR can be improved by time averaging, that is, repeatedly acquiring data under the same conditions. The NMR signal increases linearly with the number of repetitions. However, the noise is random and increases only as the square root of the number of scans. Overall, the SNR increases as the square root of the number of signal averages.

The inefficiency of time averaging as a means of increasing the SNR is a major factor in determining what is practical in vivo. For example, if an acquisition volume is decreased by a factor of 2 in each linear dimension (that is, an eightfold decrease in volume) to increase spatial resolution, the signal amplitude will also decrease by a factor of 8. However, the detected noise will be unaffected by the change in size of the selected volume (because it is generated by the coil and the patient as a whole), resulting in an overall decrease in the SNR by a factor of 8. To recover the original SNR ratio by time averaging, an increase in the experiment time by a factor of 64 would be necessary (that is, number of averages = the square of the desired factor of increase in the SNR = 8^2), which would be prohibitive in all but the most unusual circumstances.

The use of higher field strength magnets is a more efficient (if expensive) way of increasing the SNR. As stated above, the SNR is related approximately linearly to field strength in vivo. The increase at higher fields can be "traded" for time or spatial resolution, as discussed above. Heatherington et al.[3] have demonstrated that it is possible to obtain high-quality localized ^{1}H spectra from the brain at 4.1 T, and they have made use of the improved SNR to obtain remarkably high spatial resolution (nominal voxel size, 0.5 mL; compare results from 1.5-T to 2-T systems below).

In Vivo Magnetic Resonance Spectroscopy–Visible Metabolites

The following brain metabolites are present at sufficiently high concentrations to give usable signal in vivo:

1. For ^{31}P MRS, the metabolites used in epilepsy studies have included adenosine triphosphate (ATP), phosphomonoesters (PME), phosphodiesters (PDE), phosphocreatine (PCr), and inorganic phosphate (Pi). The last of these, Pi, has the useful NMR property of having a chemical shift that is pH-dependent. This is because Pi exists mainly as HPO_4 and H_2PO_4 at neutral pH. The chemical shift of these two species differs by about 2.4 ppm. However, in solution, the rapid exchange between the two causes only a single resonance to be detected, the resonance frequency of which is determined by the relative amounts of each species present. This equilibrium, in turn, depends on the concentration of H^+ ions. Thus, the effective chemical shift of Pi reflects the pH of the local environment. (The use of phosphorus MRS in the study of epilepsy is discussed in Chapter 9.)

2. For ^{1}H MRS, the metabolites that can be detected are determined partly by the conditions used for acquisition. Some molecules, such as gamma-aminobutyric acid (GABA), glutamate, glutamine, and lactate, produce NMR signals that exhibit "spin-spin coupling," which results in multiplet signals that are modulated with time. Thus, the appearance of their resonance lines is very dependent on the acquisition conditions used, in particular, the echo time. Specifically, the in vivo detection of GABA is facilitated by the use of spectral editing techniques.[4]

3. In clinical epilepsy studies, the main signals of interest have been those from N-acetyl groups (believed to be largely from N-acetylaspartate [NAA] 2.01 ppm), creatine + phosphocreatine (Cr, 3.0 ppm), choline-containing compounds (Cho, 3.2 ppm), and lactate (Lac, doublet signal centered at 1.33 ppm). Several lines of evidence, including cell culture studies,[5,6] have indicated that NAA is located primarily in neurons (although a surprising finding is that it is also present in some precursor cells known as "oligodendrocyte-type 2-astrocyte [O-2-A] progenitor cells"). Therefore, a decrease in the NAA signal is frequently interpreted as a loss or dysfunction of neurons. Such a decrease in NAA has been found in many cases in which neuronal loss would be expected clinically, such as in infarcts, tumors, and epilepsy (see below). There remains some doubt as to the proportion of the signal at 2.01 ppm that is attributable to NAA, because studies have shown that the amount of NAA extracted from excised tissue samples is less than the signal measured in vivo would suggest. Nevertheless, it is not unusual for all or almost all of this signal to be lost in circumstances in which severe neuronal depletion occurs. Cr and Cho are found in neurons and glial cells, although cell studies suggest that their concentrations are higher in glial cells.[6]

Volume Localization

The acquisition of spectroscopic data in vivo is of limited use in most studies unless the spatial origin of the signals obtained is known. This implies the need for a method of limiting the extent of the volume from which signal is acquired and for relating this volume to the anatomy of the region being studied.

Initial in vivo MRS studies used the relatively crude method of placing a surface coil directly over the region of interest and relying on the limited field of view of such a coil to provide some degree of localization.[7] Although important data were obtained, this method has many limitations, including an imprecisely defined volume, restriction to relatively superficial structures, and difficulty in relating the volume from which the signal was acquired to the relevant anatomy. Because these drawbacks were widely recognized, many different localization methods were developed. Some of these methods used RF field gradients (for example, as in rotating frame zeugmatography),[8] some were dependent on shaping the static magnetic field (for example, topical magnetic resonance),[9] and others used multiple RF excitation pulses in conjunction with surface coils (for example, as in the use of depth pulses).[10] However, the most successful type of localization methods is that in which amplitude and/or phase-modulated RF pulses are used in conjunction with linear magnetic field gradients. (This is exactly analogous to slice selection in MRI.) Such techniques have great flexibility in terms of positioning and size of volume for signal acquisition, and they are readily combined with imaging methods to provide good anatomical information for volume location. In applying these methods, two distinct approaches have been used:

1. Single voxel techniques in which data are acquired from a single region of interest (usually in the form of a cube on the order of an 8-mL volume for ^{1}H or 60- to 100-mL volume for ^{31}P) before moving to other regions where the process can be repeated.

2. Chemical shift imaging (CSI) (also called "magnetic resonance spectroscopic imaging" [MRSI]). With this method, the equivalent of many volumes can be acquired simultaneously, and the increase in efficiency can be used to obtain smaller voxels (on the order of 1 to 2 mL for ^{1}H or 25 mL for ^{31}P) than by single voxel methods. In practice, a hybrid technique usually is used in which a large region in the form of a slab of tissue is excited (equivalent to a very large single voxel) before spatially encoding the metabolite signals within that slab in a way similar to conventional imaging (Figure 8-1).

Single Voxel Localization

Most localized in vivo MRS has been performed with single voxel methods. Of these, three techniques have been widely used; all of them select cubic volumes by using three intersecting orthogonal slices. These methods are image-related in vivo spectroscopy (ISIS), spin echo (90° – 180° – 180°), and stimulated echo (90° – 90° – 90°).

ISIS[11] works on a principle different from that of the other two. Although it is often used for ^{1}H studies, ISIS was designed primarily for performing phosphorus spectroscopy, in which restrictions are imposed by the short T_2 relaxation times and spin-spin coupling properties of phosphorus metabolites. To this end, an echo signal is not excited as in the other methods, but the localized magnetization is prepared by inversion pulses in the z-direction (thus, avoiding T_2 relaxation other than during the RF pulses) before excitation with a single read-out pulse. A scheme of eight additions and subtractions is necessary to eliminate unwanted signals and to effect localization in three dimensions. The use of phase and frequency-modulated inversion pulses (such as the hyperbolic secant pulse) allows this method to be applied using transmitter coils that produce inhomogeneous fields, because above a threshold level these pulses are insensitive to pulse power. The main drawbacks of ISIS are the need for 8 cycles to achieve localization (the signal from the desired volume is acquired in each of the eight scans, so there is no signal-to-noise penalty) and the potential for subtraction errors when localizing to a small volume in the presence of a large surrounding signal. The latter problem has been reduced by the use of presaturation pulses in a later variant of the method known as OSIRIS.[12]

The two echo methods have been applied extensively in the study of ^{1}H MRS. Both methods rely on the application of an initial shaped 90° RF pulse in the presence of a magnetic field gradient to achieve the selective excitation of a slice in a manner identical to that used in MRI. This is followed by the application of two additional pulses in the presence of gradients in the other two spatial orientations to refocus only the spins in a cube at the intersection of all three slices. In the case of the spin echo method,[13] pulses 2 and 3 are 180° pulses, whereas the stimulated echo uses two 90° pulses.[14]

Although this is not the place to describe in detail the physics of spin echoes and stimulated echoes, it is helpful to consider the practical consequences of using one or the other method based on its application:

1. The stimulated echo method uses only half of the signal initially excited, whereas the spin echo method refocuses all the available signal. Therefore, for the same echo time and same acquisition conditions, the spin echo method theoretically gives twice the signal obtained with a stimulated echo.

2. With the spin echo method, the signal that eventually is acquired as an echo remains in the transverse plane during all time periods after the initial excitation pulse, where it is subject to T_2 relaxation and the effects of any magnetic field gradient pulses. In contrast, the half of the signal that is used to produce a stimulated echo is stored in the longitudinal direction in the period between pulses 2 and 3, during which time it is not subject to T_2

decay and is unaffected by gradients. Therefore, the "echo time" consists of the sum of the first and last time periods, that is, the period between pulses 1 and 2 and the period between pulse 3 and signal acquisition. This means that the echo time (TE) can be kept very short, with the middle time period used for some of the necessary switching of the various field gradients. All time periods contribute to TE in the case of a spin echo, and, thus, it is more difficult to achieve such short TE values.

Short TE is desirable for detecting metabolites that have either short T_2 relaxation times or which, through spin-spin coupling, produce complex resonances that become modulated (and, thus, often more complex) with increasing TE. (An exception to this generalization is the doublet signal from lactate, which is completely inverted at TE = 135 ms and, thus, often studied at this relatively long echo time.) Generally, stimulated echo localization is best suited to achieving short TEs, whereas the increased signal available from a spin echo becomes more important at longer TE values.

Chemical Shift Imaging

As an alternative to the sequential excitation of (and data collection from) a series of individual voxels, it is possible to select a large region of the brain equivalent to many single voxels and to produce spatial information in such a region with pulsed magnetic field gradients.[15–17] The volume excited can take the form of a single slab of tissue 1 to 2 cm thick, within which two-dimensional spatial encoding is used to produce voxels of 1- to 2-mL volume, or the CSI volume can be a larger volume requiring three-dimensional spatial encoding to produce similar voxel sizes but which can provide information on metabolite distributions over a greater region of the brain.

To preserve the spectroscopic information available from small differences in chemical shift, it is essential to maintain high homogeneity of the magnetic field during the period of signal acquisition. Therefore, it is undesirable for any magnetic field gradient to be present during the period of data collection. For this reason, spatial encoding of the spectral information obtained from large CSI volumes is achieved by a method known as "phase encoding," which is also used to produce one dimension of spatial information in conventional MRI. A pulsed magnetic field gradient is used during a time period before acquisition to produce a phase shift in the data whose magnitude for any given nucleus depends on the spatial location of that nucleus, thus producing spatial information while retaining the high-resolution chemical shift information.

The phase-encoding gradient has to be stepped through n different values to produce n spatial data points in any individual direction. Thus for a slab of tissue, to divide the region into n × n voxels, n phase-encoding steps are required in each of two gradient directions, that is, a total of n × n gradient steps. To extend the spatial information into a third dimension, so that the volume is divided into n × n × n voxels, would require a further n gradient step in the remaining direction. Because each of these gradient steps requires 1 × TR (the repetition time), where TR is 1.5 to 2 seconds, the overall time required for a CSI volume is long. However, because the whole volume is sampled each time, it is an efficient method of data acquisition and enables the maximal amount of metabolic information to be obtained in a given time.

CSI has obvious advantages over single voxel spectroscopy in terms of the amount of different regional information that can be acquired in a given time, and in many instances, it will be the technique of choice for MRS studies of the brain in the future. However, it also has several disadvantages that suggest it should be used with caution.

1. Magnetic field homogeneity is required over a region that is large with respect to the equivalent region in single voxel localization. Regional variations in field homogeneity can produce low quality spectra from some localities; in particular, resultant variability in water suppression can cause distortions in the apparent relative metabolite signals, with potentially erroneous conclusions being drawn. For this reason, spectra acquired by single voxel localization are frequently of higher quality than the equivalent CSI spectra (particularly in regions of high magnetic field inhomogeneity such as the anterior and mesial temporal regions) because the field homogeneity is optimized over the particular small region of interest.

2. Differentiation of adjacent voxels using phase encoding leads to less accurate localization than using single voxel methods because the signal from individual voxels contributes to that of their neighbors by the point spread function,[18] a process known as "voxel bleeding." This can be a particular problem with large signals from voxels spatially adjacent to those with smaller signals. For example, subcutaneous lipid may contribute not only to the immediately adjacent voxels but to more remote ones.

Sauter et al.[19] have performed a comparative study of CSI and single voxel localization. With the comparison criteria of localization, sensitivity, and resolution, their results from phantom studies suggested that single voxel methods give superior localization, although the degree of contamination from adjacent voxels in CSI decreased with increasing number of phase-encoding steps. The same observations were found to be valid for comparative volunteer studies. The spectra acquired by both single voxel and CSI methods showed virtually the same sensitivity and spectral resolution.

3. One of the main advantages of CSI is the amount of information available, but this creates problems with respect to postprocessing and display of the data. The necessary Fourier transformation of the acquired signals can be time-consuming and demanding of the hardware needed to carry out this process. In many instances, the hardware used to perform postprocessing on conventional imaging systems may be unacceptably slow in dealing with CSI data.

A related problem is that of data display. For example, a CSI acquisition matrix of 8×8 would generate 64 localized spectra. The difficulty in facilitating the inspection of such a large amount of data is overcome partly by creating metabolic maps by spectral integration over individual resonance lines (often after curve fitting) and displaying the results as contour maps or metabolic images (Figure 8-1). Such maps are easily read and understood, but they potentially can be misleading if used alone. They usually involve interpolation of the pixel data to improve the displayed resolution (for example, from a matrix of 16×16 to one of 64×64) for ease of visualization and anatomical referencing. However, it is important to keep in mind the real resolution of the acquired data when drawing conclusions about any apparent abnormalities. Also, it is possible for poor quality spectra from regions of particular difficulty (for example, poor field homogeneity or lipid infiltration from the scalp) to appear as regions of erroneous metabolite density on the metabolic maps. Therefore, it is essential to interpret such images in conjunction with careful examination of the individual spectra from which they were constructed.

It should be emphasized that if the above problems are recognized and addressed, CSI is capable of providing valuable information about the spatial distribution of metabolites which would be impractical to obtain by single voxel methods.

PROTON (^{1}H) MAGNETIC RESONANCE SPECTROSCOPY IN EPILEPSY

Of the various forms of epilepsy, the partial or focal epilepsies are typically the most intractable, and of this group, temporal lobe epilepsy is the most common type.[20] Surgical removal of the focal abnormality causing the generation of seizures can be an effective cure for this form of epilepsy in 60% to 90% of patients if the damaged region can be identified accurately.[21] Surgical outcome is improved if abnormality such as hippocampal sclerosis or a foreign tissue lesion is present in the resected tissue.[22] Recent advances in MRI have greatly improved preoperative assessment, because it increasingly is able to identify the anatomical abnormalities that often underlie partial seizure disorders. This is particularly so for hippocampal sclerosis, small discrete structural lesions such as cavernomas, and areas of cortical

dysplasia—lesions that have not been reliably visualized previously. Present methods include both qualitative and quantitative approaches.[23–29] Accurate definition of brain anatomy and the identification of regions of abnormality using MRI have also proved useful for interpreting functional imaging studies such as positron emission tomography (PET) and single-photon emission computed tomography (SPECT), which have provided valuable information about the origin of seizures. Clinical evaluation of a patient with epilepsy usually involves reaching a consensus diagnosis from the information available, largely because no technique has provided results that are always reliable. The important advantage of ^{1}H MRS is that it can be performed with MRI in a single session and can provide valuable information that is different from and complementary to that provided by MRI.

There are a number of factors which together suggested that ^{1}H MRS might be able to contribute to the study of epilepsy. Accumulation of cerebral lactate was demonstrated by ^{1}H MRS in rabbits after bicuculline-induced status epilepticus.[30] Matthews et al.[31] reported focally increased lactate in a patient who had epilepsia partialis continua. Also, several lines of evidence have suggested that decreased signal from NAA reflects neuronal loss or dysfunction, and such abnormalities have been documented in patients with intractable focal epilepsy.[32] Proton spectroscopy has a greater SNR and better spatial resolution than ^{31}P MRS and is more easily integrated with MRI in a single examination. Taken together, these data suggest a role for ^{1}H spectroscopy in the clinical investigation of epilepsy. In vivo MRS studies in epilepsy have been directed largely at the temporal lobes of patients with intractable epilepsy for whom surgical treatment is being considered.

In a series of 82 patients (children and adults) with various seizure disorders, localized water-suppressed spectra were obtained[33] on a 1.5-T system, from $2 \times 2 \times 2$-cm voxels placed individually in the left and right medial temporal lobes, including part of the hippocampus together with temporal lobe white matter and neocortex. Localization was achieved using a spin echo sequence, with an echo time of 135 ms. Signal intensities at 2.0 ppm (NAA), 3.0 ppm (Cr), and 3.2 ppm (Cho) were measured by peak integration (Figure 8-2). Multiplication of the signal intensity by the 90° pulse voltage compensated for differences in RF coil loading between individual patients and enabled corrected signal intensities to be compared between subjects. As a group, the patients with epilepsy had a decrease in the mean signal intensity of NAA and an increase in the mean signal intensities of Cho and Cr, with a consequent decrease in the NAA/Cho + Cr ratio, as compared with a population of normal subjects.

NAA in the brain is located primarily in neurons, whereas creatine, phosphocreatine, and choline-containing compounds are also found in other cell types (see above).

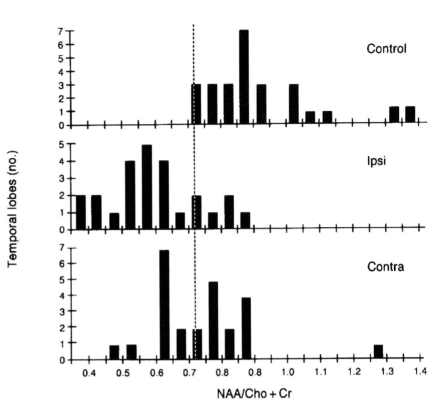

FIGURE 8-3. Ratios of N-acetylaspartate (*NAA*) to choline-containing compounds (*Cho*) and creatine + phosphocreatine (*Cr*) for 13 control subjects and for the temporal lobes ipsilateral and contralateral to the seizure focus in 25 patients with temporal lobe epilepsy. The histograms show the number of temporal lobes with the specified NAA/Cho + Cr ratios. The vertical dotted line represents the lower limit (NAA/Cho + Cr = 0.72) of the 95% reference range, which was derived from the control data. (From Connelly et al.[34] By permission of *Neurology*.)

The implication of these results is loss or dysfunction of neurons in the medial temporal lobe in patients with epilepsy. Furthermore, the concentrations of creatine, phosphocreatine, and choline-containing compounds may be higher in oligodendrocytes and astrocytes than in neurons,[6] and the increased signal from these compounds found in the above study may indicate gliosis. A detailed interpretation of such findings requires analysis of the spectral changes in relation to the localization and lateralization of the seizure focus as evidenced by more conventional techniques.

A subsequent investigation focused on 25 adults with well-characterized intractable temporal lobe epilepsy (on the basis of clinical electroencephalographic [EEG], MRI, and neuropsychologic data) and 13 age-matched control subjects.[34] On the basis of the MRI findings, 19 patients were thought to have hippocampal sclerosis and 3 to have foreign tissue lesions; one patient had widespread signal change suggestive of gliosis, and two others had no detectable abnormality. Of the 14 patients from whom surgical specimens were available, the MRI findings were confirmed histopathologically. The group data from the MRS investigations of the temporal lobes of the patients with epilepsy showed a 22% decrease in NAA, a 15% increase in Cr, and a 25% increase in Cho ipsilateral to the epileptic focus, as compared with normal subjects. The mean NAA/Cho + Cr ratios were significantly less in the patients with epilepsy than in the control subjects, both ipsilateral and con-

tralateral to the focus, with the ipsilateral side being more affected. These findings are consistent with those of Gadian et al.[33] (see above).

In comparing individual patients with the normative data, ^{1}H MRS showed abnormalities in the form of a decreased NAA/Cho + Cr ratio compared with that of controls in 22 of 25 patients (88%), with bilateral abnormalities in 10 patients (40%) (Figure 8-3). In 6 of the 10 patients with bilateral abnormalities, one temporal lobe was judged to be significantly more abnormal than the other. Overall, lateralization was possible in 18 of 22 patients with abnormal MRS findings and was concordant with the side of seizure origin in 15 of the 18 patients. Of the three patients with inconsistent findings, two also had imaging abnormalities in the contralateral temporal lobe (cystic abnormality in one and bilateral hippocampal abnormalities in the other), and the other patient had severe bilateral abnormalities on MRS. Comparison of the MRS and MRI findings showed good agreement, but the apparent anomalies are of particular interest. Two patients with unilateral hippocampal sclerosis showed unlateralized bilateral MRS abnormalities, two patients with no abnormality on MRI had abnormal MRS findings, and three patients with bilaterally normal MRS findings had hippocampal sclerosis.

Advantages of CSI are that it is able to determine the regional distribution of metabolites and to identify areas of maximal abnormality. Using ^{1}H CSI on a 1.5-T system, Cendes et al.[35] examined 10 patients with temporal lobe epilepsy who were being evaluated for surgical treatment and 5 control subjects. The spatial resolution in this study was improved with respect to single voxel studies, with an in-plane resolution of 8 mm (the plane thickness used was not stated). The echo time (TE) was 272 ms. The data were assessed in terms of the NAA/Cr ratio, which was determined for regions defined as middle and posterior temporal lobes in all cases, and for any metabolic lesions (that is, regions of maximum CSI abnormality). The left-right asymmetry of NAA/Cr ratios was significantly different from that of control subjects in at least one temporal lobe in all cases, using the difference between the two sides divided by the mean of the two sides as the asymmetry index. The metabolic lesions were generally smaller than the anatomically defined middle and posterior regions and showed a greater magnitude of asymmetry. The NAA/Cr ratio was low in the midtemporal lobe in five patients and in the posterior temporal lobes in eight. The asymmetry was greater in the midtemporal region in three patients and in the posterior temporal region in six. No information was provided about the absolute intensities of individual metabolites.

The use of an asymmetry index alone precludes the detection of bilateral abnormalities. However, comparison of the NAA/Cr ratios in the patients and control subjects indicated that two patients had a decrease in the NAA/Cr ratio in the posterior temporal region bilaterally. In all the patients, the greatest decrease in NAA/Cr was ipsilateral to the seizure focus as determined clinically and by EEG, including those patients with bilateral abnormalities. Of the 10 patients, 1 had no MRI evidence of hippocampal atrophy or signal increase on T_2-weighted imaging but had a decreased NAA/Cr ratio in the midposterior temporal lobe. Intraoperatively, this patient had evidence of mild mesial temporal sclerosis.

Another CSI study was performed on eight patients with unilateral complex partial seizures and eight control subjects, using a 2-T MR system.[36] A CSI volume of $10 \times 10 \times 5$ cm was selected using a spin echo sequence, with a TE of 272 ms. Three-dimensional phase encoding was performed with $16 \times 16 \times 12$ gradient steps over a field of view of $16 \times 16 \times 14$ cm. Elliptical voxels were produced of calculated "nominal" size 1.7 cm^3 (effective in-plane resolution, about 1.25 cm; effective slice thickness, 1.1 cm).

The signal intensities for NAA, Cr, and Cho were obtained from 10 bilaterally paired individual voxels from each subject and examined for the presence of asymmetry. The only significant asymmetry observed was in the ipsilateral/contralateral NAA ratios obtained from the hippocampal regions of patients with epilepsy. The side-to-side difference in NAA signal intensity was on average 21% (compared with a 22% reduction with respect to control data reported by Connelly et al.[34]). The left/right ratios of the other metabolites in patients

showed bilateral symmetry, as did all metabolites in the control group. In all the patients, the lower NAA corresponded to the side of seizure focus as determined by EEG. MRI demonstrated abnormalities in seven of the eight patients; in each patient, the abnormality was ipsilateral to both the seizure focus and the NAA abnormality. An assessment of the presence of bilateral damage is not possible from the MRS data presented because only an asymmetry index was used.

Ng et al.[37] used a 1.5-T MR system to perform ^{1}H CSI examinations on 25 patients with clinical or EEG evidence of temporal lobe epilepsy but with no lesions demonstrated on MRI and on 12 control subjects. Seventeen patients had unilateral abnormalities on EEG and eight had evidence of bilateral temporal lobe epilepsy (most of these eight patients had depth electrodes inserted in addition to the investigation with surface/sphenoidal electrodes as carried out in all other cases). MR spectra were obtained from eight 1- to 2-mL voxels in each temporal lobe in 21 patients, with only one temporal lobe examined successfully in each of 4 patients. A volume of interest was selected using spin echo localization, with a TE of 135 ms.

In all patients, a region was identified that was characterized by a decrease in the NAA signal and either an increase or no change in the signal from Cho. For this reason, the NAA/Cho ratio was used as a sensitive marker of metabolic abnormality.[34] There were no significant differences in the NAA/Cho ratio between the temporal lobes in control subjects or between the temporal lobes in control subjects and the uninvolved temporal lobe in 14 of 17 patients with unilateral abnormalities. However, all 17 patients with unilateral abnormalities had a significant decrease in the NAA/Cho ratio in the temporal lobe ipsilateral to the EEG-determined seizure focus, with additional contralateral abnormalities in 3 patients. Of the eight patients with bilateral EEG abnormalities, six showed bilaterally reduced NAA/Cho ratio and one had a unilateral NAA/Cho abnormality. Spectra were acquired from only one temporal lobe in the other patient. An increase in lactate was observed in two patients examined shortly after a seizure.

The neurobiologic implication common to the above findings is that neuronal loss or dysfunction and possibly astrocytosis occur in the temporal lobes of patients with temporal lobe epilepsy. The magnitude of the decrease in NAA in many cases is such that the abnormality could not be confined to the hippocampus, because it occupies only a small proportion of the MRS volume. This is particularly so for the single voxel studies[33,34] in which 8-mL volumes were used, but it has also been reported with CSI.[38] Therefore, the abnormality detected with MRS is presumably more diffuse and widespread than is often apparent from MRI. This finding is consistent with PET data on cerebral glucose metabolism, in which the area of hypometabolism commonly is larger than the anatomically defined focus,[39] and with similar regional abnormalities reported with SPECT (see Lancet editorial[40]). The cellular mechanisms underlying regional hypometabolism and, by inference, of the decreased NAA and increased Cho and Cr, are not certain. The above conclusions are based partly on cell culture studies.[5,6] However, further clarification may be possible by means of correlative neuropathologic studies, although it would not be straightforward to relate accurately the MRS-selected volume to the pathology samples.

Bilateral lesions occur in up to 50% of patients with temporal lobe epilepsy.[41] The significance of this is not well understood, particularly with respect to the likely seizure outcome or expected cognitive performance postoperatively if contralateral abnormalities are present. In part, this has been due to the difficulty in identifying contralateral lesions preoperatively. Now, ^{1}H MRS is able to demonstrate the presence of a high proportion of bilateral abnormalities; for example, Connelly et al.[34] found 40% (10 of 25 patients) bilaterally abnormal NAA ratios (Figure 8-3), and Ng et al.[37] found 42% (9 of 21 patients) in a CSI study. These results suggest that ^{1}H MRS can provide a quantitative means of identifying contralateral problems that because of their often diffuse nature are difficult to visualize on conventional imaging. In a postoperative study of 34 patients with temporal lobe epilepsy who had undergone amygdalohippocampectomy, Incisa della Rocchetta et al.[42] acquired data from single 8-mL cubic volumes located in the unoperated temporal lobes. Seventeen of the 34 patients (50%) had abnormal spectra on the unoperated side. No systematic relationship was found between the presence of such damage and seizure outcome. However, it was shown that statistically significant verbal memory deficits were present on delayed recall in the group data of those patients who had right-sided excisions only if they also had MRS abnormalities on the contralateral (left) side. (Patients with left-sided excisions showed verbal memory deficits regardless of the presence or absence of abnormalities on the other side.)

It is important to note that although various authors have reported the concordance/discordance between their MRS and MRI findings,[34–36] there is no consensus about what an MRI investigation should involve in the context of epilepsy. Thus, such comparative findings are not in general transferable across MR sites at present, because the MRI studies do not necessarily provide a consistent reference with respect to either the type of imaging performed or the criteria used in reporting the images. In particular, the visual assessment of images of variable quality at different medical centers can produce widely varying results with relation to the identification of, for example, hippocampal sclerosis.[28] Quantitative investigations of hippocampal signal change[29] and atrophy[25,27] are likely to give more uniform results, and some preliminary work has been done in

comparing such results with those of MRS.[38,43,44] These studies generally have shown good agreement with respect to lateralization of abnormality. However, quantitative studies also allow a comparison of the degree of abnormality, at least as evidenced by the particular variables in question. To date, studies have found good quantitative correlation between MRS findings and the results of volumetric[38] and T_2[44] measurements. This suggests that focal structural lesions may be associated with more diffuse abnormalities in many cases.

The information provided by the NAA signal in MRS is analogous to, but different from, that available from conventional MRI in that it is indicative of the presence of abnormality but not necessarily informative about transient functional events. Such findings need to be related either directly or by association to seizure activity. However, the observation of a focal increase in brain lactate levels in the postictal period suggests potential for a more direct marker of seizure activity.[37] Another study by the same investigators[45] compared the regional lactate levels in the temporal lobes of eight patients who had intractable temporal lobe epilepsy with the NAA/Cho ratios and video-EEG monitoring findings. On the basis of the EEG findings, three patients had unilateral temporal lobe epilepsy and the five others showed evidence of the condition bilaterally. ^{1}H CSI studies were performed 1.5 and 7 hours postictally, and interictal CSI scans were performed in two patients. For all the patients with unilateral disease, lactate was increased in the ipsilateral temporal lobe. Lactate was increased in one temporal lobe only in patients with bilateral disease. In six of the eight patients, lactate was increased in a focal region that also showed a low NAA/Cho ratio; in the two other patients, the NAA levels were normal. The unilateral increases in lactate suggest that the increase occurs in the region of the seizure focus in patients with unilateral temporal lobe epilepsy, but for patients with bilateral disease, the increase may indicate only the site of the most recent seizure. These findings suggest that it may be possible to map out the region of tissue that has been involved directly in seizure activity. The investigation of suspected bilateral temporal lobe epilepsy would require repeated CSI investigations to determine whether one side is consistently associated with seizure activity or whether different seizures show different lactate distributions. However, because MRS is noninvasive, it appears ideally suited to the investigation of such difficult cases.

CSI has distinct advantages over single voxel techniques with respect to coverage of the brain and spatial resolution; thus, it is becoming the method of choice in several medical centers for the study of epilepsy. However, as discussed above, CSI is technically more demanding than single voxel MRS, particularly in respect to magnetic field homogeneity (shimming), water suppression, and voxel bleeding (especially infiltration of subcutaneous fat signal into voxels other than those adjacent to the scalp). Cendes et al.[38] noted that anterior temporal lobe structures were more accessible to single voxel methods and reported only posterior and midtemporal lobe results. Ng et al.[37] reported problems with suboptimal shimming when performing CSI in a large region that included both temporal lobes; therefore, they have adopted the strategy of acquiring smaller CSI volumes from each temporal lobe consecutively. For similar reasons, Heatherington et al.[3] have used a CSI slice angulated upward from the transaxial plane, intersecting the hippocampus just posterior to the red nuclei, to avoid the anterior temporal region. Nevertheless, in the long term, it seems likely that CSI will provide information that cannot be obtained in any other fashion.

Further work needs to be done to validate the clinical usefulness of temporal lobe ^{1}H MRS, including examination of the temporal lobes of patients with epilepsy of extratemporal onset, before the data can be used with confidence in assessing patients with partial epilepsy of uncertain lateralization and localization. The use of single voxel ^{1}H MRS to identify seizure foci in extratemporal epilepsy without structural abnormalities on MRI to guide voxel placement is unlikely to be useful. Indeed, it was not helpful in one study that examined spectra acquired from 8-mL cubic volumes in the supplementary motor area in patients whose seizures were believed on clinical grounds to involve this region.[46] CSI is clearly more appropriate than single voxel localization for investigating nonlesional extratemporal epilepsy. Garcia et al.[47] performed a ^{1}H CSI study in eight patients with frontal lobe epilepsy and found focally decreased NAA in the frontal lobe ipsilateral to the seizure focus in each patient. More work is needed to confirm such findings, but it might be expected that with further advances in MR hardware and software, CSI could be used to localize focal abnormalities underlying seizure disorders in the temporal lobe and extratemporally in cases in which MRI does not reveal any structural abnormality.

As improvements in MR techniques and hardware become more widely available, metabolites other than those discussed above may become important in investigating epilepsy. For example, in a proton MRS study at 2.1 T, Rothman et al.[4] demonstrated an increase in cerebral GABA in control subjects and in patients with epilepsy after administration of vigabatrin. Subsequent work from the same group[48] showed that GABA levels could be monitored during continued use of the drug. Although these studies were performed with spectral editing techniques that cannot be done with routine clinical MR scanners, the studies demonstrate the possibility of noninvasively determining cerebral neurometabolic profiles of patients before and during the application of drug therapy. Such information could aid considerably in selecting the therapy most likely to be helpful in a patient and in monitoring the effects of treatment.

CONCLUSIONS

Currently, ^{1}H MRS appears to be a sensitive method for detecting regional cerebral metabolic disturbance. It can contribute to the lateralization of the epileptic focus and to the identification of bilateral abnormalities. In providing information on static metabolic abnormalities, primarily through the NAA signal, and on dynamic changes associated with seizure activity through the lactate signal, MRS offers potential for reducing dependence on expensive and time-consuming invasive EEG studies. However, definitively establishing this role for ^{1}H MRS may be difficult to achieve because the presurgical evaluation depends on finding a consensus between different strands of data, and the tendency for decisions to be weighted toward the more established techniques will remain. For example, if a patient is found to have a well-characterized unilateral EEG abnormality, it is unlikely with our present state of knowledge that a unilateral MRS abnormality on the other side would be deemed more significant; the likelihood is that either an operation would be performed on the side indicated by EEG or no operation would be performed. In the event of such a patient having a poor seizure outcome postoperatively, it would not be known if the EEG localization was misleading and the MRS localization was correct or if the patient had bilateral temporal lobe epilepsy. Examination of a larger number of patients is needed to determine the strength of the associations between MRS and other investigatory data and the clinical significance of MRS data that may appear to be discordant with those from more established methods. Nevertheless, it is apparent from the data available that MRS offers a noninvasive method for obtaining information on cerebral metabolism that is likely to have significant consequences for the medical and surgical management of patients with epilepsy.

REFERENCES

1. Rothman DL, Novotny EJ, Shulman GI, et al. 1H-[13C] NMR measurements of [4-13C]glutamate turnover in human brain. Proc Natl Acad Sci USA 1992;89:9603–6.

2. Chen W, Novotny EJ, Boulware SD, et al. Quantitative measurements of regional TCA cycle flux in visual cortex of human brain using 1H-[13C] NMR spectroscopy (abstract). Proc Soc Magn Reson Med 1994;1:63.

3. Heatherington HP, Kuzniecky R, Pan JW, et al. Identification of the epileptic focus in temporal lobe epilepsy by high resolution spectroscopic imaging at 4.1T (abstract). Proc Soc Magn Reson Med 1994;1:396.

4. Rothman DL, Petroff OA, Behar KL, et al. Localized ^{1}H NMR measurements of gamma-aminobutyric acid in human brain in vivo. Proc Natl Acad Sci USA 1993;90:5662–6.

5. Urenjak J, Williams SR, Gadian DG, et al. Specific expression of N-acetylaspartate in neurons, oligodendrocyte-type-2 astrocyte progenitors, and immature oligodendrocytes in vitro. J Neurochem 1992; 59:55–61.

6. Urenjak J, Williams SR, Gadian DG, et al. Proton nuclear magnetic resonance spectroscopy unambiguously identifies different neural cell types. J Neurosci 1993;13:981–9.

7. Ackerman JJ, Grove TH, Wong GG, et al. Mapping of metabolites in whole animals by 31P NMR using surface coils. Nature 1980;283:167–70.

8. Hoult DI. Rotating frame zeugmatography. J Magn Reson 1979;33:183–97.

9. Gordon RE, Hanley PE, Shaw D. Topical magnetic resonance. Prog NMR Spectroscopy 1982;15:1–47.

10. Bendall MR, Gordon RE. Depth and refocusing pulses designed for multipulse NMR using surface coils. J Magn Reson 1983;53:365–85.

11. Ordidge RJ, Connelly A, Lohman JB. Image-selected in vivo spectroscopy (ISIS): a new technique for spatially selective NMR spectroscopy. J Magn Reson 1986;66:283–94.

12. Connelly A, Counsell C, Lohman JAB, et al. Outer volume suppressed image related in vivo spectroscopy (OSIRIS): a high-sensitivity localization technique. J Magn Reson 1988;78:519–25.

13. Ordidge RJ, Bendall MR, Gordon RG, et al. Volume selection for in-vivo biological spectroscopy. In: Govil, Khetrapal, Saran, eds. Magnetic resonance in biology and medicine. New Delhi: Tata-McGraw-Hill, 1985:387–97.

14. Frahm J, Bruhn H, Gyngell ML, et al. Localized high-resolution proton NMR spectroscopy using stimulated echoes: initial applications to human brain in vivo. Magn Reson Med 1989;9:79–93.

15. Kumar A, Welti D, Ernst RR. NMR Fourier zeugmatography. J Magn Reson 1975;18:69–83.

16. Brown TR, Kincaid BM, Ugurbil K. NMR chemical shift imaging in three dimensions. Proc Natl Acad Sci USA 1982;79:3523–6.

17. Maudsley AA, Hilal SK, Perman WH, et al. Spatially resolved high resolution spectroscopy by "four-dimensional" NMR. J Magn Reson 1983;51:147–52.

18. Bottomley PA, Hardy CJ, Roemer PB. Phosphate metabolite imaging and concentration measurements in human heart by nuclear magnetic resonance. Magn Reson Med 1990;14:425–34.

19. Sauter R, Schneider M, Wicklow K, et al. Localized H-1 MR spectroscopy of the human brain: single-voxel versus chemical shift imaging techniques (abstract). J Magn Reson Imaging 1991;1:241–2.

20. Hauser W. The natural history of temporal lobe epilepsy. In: Lüders HO, ed. Epilepsy surgery. New York: Raven Press, 1992:133–41.

21. Engel J Jr, Van Ness PC, Rasmussen TB, et al. Outcome with respect to epileptic seizures. In: Engel J Jr, ed. Surgical treatment of the epilepsies. 2nd ed. New York: Raven Press, 1993:609–21.

22. Cascino GD, Jack CR Jr, Parisi JE, et al. MRI in the presurgical evaluation of patients with frontal lobe epilepsy and children with temporal lobe epilepsy: pathologic correlation and prognostic importance. Epilepsy Res 1992;11:51–9.

23. Bergen D, Bleck T, Ramsey R, et al. Magnetic resonance imaging as a sensitive and specific predictor of neoplasms removed for intractable epilepsy. Epilepsia 1989;30:318–21.

24. Brooks BS, King DW, el Gammal T, et al. MR imaging in patients with intractable complex partial epileptic seizures. AJNR Am J Neuroradiol 1990; 11:93–9.

25. Jack CR Jr, Sharbrough FW, Twomey CK, et al. Temporal lobe seizures: lateralization with MR volume measurements of the hippocampal formation. Radiology 1990;175:423–9.

26. Jack CR Jr, Sharbrough FW, Cascino GD, et al. Magnetic resonance image-based hippocampal volumetry: correlation with outcome after temporal lobectomy. Ann Neurol 1992;31:138–46.

27. Cook MJ, Fish DR, Shorvon SD, et al. Hippocampal volumetric and morphometric studies in frontal and temporal lobe epilepsy. Brain 1992;115:1001–15.

28. Jackson GD, Berkovic SF, Duncan JS, et al. Optimizing the diagnosis of hippocampal sclerosis using MR imaging. AJNR Am J Neuroradiol 1993;14:753–62.

29. Jackson GD, Connelly A, Duncan JS, et al. Detection of hippocampal pathology in intractable partial epilepsy: increased sensitivity with quantitative magnetic resonance T2 relaxometry. Neurology 1993; 43:1793–9.

30. Petroff OA, Pritchard JW, Ogino T, et al. Combined ^{1}H and 31P nuclear magnetic resonance spectroscopic studies of bicuculline-induced seizures in vivo. Ann Neurol 1986;20:185–93.

31. Matthews PM, Andermann F, Arnold DL. A proton magnetic resonance spectroscopy study of focal epilepsy in humans. Neurology 1990;40:985–9.

32. Connelly A, Cross JH, Gadian DG, et al. Focal brain abnormalities in intractable epilepsy of childhood (abstract). Proc Soc Magn Reson Med 1991;1:224.

33. Gadian DG, Connelly A, Duncan JS, et al. [1]H magnetic resonance spectroscopy in the investigation of intractable epilepsy. Acta Neurol Scand Suppl 1994; 152:116–21.

34. Connelly A, Jackson GD, Duncan JS, et al. Magnetic resonance spectroscopy in temporal lobe epilepsy. Neurology 1994;44:1411–7.

35. Cendes F, Andermann F, Preul MC, et al. Lateralization of temporal lobe epilepsy based on regional metabolic abnormalities in proton magnetic resonance spectroscopic images. Ann Neurol 1994;35:211–6.

36. Hugg JW, Laxer KD, Matson GB, et al. Neuron loss localizes human temporal lobe epilepsy by in vivo proton magnetic resonance spectroscopic imaging. Ann Neurol 1993;34:788–94.

37. Ng TC, Comair YG, Xue M, et al. Temporal lobe epilepsy: presurgical localization with proton chemical shift imaging. Radiology 1994;193:465–72.

38. Cendes F, Andermann F, Dubeau F, et al. Combined MRI volumetric studies and MR spectroscopic imaging for lateralization of temporal lobe epilepsy (abstract). Proc Soc Magn Reson Med 1994;1:397.

39. Sackellares JC, Siegel GJ, Abou-Khalil BW, et al. Differences between lateral and mesial temporal metabolism interictally in epilepsy of mesial temporal origin. Neurology 1990;40:1420–6.

40. SPECT and PET in epilepsy. Lancet 1989;1:135–7. (Editorial)

41. Margerison JH, Corsellis JAN. Epilepsy and the temporal lobes: a clinical, electroencephalographic and neuropathological study of the brain in epilepsy, with particular reference to the temporal lobes. Brain 1966;89:499–530.

42. Incisa della Rocchetta A, Gadian DG, Connelly A, et al. Verbal memory impairment after right temporal lobe surgery: role of contralateral damage as revealed by ^{1}H magnetic resonance spectroscopy and T2 relaxometry. Neurology 1995;45:797–802.

43. Ng TC, Najm I, Xue M, et al. Lateralization of temporal lobe epilepsy: a comparison of proton CSI and MRI volumetry measurements (abstract). Proc Soc Magn Reson Med 1994;10:610.

44. Connelly A, Jackson GD, Duncan JS, et al. ^{1}H MRS and T2 relaxometry in adults with intractable partial epilepsy (abstract). Proc Soc Magn Reson Med 1994;1:403.

45. Comair YG, Ng TC, Xue M, et al. Early postictal lactate detection in temporal lobe epilepsy for localisation of seizure focus: a proton chemical shift imaging study (abstract). Proc Soc Magn Reson Med 1994;1:401.

46. Cook MJ, Manford M, Gadian DG, et al. Proton magnetic resonance spectroscopy in supplementary motor area seizures (abstract). Epilepsia 1991;32 Suppl 3:78.

47. Garcia PA, Laxer KD, van der Grond J, et al. [1]H magnetic resonance spectroscopic imaging in patients with frontal lobe epilepsy (abstract). Epilepsia 1993;34:122.

48. Petroff OAC, Rothman DL, Behar KL, et al. Evidence for tachyphylaxis with increasing vigabatrin dosage on GABA levels in human brain measured in vivo with ^{1}H NMR spectroscopy (abstract). Proc Soc Magn Reson Med 1994;1:404.

^{31}P Magnetic Resonance Spectroscopy of Epilepsy

Kenneth D. Laxer

Despite the medications that are available, about 25% of epilepsy patients have seizures that are refractory to medical treatment.[1] Half of these patients are potential candidates for neurosurgical removal of the epileptogenic focus (about 100,000 patients in the United States).[2] The best surgical results are obtained when the various preoperative localizing examinations (videoelectroencephalographic telemetry, magnetic resonance imaging [MRI], positron emission tomography [PET], single-photon emission computed tomography [SPECT], etcetera) are concordant, implicating the same brain region. However, there is still a large population of patients with medically refractory seizures in whom MRI, SPECT, or PET imaging fails to confirm the epileptogenic region as defined by electroencephalography (EEG). Patients without imaging concordance have a significantly poorer outcome from seizure surgery. For example, patients with mass lesions detected with MRI usually have a good surgical outcome.[3] The difference in outcome between "lesional" and "nonlesional" patients is particularly noticeable for patients with extratemporal foci; 67% of extratemporal "lesionectomy" patients become seizure-free, in comparison with only 44% of "nonlesional" patients.[4] Similarly, concordance between subtle changes in the hippocampal formation on MRI and telemetry predicts a good outcome. Patients with unilateral hippocampal atrophy or increased signal concordant with the ictal EEG have a 95% chance of becoming seizure-free after temporal lobectomy; however, in patients with normal MRI findings (that is, non-

concordance), the prognosis for seizure-free outcome decreases to about 50%.[5,6]

It is clear that with PET and high-resolution and volumetric MRI the temporal lobes can be imaged effectively. The imaging of extratemporal lobe epilepsy has not been as successful. This partly explains why typically more than 75% of patients become seizure-free after temporal lobectomy, whereas only 50% of those undergoing frontal lobectomy do.[4] Better imaging techniques for nonlesional nontemporal lobe epilepsy need to be developed.

MAGNETIC RESONANCE SPECTROSCOPY

Magnetic resonance spectroscopy (MRS) is the only noninvasive technique capable of measuring chemicals within the body. It can be performed on many conventional MRI systems. MRS exploits the principle that every chemically distinct nucleus in a compound resonates at a slightly different frequency. This allows the detection of various proton signals on a given protein, the different phosphates of adenosine triphosphate (ATP), and carbon signals in organic molecules.[7] In addition, the nuclear magnetic resonance signals from many compounds can be detected simultaneously in one MRS experiment and MRS imaging (MRSI) has the ability to obtain MRS signals from multiple regions simultaneously.[8] MRS single-volume localization techniques, using selective pulses and gradients, offer the advantages of sharp spatial resolution and high sensitivity.

Spectroscopic imaging techniques (using phase encoding) have the important advantage that multiple regions are sampled simultaneously at a cost of some spectral resolution.

^{1}H MRS detects N-acetylaspartate, lactate, choline, creatinine/phosphocreatine, and amino acids, including glutamate, glutamine, aspartate, and taurine (Chapter 8).^{31}P MRS detects phosphocreatine (PCr), ATP, inorganic phosphate (Pi), pH (from the chemical shift of Pi), free Mg^{2+} (from the chemical shift of ATP), phosphomonoesters (PME) (largely phosphorylcholine and phosphorylethanolamine), and phosphodiesters (PDE) (largely glycerophosphorylcholine, glycerophosphorylethanolamine), and mobile phospholipids.[7] PCr, ATP, Pi, pH, and lactate provide information about bioenergetics, and PDE, PME, and choline provide information about lipid metabolism.

ICTAL MAGNETIC RESONANCE SPECTROSCOPY

Experimental seizures in animals produced by various methods consistently demonstrate alteration of energy metabolism, including the depletion of PCr, ATP, and increased levels of Pi, lactate, and H^+.[9] These ictally induced metabolic changes have been verified with MRS in animals.[10–12] Yaksh and Anderson[11] demonstrated a marked decrease in pH from 7.11 to 6.85 during seizures in cats; the brain tissue remained acidotic for more than 20 minutes postictally. By using ^{31}P MRS, similar changes were found in energy metabolism in human neonates during seizures, with diminished PCr and increased Pi and H^+ intraictally on the side of the seizure focus.[13,14]

Although the ictal events per se have a short duration, the induced metabolic changes may persist for hours. After completion of a seizure, recovery from acidosis is slower than recovery of high energy phosphates. Furthermore, brain levels of lactate may remain increased for a considerable time postictally, probably due to continuing enhanced glycolysis. Following seizures induced in rats with flurothyl, acidosis persists for more than 45 minutes.[15] Postictally, intracellular pH increased to normal and subsequently to supernormal values at a time when tissue levels of lactate had not normalized.[15]

INTERICTAL MAGNETIC RESONANCE SPECTROSCOPY

Interictally, seizure foci of epileptic patients have decreased glucose uptake and decreased perfusion, as demonstrated with PET scanning.[16–19] These data suggested that metabolic abnormalities, such as an asymmetry of high-energy phosphates or pH, might be detected with MRS interictally in patients with epilepsy. We initially used a single-volume technique (ISIS) to study eight patients with refractory temporal lobe epilepsy.[20] All the patients had normal computed tomographic (CT) findings, and four of the eight patients had normal findings on MRI. MRI-guided ^{31}P MRS was used to measure brain levels of PCr, ATP, Pi, Mg^{2+}, and pH in the temporal lobes. The ^{31}P MRS spectra were obtained in vivo before temporal lobectomy. All the patients have been seizure-free postoperatively. Electrocorticography, gross surgical findings, and microscopic pathologic findings were consistent with mesial temporal sclerosis.

The ^{31}P spectra were obtained at 2 T, and the person performing and processing the MRS was blinded to the side of the seizure focus. Volumes of interest (84 to 105 mL) in the right and left anterior temporal lobes were studied (Figure 9-1). No significant difference was found between ipsilateral and contralateral temporal lobe concentrations of ATP, PCr, or PDE. The interictal pH was significantly more alkaline on the side of the seizure focus than on the contralateral side (7.25 versus 7.08; $P < 0.05$). Seven of the eight patients had this pH asymmetry.

Also, the Pi concentration was increased significantly in the anterior temporal lobe on the side of the seizure focus (1.9 mM versus 1.1 mM; $P < 0.05$). The seven patients with ipisilateral temporal lobe alkalosis also demonstrated a greater Pi on the side of the focus. There also was a trend for PME to be decreased in the focus. The pH and Pi changes were not related to the age of the patient, seizure duration, or seizure frequency, and there was no relationship between the presence or absence of MRI or SPECT asymmetries and the degree of asymmetry of the phosphate variables. Using the same technique (ISIS), Kuzniecky et al.[21] found a decrease in the PCr/Pi ratio on the side of the seizure focus in temporal lobe epilepsy and a trend for the pH to be decreased on the contralateral side.

The results described above were obtained on preselected volumes using ISIS. Whole-brain MRSI simultaneously obtains spectra from multiple regions throughout the field of view, and metabolite images can be reconstructed from these spectra. The advantage is that the hippocampus or any other region can be selected after acquisition. Recently, the clinical feasibility of ^{31}P MRSI with effective voxel sizes of 16 to 25 mL has been demonstrated.[8,22–28]

With ^{31}P MRSI, patients with medically refractory temporal lobe epilepsy were tested to confirm the ISIS results of increased Pi and pH in the epileptogenic focus (that is, the voxel containing the anterior hippocampus). The spectra were obtained interictally and revealed that the seizure foci were more alkaline (7.17 ± 0.03 versus 7.06 ± 0.02; $P < 0.01$) and had increased Pi (1.2 ± 0.2 mM versus 0.6 ± 0.1 mM; $P < 0.01$) and decreased PME (2.1 ± 0.03 mM versus 3.3 ± 0.5 mM; $P < 0.01$), as compared with the contralateral homologous region (Figure 9-2).[29] No asymmetry was found between the hemispheres for any phosphorus metabolite or pH in a normal control population. The patients had normal CT findings, and two of seven patients with temporal lobe epilepsy had normal MRI findings. One patient with a medial frontal focus had normal CT and MRI findings; however, the interictal

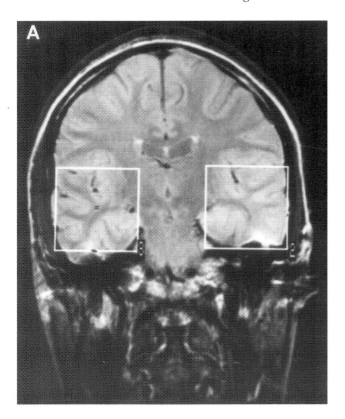

SPECT scan implicated the contralateral frontal region in this patient. The seizure focus was correctly lateralized with ³¹P MRSI in all the patients with temporal lobe epilepsy and in the patient with the medial frontal focus.

On the basis of this constellation of findings (that is, increased Pi and pH and decreased PME), an asymmetry variable that combined these values was determined in normal control subjects and patients.[29] For all the patients with complex partial seizures, the values were outside the normal range, pointing in the direction of the seizure focus. Therefore, with knowledge of the focus from EEG telemetry, MRSI can accurately lateralize the seizure focus in temporal lobe epilepsy by using only the data from the hippocampi.

Accepting that MRSI could accurately lateralize the seizure focus in patients with refractory temporal lobe epilepsy, the next question was whether by using these asymmetries MRSI could localize the seizure focus in temporal lobe epilepsy arising from the anterior hippocampus. In 11 patients, the ³¹P spectra were analyzed from eight regions in each hemisphere (anterior hippocampus, posterior hippocampus, summed hippocampus, lateral temporal lobe, summed temporal lobe, frontal lobe, parietal lobe, and occipital lobe).[30] Again, the seizure focus was more

FIGURE 9-1. A. T₁-weighted coronal slice MRI showing the volumes of interest in the temporal lobes.
B. Normal control ³¹P magnetic resonance spectrum demonstrating resonances for phosphomonoesters (*PME*), inorganic phosphate (*Pi*), phosphodiesters (*PDE*), phosphocreatine (*PCr*), and ATP (*a,ß,γ*).
C. Overlap of curve-fitted spectra revealing a shift in the Pi resonance consistent with ipsilateral alkalosis. (From Laxer et al.[20] By permission of the International League Against Epilepsy.)

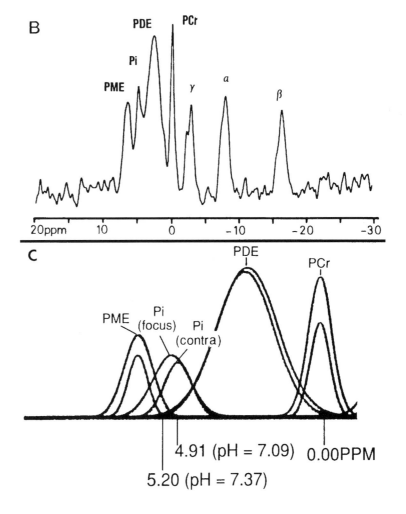

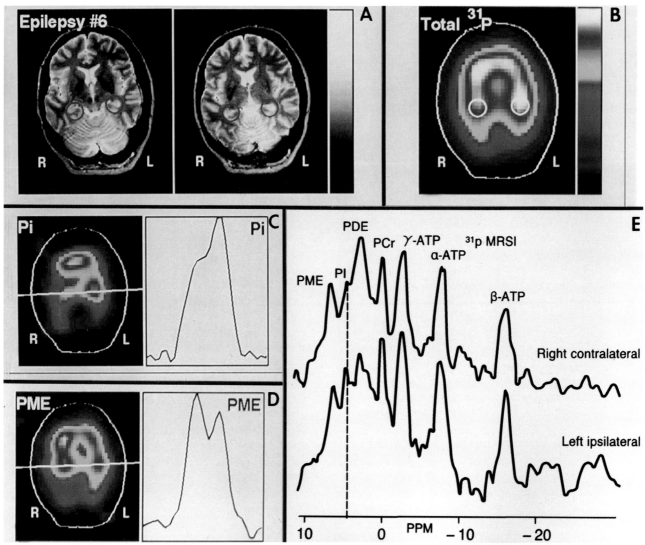

FIGURE 9-2. [31]P magnetic resonance spectroscopic imaging of temporal lobe epilepsy in a patient with a left hippocampal focus. A. Two T_2-weighted transaxial MRI slices corresponding to the magnetic resonance spectroscopic slices in B–D. B. Total phosphorus (^{31}P) metabolite map with MRI skull outline (25-mL effective voxel size). C. Inorganic phosphorus (*Pi*) metabolite map and region profile line showing increased Pi in left hippocampus. D. Phosphomonoester (*PME*) metabolite map and region profile line showing decreased PME in left hippocampus. E. Single voxel spectra from left (*L*) (ipsilateral) and right (*R*) (contralateral) hippocampi, indicated by *circles* in A, showing increased Pi, decreased PME, and increased pH (leftward shift of Pi peak). (From Hugg et al.[29] By permission of *Neurology*.)

alkaline (7.13 ± 0.04 versus 6.97 ± 0.03; *P* < 0.01) and had a higher level of Pi (0.12 ± 0.01 mM versus 0.07 ± 0.01 mM; *P* < 0.01) and a lower level of PME (0.15 ± 0.01 mM versus 0.21 ± 0.02 mM; *P* < 0.01) in comparison with the contralateral anterior hippocampus. Regions outside the anterior hippocampus but within the temporal lobe demonstrated similar asymmetries for PME and Pi but not for pH. Regions outside the temporal lobe did not have significant metabolite asymmetries (Figure 9-3). The seizure focus was the only region in the brain that demonstrated all three abnormalities (that is, increased pH and Pi and decreased PME). With an asymmetry score that included the three

variables, the seizure focus was lateralized correctly in 11 of 11 patients: the focus was localized to the correct temporal lobe in 7, but to the anterior hippocampus in only 5.

[31]P MAGNETIC RESONANCE SPECTROSCOPY OF TEMPORAL LOBE EPILEPSY COMPARED WITH THAT OF CONTROLS

Spectra from normal control subjects were analyzed to determine whether there were asymmetries between the left and right sides, whether pH and Pi were significantly increased and PME significantly decreased in the epileptogenic hemispheres compared with controls, and whether there were asymmetries in pH, PME, or Pi in the contralateral sides of epileptic brains compared with controls. No hemispheric asymmetry was found for any of the metabolites in any of the regions in control subjects. Pi and pH were significantly increased and PME was significantly decreased in the epileptogenic anterior hippocampus in the 11 patients as compared with control subjects. The values determined in the hippocampus contralateral to the seizure focus were not significantly different from controls. However, the mean values for all brain regions suggest changes in the contralateral side that are opposite to those in the epileptogenic region.[30] The regional means for pH, Pi, and PME in the control subjects were consistently between those for the epileptogenic and contralateral regions (Figure 9-3). Using changes in both the ipsilateral and contralateral hemispheres may increase the sensitivity of ^{31}P MRS for localizing the seizure focus.

^{31}P MAGNETIC RESONANCE SPECTROSCOPY IN FRONTAL LOBE EPILEPSY

On the basis of the results obtained with ^{31}P MRSI in temporal lobe epilepsy, a similar approach was used for patients with frontal lobe epilepsy.[31] In all the patients, alkalosis was found in the epileptogenic frontal lobe, as compared with the contralateral lobe (7.10 ± 0.05 versus 7 ± 6; $P < 0.001$). Seven of eight patients also exhibited decreased PME in the epileptogenic frontal lobe (16 ± 6 mM versus 23 ± 4 mM; $P < 0.01$). In contrast to temporal lobe epilepsy, Pi was not increased in the epileptogenic frontal lobe. These patients were chosen because they had well-defined frontal foci without evidence of focal lesions on MRI. Furthermore, five of the eight patients also had undergone PET studies, all of which were normal. Despite the absence of concordant imaging data (MRI or PET), MRSI was able to accurately predict the lateralization of the seizure focus. Studies are under way to investigate the ability of ^{31}P MRSI to accurately predict seizure localization in frontal lobe epilepsy.

CONCLUSIONS

Preliminary studies with MRS have demonstrated metabolic abnormalities in the epileptogenic zone, with the focus defined by increased Pi and pH and decreased PME. These changes accurately predict the side and site of seizure onset. In temporal lobe epilepsy, the sensitivity of MRS is as good as or better than that of PET. These findings need to be verified in large patient populations. It needs to be determined whether MRSI can accurately predict seizure localization in cases of nontemporal lobe epilepsy. Although MRSI is still in its infancy, it holds promise as an imaging technique for localizing a seizure focus preoperatively.

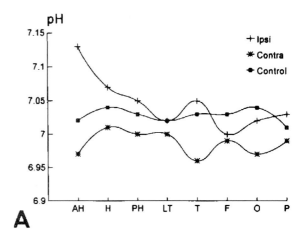

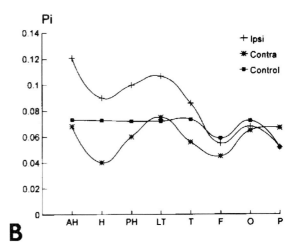

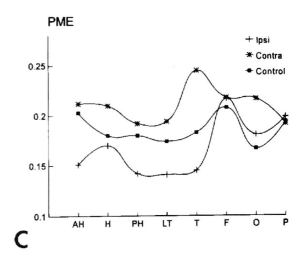

FIGURE 9-3. Regional (A) *pH*, (B) inorganic phosphorus (*Pi*), and (C) phosphomonoester (*PME*) metabolite concentrations in hemispheres ipsilateral and contralateral to anterior hippocampal seizure foci and in normal control subjects. (*AH*) anterior hippocampus, (*F*) summed frontal lobe, (*H*) hippocampus, (*LT*) lateral temporal lobe, (*O*) occipital lobe, (*P*) parietal lobe, (*PH*) posterior hippocampus, (*T*) temporal lobe.

REFERENCES

1. United States Commission for the Control of Epilepsy and Its Consequences. Plan for nationwide action on epilepsy (DHEW Publication No. [NIH] 78–276). Vol 1. Bethesda, Maryland: United States Department of Health, Education, and Welfare, Public Health Service, 1978.

2. Surgery for epilepsy (National Institutes of Health Consensus Conference). JAMA 1990;264:729–33.

3. Spencer DD, Spencer SS, Mattson RH, et al. Intracerebral masses in patients with intractable partial epilepsy. Neurology 1984;34:432–6.

4. Engel J Jr, Van Ness PC, Rasmussen TB, et al. Outcome with respect to epileptic seizures. In: Engel J Jr, ed. Surgical treatment of the epilepsies. 2nd ed. New York: Raven Press, 1993:609–21.

5. Jack CR Jr, Sharbrough FW, Cascino GD, et al. Magnetic resonance image-based hippocampal volumetry: correlation with outcome after temporal lobectomy. Ann Neurol 1992;31:138–46.

6. Garcia PA, Laxer KD, Barbaro NM, et al. Prognostic value of qualitative magnetic resonance imaging hippocampal abnormalities in patients undergoing temporal lobectomy for medically refractory seizures. Epilepsia 1994;35:520–4.

7. Matson GB, Weiner MW. Spectroscopy. In: Stark DD, Bradley WG Jr, eds. Magnetic resonance imaging. St. Louis: Mosby Year Book, 1992:438–78.

8. Hugg JW, Matson GB, Twieg DB, et al. Phosphorus-31 MR spectroscopic imaging (MRSI) of normal and pathological human brains. Magn Reson Imaging 1992;10:227–43.

9. Siesjö BK. Brain energy metabolism. Chichester, New York: John Wiley & Sons, 1978:345–79.

10. Schnall MD, Yoshizaki K, Chance B, et al. Triple nuclear NMR studies of cerebral metabolism during generalized seizure. Magn Reson Med 1988;6:15–23.

11. Yaksh TL, Anderson RE. In vivo studies on intracellular pH, focal flow, and vessel diameter in the cat cerebral cortex: effects of altered CO_2 and electrical stimulation. J Cereb Blood Flow Metab 1987;7:332–41.

12. Young RS, Osbakken MD, Briggs RW, et al. 31P NMR study of cerebral metabolism during prolonged seizures in the neonatal dog. Ann Neurol 1985;18:14–20.

13. Younkin DP, Delivoria-Papadopoulos M, Maris J, et al. Cerebral metabolic effects of neonatal seizures measured with in vivo ^{31}P NMR spectroscopy. Ann Neurol 1986;20:513–9.

14. Young RS, Cowan BE, Petroff OA, et al. In vivo 31P and in vitro 1H nuclear magnetic resonance study of hypoglycemia during neonatal seizure. Ann Neurol 1987;22:622–8.

15. Siesjö BK, von Hanwehr R, Nergelius G, et al. Extra- and intracellular pH in the brain during seizures and in the recovery period following the arrest of seizure activity. J Cereb Blood Flow Metab 1985;5:47–57.

16. Engel J Jr. Surgical treatment of the epilepsies. New York: Raven Press, 1987.

17. Engel J Jr, Rausch R, Lieb JP, et al. Correlation of criteria used for localizing epileptic foci in patients considered for surgical therapy of epilepsy. Ann Neurol 1981;9:215–24.

18. Engel J Jr, Kuhl DE, Phelps ME. A comparison of electrical and metabolic studies of brain function in epileptic patients: simultaneous EEG and positron emission computed tomography. Trans Am Neurol Assoc 1980;105:74–6.

19. Engel J Jr, Kuhl DE, Phelps ME, et al. Interictal cerebral glucose metabolism in partial epilepsy and its relation to EEG changes. Ann Neurol 1982;12:510–7.

20. Laxer KD, Hubesch B, Sappey-Marinier D, et al. Increased pH and inorganic phosphate in temporal seizure foci demonstrated by [31P]MRS. Epilepsia 1992;33:618–23.

21. Kuzniecky R, Elgavish GA, Hetherington HP, et al. In vivo 31P nuclear magnetic resonance spectroscopy of human temporal lobe epilepsy. Neurology 1992;42:1586–90.

22. Maudsley AA, Twieg DB, Sappey-Marinier D, et al. Spin echo 31P spectroscopic imaging in the human brain. Magn Reson Med 1990;14:415–22.

23. Maudsley AA, Hilal SK, Simon HE, et al. In vivo MR spectroscopic imaging with P-31. Work in progress. Radiology 1984;153:745–50.

24. Meyerhoff DJ, Maudsley AA, Schaefer S, et al. Phosphorus-31 magnetic resonance metabolite imaging in the human body. Magn Reson Imaging 1992;10:245–56.

25. Tropp JS, Sugiura S, Derby KA, et al. Characterization of MR spectroscopic imaging of the human head and limb at 2.0 T. Radiology 1988;169:207–12.

26. Twieg DB, Meyerhoff DJ, Hubesch B, et al. Phosphorus-31 magnetic resonance spectroscopy in humans by spectroscopic imaging: localized spectroscopy and metabolite imaging. Magn Reson Med 1989;12:291–305.

27. Vigneron DB, Nelson SJ, Murphy-Boesch J, et al. Chemical shift imaging of human brain: axial, sagittal, and coronal P-31 metabolite images. Radiology 1990;177:643–9.

28. Bailes DR, Bryant DJ, Bydder GM, et al. Localized phosphorus-31 NMR spectroscopy of normal and pathological human organs in vivo using phase-encoding techniques. J Magn Reson 1987;74:158–70.

29. Hugg JW, Laxer KD, Matson GB, et al. Lateralization of human focal epilepsy by ^{31}P magnetic resonance spectroscopic imaging. Neurology 1992;42:2011–8.

30. Laxer KD, van der Grond J, Gerson JR, et al. Temporal lobe epilepsy localization by ^{31}P magnetic resonance spectroscopic imaging (abstract). Epilepsia 1993;34 Suppl 6:122.

31. Garcia PA, Laxer KD, van der Grond J, et al. Phosphorus magnetic resonance spectroscopic imaging in patients with frontal lobe epilepsy. Ann Neurol 1994;35:217–21.

Functional Magnetic Resonance Imaging

Clifford R. Jack, Jr., Christine C. Lee, and Stephen J. Riederer

PHYSIOLOGY AND MAGNETIC RESONANCE IMAGING OF MENTAL TASK ACTIVATION

In functional magnetic resonance imaging (*f*MRI), it is important to distinguish clearly between regional alterations in cerebral hemodynamics that exist in a "resting," or baseline, state and those that result from a transient increase in local neuronal depolarization rate during the performance of certain mental tasks. During baseline conditions in normal brains, local cerebral blood flow is directly linked to local tissue metabolic rate. Conversely, a transient increase in the rate of neuronal depolarization induced by cognitive tasks produces a change in cerebral hemodynamics in and around the activated cerebral region or regions.[1-3] Positron emission tomography (PET) experiments in the mid-1980s demonstrated that sensory-motor or visual stimulation tasks produce the following local physiologic changes: increase in cerebral blood flow (up to 50%), increase in cerebral blood volume (approximately 7%), increase in glucose consumption (up to 50%), and a negligible increase in O_2 consumption (5%). The uncoupling of O_2 delivery (that is, cerebral blood flow) from O_2 metabolism leads to a decrease in the oxygen extraction fraction of about 30% and an increase in distal capillary and venous blood oxygenation.[1-3] ^{1}H magnetic resonance spectroscopic (MRS) studies of functional activation (not discussed in this chapter) have also demonstrated a local increase in brain lactic acid concentration during mental activation tasks.[4] The physiologic events described above provide two potential mechanisms for detection by MRI: (1) contrast based strictly on changes in local tissue perfusion, and (2) contrast based on local changes in blood oxygenation level. In this context, "contrast" refers to the sensitivity with which those areas of the brain in which a change in MR signal occurs as a result of mental activation can be identified.

Blood Oxygen Level–Dependent Contrast

The more widely studied of the two mechanisms has been blood oxygen level–dependent (BOLD) contrast, which is based on the local decoupling of oxygen delivery from metabolism during mental task activation.[5-7] That is, mental task activation leads to a local *increase* in the concentration of oxyhemoglobin. Deoxyhemoglobin is paramagnetic, whereas oxyhemoglobin is diamagnetic. In tissue, deoxyhemoglobin, like any paramagnetic substance, produces microscopic inhomogeneities in an externally applied magnetic field. These field inhomogeneities lead to more rapid loss of coherent precession of tissue protons during an image acquisition, that is, the effective T_2 relaxation time (T_2 eff) is shortened.[8-10] More specifically, the effective T_2 relaxation time is the sum of the relaxation effects of static field inhomogeneities (T_2*) in the absence of proton diffusion plus the effect of protons diffusing through a nonhomogeneous field (T_2), such that $1/T_2$ eff = $1/T_2$ + $1/T_2$*. The importance of these concepts is apparent below in the discussion of appropriate MR pulse sequences for fMRI imaging. Suffice it to say here that gradient echo sequences do not refocus or compensate for the effect of static field inhomogeneities during imaging and, thus, are T_2*-weighted, whereas spin echo pulse sequences do refocus and, thus, are T_2-weighted. BOLD contrast was first described by Ogawa et al.,[5-7] who suggested that this contrast mechanism could be used to image functionally active areas of the brain with MRI.[5,6] Several groups quickly extended this concept to in vivo identification of human brain function.[7,11,12] Although much of the initial work in fMRI with BOLD contrast was performed using high field strength magnets (4 T), high-speed imaging techniques, or both, it became apparent that fMRI could be performed at virtually any site with standard commercial MRI equipment.

This explanation of BOLD contrast is likely an oversimplification of the actual physiologic events that accompany activation of mental tasks. Optic imaging studies indicate that the initial response to sensory stimulation occurs from 200 ms to 400 ms after the onset of the stimulus.[13] This same early response has been observed at 500 ms with functional MR spectroscopic studies that show a decrease in the MR signal. This has been interpreted to be consistent with a local increase in the deoxyhemoglobin.[14] Optic imaging and functional spectroscopic studies both show that the early response is followed by a distinct and qualitatively different late response that consists of an increase in cerebral blood volume and a decrease in deoxyhemoglobin 1 to 3 seconds after stimulus onset.[13,14] The initial response is smaller in magnitude and confined to a more localized area of cerebral cortex than the late response. The initial response may represent increased O_2 utilization, whereas the late response may represent the "overshoot" of cerebral blood flow that provides the basis for the BOLD effect exploited in fMRI. This area is under active investigation.

Contrast Based on Blood Inflow

The second major mechanism of fMRI contrast is based solely on the change in cerebral blood flow/cerebral blood volume due to cerebral activation (that is, accompanying changes in blood oxygenation level are not a factor in image contrast of this type). Two broad classes of MR techniques have been used to image the local increase in cerebral blood flow/cerebral blood volume that occurs during activation of mental tasks: exogenous contrast bolus tracking and flow-sensitive MR imaging techniques.

Bolus Tracking

Imaging of mental task activation with MRI was described first by Belliveau et al.,[15] who used the contrast bolus tracking technique. This technique uses an exogenously administered MR contrast agent (the same contrast routinely used for diagnostic MRI). As the contrast bolus passes through the cerebral microcirculation, it increases local tissue magnetic susceptibility and leads to a transient decrease in tissue signal intensity, the magnitude of which is directly proportional to the dose of contrast *and* local cerebral blood volume.[16-18] The change in cerebral blood volume between active and nonactive mental states produces the "task activation contrast." The contrast bolus tracking technique is probably better suited to imaging static hemodynamic abnormalities (for example, those associated with tumor or stroke). It has been supplanted largely by techniques that exploit endogenous contrast mechanisms (BOLD or inflow effects).

Inflow

Inflow effects can be visualized noninvasively in two ways. The repeated radiofrequency excitation of a tissue slice during MR imaging decreases the number of spins aligned perpendicular to the plane of imaging (that is, decreases the longitudinal magnetization to a "steady state" level) during image acquisition. Thus, fully magnetized blood flowing into the slice of tissue (that is, the direction of flow is perpendicular to the slice) that is being imaged has a larger net longitudinal magnetization than the tissue in the imaging slice that has received a number of radiofrequency excitations. Inflow leads to increased signal intensity in the vessel itself, which is proportional to cerebral blood flow. Because intravascular water exchanges with extravascular tissue water during the imaging time, inflow produces an increase in the signal intensity of the tissue slice. The regional change in cerebral blood flow between active and nonactive mental states is the basis of the contrast in fMRI imaging techniques that use inflow effects.[11] Subtraction of images obtained without and with mental task activation reveals the change in signal intensity in those pixels having an increase in cerebral blood flow. Because no change in signal intensity occurs in those pixels that are not activated, the subtraction process results in cancellation or removal of inactive tissue pixels from the final functioning image. This is the same inflow effect that is exploited to produce time-of-flight MR angiographic images.

Alternatively, the longitudinal magnetization of "upstream" blood flowing into the imaging slice can be inverted or "tagged" by a radiofrequency pulse placed proximally in the direction of arterial flow and perpendicular to the imaging slice of interest.[19–21] "Tagged" spins, which have decreased longitudinal magnetization, flow into the imaging slice and replace the spins in the imaging slice that have a larger net longitudinal magnetization vector. This exchange *decreases* the net longitudinal magnetization of the tissue and, thus, effectively decreases the signal intensity of the tissue in the imaging slice in proportion to cerebral blood flow. The local increase in cerebral blood flow during task activation (change in cerebral blood flow) theoretically can be imaged at various points along the continuum of the vascular tree from artery to capillary to venous level. Visualization at the microvascular level (capillaries or microvenular level) is most desirable, because this is spatially specific for the area of cortex functionally activated. A potentially significant advantage of inflow over BOLD contrast mechanisms is that with proper attention to the timing of the inverting pulse, inflow techniques can localize the point source of *f*MRI contrast to the capillary tissue bed in the cerebral cortex, whereas BOLD techniques are weighted toward visualization of venous elements.

Blood Oxygen Level–Dependent vs Inflow

Several *f*MRI studies have indicated that in using the BOLD technique the *f*MRI signal is located partly or even predominantly in cortical veins rather than in the parenchyma, particularly at field strengths ≤1.5 T and when using gradient echo sequences.[22,23] However, several recent studies have indicated that much of what was labeled venous BOLD contrast in earlier *f*MRI studies was due to inflow effects.[24–27] Pulse sequence variables that accentuate inflow effects are those that tend to saturate the longitudinal magnetization of stationary tissue relative to that of fresh blood flowing into the imaging slice. Several early *f*MRI studies used precisely these imaging variables; as a result, activated pixels thought to reflect the BOLD contrast mechanism were most likely due partly to BOLD and partly to inflow (depending on the precise imaging variables used). A major operator-controlled determinant of BOLD contrast is the TE (BOLD is optimized at TE = T_2^* for GRE sequences and TE = T_2 for spin echo sequences). Conversely, short TR (relative to the T_1 of tissue), large flip angle, and thin slices accentuate inflow effects.

APPLICATIONS OF FUNCTIONAL MAGNETIC RESONANCE IMAGING

Initial *f*MRI demonstrations of human in vivo brain mapping used normal volunteers, who performed tasks that activated primary cortical areas of sensorimotor, visual, and auditory functions[7,11,12,28–39] (Figure 10-1). Subsequent studies demonstrated that the known somatotopic and retinotopic organization of these primary cortical

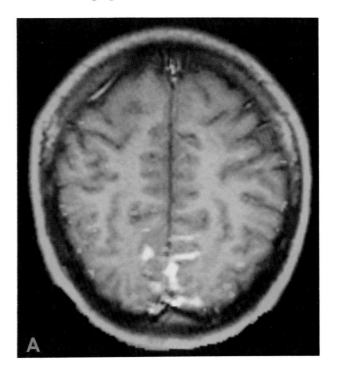

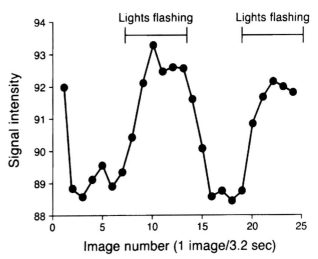

FIGURE 10-1. Functional MRI of visual activation. A. Results of full-field photic stimulation task obtained at 1.5 T using a standard radiofrequency spoiled gradient echo pulse sequence (60 ms TE). Images were acquired in an oblique plane parallel to the calcarine fissure. Pixels demonstrating significant activation were clustered in the calcarine cortex and are indicated in red. The functional map is superimposed on a matching T_1-weighted anatomical image. B. Plot of signal intensity in a region of interest encompassing the calcarine cortex versus time/image number. Note that signal intensity in the calcarine cortex increases during visual stimulation and decreases in darkness, that is, rest. (From Thompson et al.[74] By permission of the Radiological Society of North America.)

areas could be faithfully reproduced.[40–42] Ipsilateral cortical activation and hemispheric differences in activation that vary with handedness have been shown with a finger tapping task.[24,43] A number of functional systems have now been studied with fMRI. These include the supplementary and premotor cortical areas, the basal ganglia, and the cerebellum during sensorimotor tasks[44,45]; the primary and secondary motor and visual cortical areas activated during ideation and planning[46]; the visual cortex with changing stimulus patterns[47,48]; Broca's area and dorsolateral prefrontal cortex with word generation, semantic monitoring, and word fluency tasks[49]; the prefrontal areas activated during working memory[50]; and the hippocampus with declarative memory tasks.[51] Other functional systems studied include those involved with gustatory and olfactory processing, auditory recognition, linguistic and attention processing,[47] and sex-based differences in cerebral hemisphere specificity for information processing.[52] In vivo and mathematical modeling studies have been performed that probe basic mechanisms of fMRI contrast, its physiologic basis, the anatomical location of the fMRI activation signal, image processing strategies for signal localization, and the effect of a number of imaging parameters on the fMRI signal.[53–61] Hemodynamic changes that occur during seizures have been demonstrated.[62] Specific applications of fMRI to epilepsy are discussed below.

CURRENT ISSUES

A number of issues, many of which are related, are under active investigation in fMRI.

Sensitivity and Specificity

Which fMRI imaging method provides the greatest sensitivity and specificity? Ideally, the point source of the functional activation signal is located only within the neurons that are activated by a particular mental task. Instead, fMRI contrast is derived from the local hemodynamic changes that accompany task activation. The point source of the activation signal with fMRI is located in the vascular bed and surrounding perivascular tissues. The most desirable functional anatomical specificity would occur for an fMRI point source located in the microcirculation (capillary bed) that perfuses only those neurons responsible for performing a given mental task. BOLD contrast is dependent on differing levels of deoxyhemoglobin between the active and the nonactive states. The percentage of hemoglobin molecules that have exchanged O_2 for CO_2 increases as a bolus of blood traverses the capillary bed and is maximum when capillaries coalesce into venules. Therefore, the BOLD effect is most pronounced at the distal capillary and venous level. A concern with BOLD imaging has been that the point source of fMRI contrast may be located predominantly in macroscopic draining veins rather than in the microcirculation. This should not present a problem if the point source of the BOLD activation signal is located in the pial venules immediately adjacent to the set of activated neurons. However, it does become a significant problem if the "bolus of oxyhemoglobin" produced by mental activation has moved downstream in the venous drainage system away from the activated neurons. To the extent that this latter mechanism occurs, there is a loss of spatial and temporal resolution with BOLD fMRI and a concomitant loss of precision for functional brain mapping. The precise location of the point source of fMRI activation with the BOLD technique (microcirculation, pial venous structures, or large cortical veins, or some combination of the three) is currently an area of significant interest in fMRI. This "vein vs brain" discussion is intimately related to the issues of field strength, imaging methods, and pulse sequence discussed below.

Field Strength

Interest in fMRI has produced an interesting phenomenon in the field of MR, where high-field diagnostic MR imagers (1.5 T) are considered to represent low-field fMRI imagers, and high-field fMRI studies are those performed at 3 T or 4 T. Image contrast-to-noise increases about linearly with field strength, thus conferring an obvious advantage to high-field systems. More importantly, modeling and in vivo studies suggest that the susceptibility effects that are the basis for BOLD contrast increase exponentially with field strength.[53,54,59] Susceptibility effects are pronounced at the level of the cerebral microcirculation at high field but at the macrocirculation level in magnets operating at field strengths used in clinical imaging (< 2.0 T). Therefore, high field strength confers a significant advantage over magnets operating at standard clinical field strengths *both* in fMRI sensitivity and specificity. Currently, only a few high-field whole-body imagers are in operation in the world, and these systems are quite expensive. There is great interest in identifying techniques that would improve both the sensitivity and specificity of fMRI at the widely available field strengths in the 1 T to 2 T range.

Pulse Sequence

Spin echo pulse sequences weight the fMRI signal toward the level of the microcirculation, whereas gradient echo sequences weight the signal toward vascular structures 10 μm and greater (that is, venous structures).[53–58] Echo-shifted sequences (these use a 180° refocusing pulse, but the gradient echo is shifted away from the center of the spin echo) lie between these two.[58] The fMRI activation signal is significantly greater with gradient echo than with spin echo techniques. Therein lies the problem. At 1.5 T, the magnitude of the fMRI signal using a BOLD gradient echo technique, although small (2% to 5%), is nonetheless reliably detectable. However, the point source of this signal is weighted toward a less desirable location, larger veins. Conversely, with spin echo techniques, the point source of the signal is weighted more toward the microcirculation, but it is so small that detection is a problem. Investigators working at 1.5 T may be limited to gradient-recalled echo or echo-shifted techniques for some applications and, thus, create ƒMRI images weighted toward the venous system. Investigators working at high fields have greater inherent ƒMRI contrast-to-noise and, thus, have the luxury of using spin echo sequences to improve specificity, if so desired.

Imaging Method

What is the optimal way to image mental task activation? As mentioned above, much of the effort in ƒMRI has focused on the BOLD approach. Contrast is weighted toward the venous circulation with BOLD. With correct timing of the "tagging" pulse, contrast can be weighted toward the capillary/tissue level with inflow techniques measuring induced perfusion changes. However, some limitations exist with inflow techniques. Spin tagging requires that arterial flow perpendicular to the anatomical slice of interest exists and can be identified readily for proximal spin tagging. This may not always be the case in brain regions with complex and overlapping routes of arterial supply. Three-dimensional or whole brain functional imaging may also be a problem for the above reason.

Imaging Speed and Gradient Hardware

Several of the pioneering groups of investigators in ƒMRI have used echo planar imaging (EPI) techniques.[11] EPI is the fastest MR imaging technique available. After radiofrequency excitation, the readout gradient is rapidly modulated to create a series of echoes. All the data necessary for reconstructing a complete image can be acquired in a single excitation or "shot." EPI is usually associated with high-performance gradient systems; the combination of the EPI pulse sequence and the high-performance gradients enable production of a complete cross-sectional image in less than 100 ms. Standard imagers use whole-body gradient coils with a maximum gradient strength of roughly 10 mT/m and a rise time from zero to maximum on the order of 0.5 ms. This is distinguished from high-performance gradient systems used for single-shot EPI, which may have strengths of 20 mT/m or higher and rise times as short as 50 µs. At least two significant advantages exist for single-shot EPI with high-performance gradients in comparison with non-single-shot pulse sequences using standard imaging gradients. One is related to the problem of motion artifacts discussed below, and the other is related to anatomical coverage per unit of time. Investigators performing non-

single-shot ƒMRI acquisition protocols are relegated to producing ƒMRI examinations that have either limited anatomical coverage (perhaps four or fewer anatomical imaging slices) or excessively long acquisition protocols. This has led, in our hands at least, to the approach of carefully identifying normal anatomical landmarks and acquiring single-slice ƒMRI acquisitions in a few well-chosen anatomical planes. Unfortunately, this approach is predicated on "knowing where to look" in advance in order to appropriately place the imaging slices for functional acquisition. This is intellectually unsatisfactory. It also leads to practical difficulties. However, by virtue of greater imaging speed, EPI ƒMRI examinations performed with high-performance gradients can cover most or all the brain in a reasonable imaging time. The principal disadvantage of high-performance gradient systems is that to exploit the speed capability the bandwidth of the signal must be increased, thereby decreasing the signal-to-noise ratio (SNR).[63] Depending on the specific experiment performed, this may or may not be important. This issue of high-performance versus standard gradients may not be significant in the future because the major MR manufacturers have (or soon will have) commercially available high-performance gradient systems. Whole-body high-performance gradient systems or head-only insert subsystems[64] that can be retrofitted to existing scanners are now commercially available. Therefore, it seems likely that in the future most fMR imaging may be performed with high-performance gradient systems that permit single-shot acquisitions.

Single-shot EPI requires specialized high-performance gradient hardware and must be distinguished from interleaved EPI, which can be performed with slower standard gradient systems.[65] With interleaved EPI, the basic concept of a rapidly modulating readout gradient remains intact. However, because of the slower gradient slew rate, a limited number of readout gradient modulations can occur during the $T_2{}^*$ decay envelope of a single excitation. Thus, multiple interleaves or shots through k-space are necessary to acquire sufficient data to reconstruct a single imaging slice. This is the approach currently used at our institution on a standard 1.5 T GE Signa system.

Motion

A major problem in ƒMRI is movement by the subject. In our experience, this problem is significantly more pronounced with imaging patients than with imaging normal volunteer subjects. It is necessary to limit head motion as much as possible during the acquisition of a series of images. Techniques for fixing the head in the magnet more rigidly than is normally done during clinical imaging include suction devices, custom-fit bite bars, and molded face mask restraints. Although these techniques are effective to some degree, they do not entirely eliminate motion. Three main types of motion occur in the head: bulk voluntary head movement unassociated with respiration, head movement associated with respiration, and heart-driven pulsatile motion of the brain, the overlying vessels, and the cerebrospinal fluid.[66,67] Another source of motion-related fMRI artifact is respiratory diaphragmatic movement that appears to induce cyclic phase shifts in brain images, presumably due to changes in the static magnetic field.[67] Motion-related imaging artifacts can be divided conceptually into two categories: intraimage motion and interimage motion. Intraimage motion refers to motion that occurs during the period of time that the views needed to reconstruct a single image are being acquired. With non–single-shot fMRI techniques, it is inevitable that different views near the center of k-space (lines of data that contribute most of the image contrast) occur during different brain "physiologic" states. For example, some echoes are collected in full inspiration, some in full expiration, and others at all points in between. This creates image blurring. The major advantage of single-shot EPI over all non–single-shot techniques is that with the former technique a complete image can be generated in as little as 100 ms. This is rapid enough to "freeze" nonrandom physiologic brain and vessel motion produced by the cardiac and respiratory cycles.[68] Conversely, non–single-shot EPI techniques require that a single image be created or built up over many cardiac/respiratory cycles. Thus, fluctuations in pixel intensity due to these physiologic cycles are unavoidably built into non–single-shot EPI images and may present as significant artifacts when an fMRI time series is analyzed.

Interimage motion occurs between successive images in an fMRI time series. This problem cannot be solved by using single-shot EPI acquisition. Although single-shot EPI is useful for eliminating the effects of periodic brain motion such as that induced by the systolic cardiac pulse, it is not effective at correcting for the effects of bulk head motion in which the position of the head is shifted over a period of several minutes while the activation task is cycled off and on. If the subject's head moves on successive images through a time series, then spatial realignment of the images in the series is necessary to extract meaningful functional information. Techniques such as navigator echoes or retrospective registration of a series of images have been proposed to deal with the problem of interimage misregistration.[69–71]

Data Processing

With fMRI, several images are produced over time as a mental task is alternated off, on, off, on, etc. Different ways of processing these serial time course images have been proposed. Initially, processing of the fMRI time course data was accomplished by simply subtracting the active from nonactive images or by using maps based on the t statistic or z statistic.[72] These were later supplemented by algorithms implementing cross-correlation, autocorrelation, cluster detection, and various statistical nonparametric mapping approaches.[32,60] The "best" approach has not been determined.

Stimulus Delivery

A significant challenge for fMRI is the development of appropriate activation stimulus paradigms. Many mental tasks, particularly those involving higher cognitive function, activate a distributed network of brain processing centers. To produce a functional image that localizes the discrete brain areas responsible for a specific higher order processing activity, the stimulus paradigm must be designed carefully. Images obtained during control conditions should contain a stimulus that includes all cognitive processing activity except the targeted higher order function, and the "active" stimulus task should contain baseline activity in conjunction with the desired targeted functional task. This has been recognized by PET researchers for years. The delivery of specific stimuli and the recording of a subject's responses are considerably more difficult for MRI than for PET. Compared with PET, the MRI environment is physically constrained and extremely noisy, and the delivery of stimuli, the recording of physiologic data, and the recordings of the subjects' responses are difficult, requiring complex electromagnetic shielding schemes, because videoscreens commonly used to display stimuli in PET cannot be used in the MRI environment. Consequently, the development of appropriate stimulus paradigms and the tools with which to deliver stimuli and to record responses in coordination with the MR imaging pulse sequences is a major challenge for fMRI.

Functional Magnetic Resonance Imaging and Other Brain Mapping Modalities

Currently, several different techniques are used for brain mapping, including PET, magnetic source imaging (MSI), fMRI, event-related potential (ERP), mapping transcranial magnetic stimulation, direct intraoperative cortical stimulation in awake patients, extraoperative stimulation mapping after subdural grid insertion, operatively recorded sensory evoked potentials, and optic imaging.[31] Applications for in vivo brain mapping can be divided roughly into those that are primarily for research and those that are used for clinical management of patients, mainly neurosurgical planning. Brain mapping techniques applicable to neurobiologic research in volunteer subjects obviously are limited to noninvasive ones. These are primarily ERP/MSI (which are considered together), PET, and fMRI (Table 10-1). PET has an advantage over fMRI in terms of flexibility, quantitation, and sensitivity. Applications demanding high sensitivity and specificity, such as neuroreceptor density, or the ability to quantify physiologic variables are best accomplished with PET. As yet, fMRI is quantified in terms of percent signal change, which bears

TABLE 10-1. Noninvasive Functional Imaging Modalities*

	PET	ƒMRI	ERP/MSI
Sensitivity	+	−	−
Spatial resolution†	−	+	−
Temporal resolution	−	−	+
Specificity for neuronal activation	−	−	+
Cost/availability‡	−	+	−
Flexibility§	+	−	−
Quantification	+	−	−
Ease of registration with magnetic resonance image anatomical template	−	+	−
Repeatability in single subject	−	+	+

ERP, event-related potential; ƒMRI, functional magnetic resonance imaging; MSI, magnetic source imaging; PET, positron emission tomography.

*"+" indicates that the modality has a clear advantage over the others.

†See discussion of vein versus brain with BOLD ƒMRI contrast.

‡See discussion of field strength with ƒMRI.

§Ability to identify and measure different physiologic variables associated with activation such as with PET, O_2 and glucose metabolism, cerebral blood volume, cerebral blood flow, and receptor imaging.

no direct relationship to any single physiologic variable. Because a radioisotope is administered in PET, this method is hampered by limited repeatability in single subjects, thus requiring intersubject data pooling. Also, because $H_2^{15}O$ is required and ^{15}O has a 2-minute half-life, a cyclotron must be on site to perform functional activation studies. The advantages of ƒMRI are greater spatial resolution, the greatest ease of registration with an MRI anatomical template, the lowest cost, and the greatest availability. The temporal resolution of ERP/MSI exceeds that of both PET and ƒMRI by several orders of magnitude. Neurobiologic research applications that demand extremely high temporal resolution would therefore be accommodated best with ERP/MSI. However, the inverse problem in ERP/MSI renders spatial resolution/anatomical specificity a problem.

FUNCTIONAL MAGNETIC RESONANCE IMAGING IN EPILEPSY

The obvious application of ƒMRI to epilepsy is for presurgical planning, that is, identification of the anatomical relationships between functionally important areas and the cortical area or areas targeted for surgical resection. The primary functional areas critical for neurosurgical planning are sensorimotor, speech, language, and memory function. Currently, most brain mapping for neurosurgical purposes is performed with electrical recording. Amytal testing could also be considered a brain mapping technique for memory, speech, and language, albeit with crude spatial resolution. Both of these methods are invasive and, at least in the case of electrical brain mapping, expensive. Replacing invasive or expensive (or both) tech-

niques with ones that are equally accurate, less expensive, and less invasive is a rational objective. In the clinical setting, expediency, cost, and availability take on increased importance, and ƒMRI has considerable advantages over both PET and MSI in this regard. It may be that ƒMRI at standard clinical field strengths will have its greatest impact clinically for surgical brain mapping.

To date, we have performed ƒMRI studies for preoperative mapping of the sensorimotor area in 20 patients with epilepsy.[73,74] We perform single-slice functional acquisition series, using an interleaved EPI sequence.[65] A functional examination consists of two to four different series acquisitions at each of three to four anatomical slice locations. The success of the procedure can be defined on two levels. At the first level, one can ask whether the study produced a reasonable functional map of the sensorimotor activation; specifically, from the surgeon's point of view, was the functional central sulcus identified? We have been able to accomplish this unequivocally in 9 of 20 patients (Figure 10-2). The reasons for failure in the other 11 patients are as follows: The ƒMRI studies were corrupted by patient head motion in nine and markedly degraded by bulk susceptibility artifacts at the site of a previous craniotomy in one. We assumed that these artifacts were due to small bits of ferrous metal embedded in the skull during the craniotomy (Figure 10-3). The artifacts resembled those occasionally seen in the cervical spine after anterior diskectomy. On the basis of anatomical criteria, one other patient had a tumor near the face-tongue portion of the sensorimotor homunculus.[75] Although several motion-free ƒMRI series were generated, we were

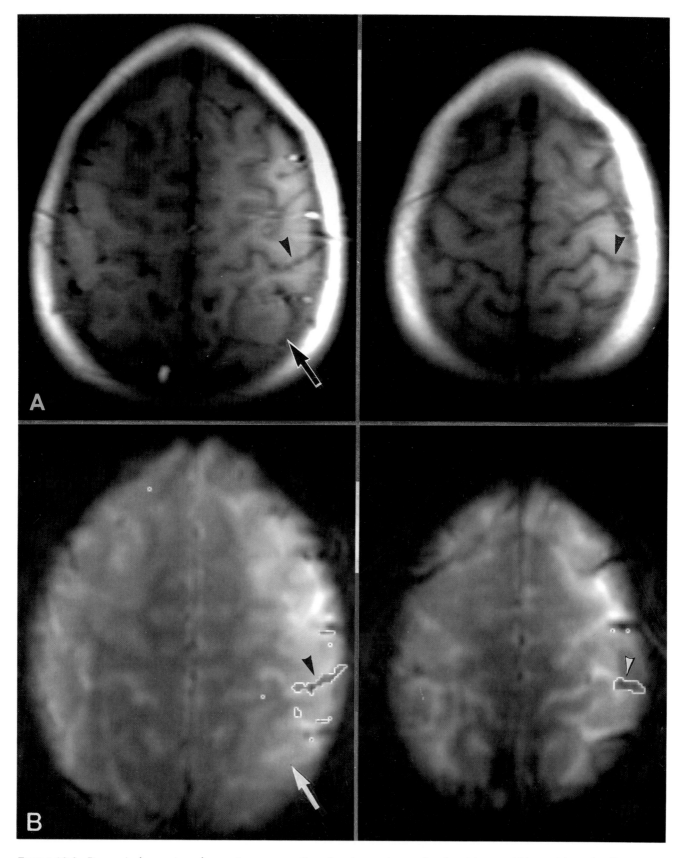

FIGURE 10-2. Presurgical mapping of sensorimotor area. Functional mapping study of an 11-year-old boy with medically intractable seizures of left hemispheric onset. A. Two short TR/TE anatomical images; the more inferior slice (*left*) shows a structural lesion (presumably a cortical tuber) in the left perirolandic region (*arrow*). B. Functional MRI study (*f*MRI)   (*continued*)

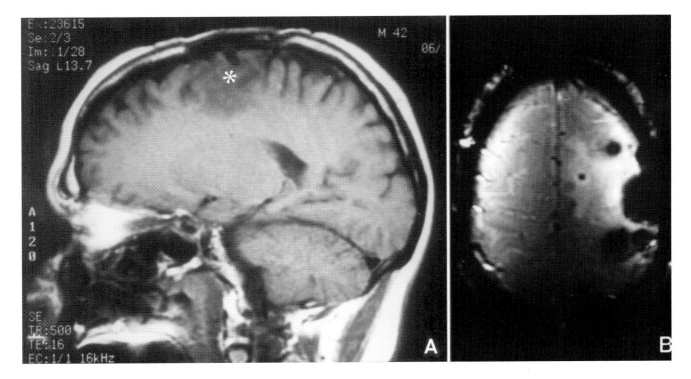

FIGURE 10-3. Postsurgical susceptibility artifact. The patient had a left perirolandic low-grade tumor producing intractable seizure disorder. Biopsy of the tumor had been performed 10 years before our attempted functional MRI mapping study. A. Parasagittal short TE/TR image showing the tumor (*asterisk*) and overlying craniotomy. B. A single interleaved echo planar image from a functional MRI time series (using phased array surface coils) showing several large areas of signal loss due to bulk susceptibility artifact that obscured the area of interest for functional mapping. Plain film radiography revealed no metal fragments in the skull or scalp. We hypothesized that microscopic metallic fragments were embedded in the skull at the time of the previous craniotomy, producing susceptibility artifacts. The effect was subtle enough that no artifact was seen with a short TE spin echo sequence (A) but was evident with a long TE gradient echo sequence (B).

FIGURE 10-2 (*continued*).   performed at the same two slice locations as the images in A, using an interleaved echo planar imaging acquisition in single-slice mode to assess the relationship of the functional central sulcus to this lesion. The activation stimulus was brushing of the right palm; 96 serial images were processed using cross-correlation analysis with a threshold value of 0.48.[32] The functional map, consisting of pixels whose correlation coefficient exceeded 0.48 (*in red*), was then superimposed on one of the interleaved echo planar images from the time series. Homemade dual-phased array surface coils were used for the *f*MRI study, which accounts for the shading toward the center of the head. In the inferior slice (*left*), activation signals that met criteria for significance were located in three left hemispheric sulci, although most of the significantly activated pixels were concentrated in the middle sulcus (*arrowheads in A and B*). This middle sulcus was contiguous with the only sulcus demonstrating significant activation (*arrowheads*) on the superior slice (*right*). We presumed that this was the central sulcus; therefore, the central sulcus was anterior to the lesion (*arrow*).

unable to demonstrate any obvious area of functional activation. We attributed this failure to constraints imposed by operating with standard gradient hardware in single-slice mode; we were unable to pick an anatomical slice based on a priori anatomical landmarks that included the tumor plus an activated area.

The second level at which presurgical sensorimotor mapping with *f*MRI in patients with epilepsy can be evaluated is the degree to which the *f*MRI result is concordant with electrical methods of functional cortical mapping. Of the nine patients in whom a satisfactory map of the sensorimotor area was generated, three subsequently had invasive cortical mapping that was sufficient to allow precise correlation between electrical and *f*MRI localization. In two of the three patients, the method of electrical localization was intraoperative sensory evoked potential recording. In the third patient, electrical localization was accomplished by intraoperative sensory evoked potential recording and by implantation of subdural electrode strips with extraoperative cortical stimulation mapping (Figure 10-4). In all three patients,

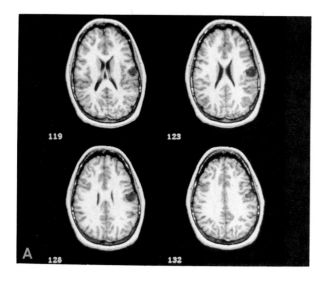

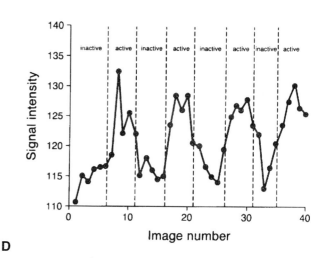

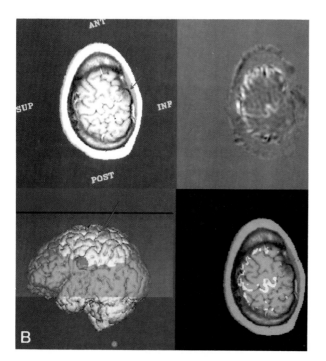

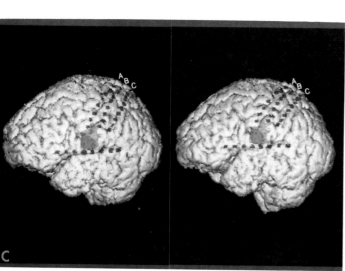

FIGURE 10-4. Sensorimotor mapping with invasive electroencephalographic correlation. A. Axial T_1-weighted images showing low-grade neoplasm in left perirolandic region (biopsy-proved grade 2 oligodendroglioma). B. Four-panel collage. *Upper left,* obliquely oriented T_1-weighted anatomical template of the cross-section in which the corresponding functional MRI sequence was obtained (*red arrow indicates the tumor*). (*ANT*) anterior, (*POST*) posterior, (*SUP*) superior, and (*INF*) inferior. *Upper right,* results of the functional activation study (self-paced finger-to-thumb tapping plus tongue movement). *Lower right,* created by assigning a color map to the functional image and superimposing that onto T_1-weighted anatomical template. The serpiginous functional activation signal observed in upper and lower right panels represented the functional central sulcus on the basis of functional MRI study (*red arrows in both panels*). *Lower left,* a volume rendering of the brain surface, with the tumor rendered as a separate green object and with the oblique plane in which functional MRI was obtained, indicated as a shaded gray planar surface. C. Three-dimensional rendering of the brain surface, with positions of the electrodes of four different subdural strips in red (corresponding to A–D) and the tumor in green. Invasive mapping with subdurally implanted electrode strips and operative sensory evoked potential recording documented that the central sulcus was located between vertically oriented strips A and B. Comparison of the surface rendering of the brain in C and B proves that central sulcus location predicted by functional MRI matched that determined with invasive electrical recording. D. Time-course plot of signal intensity from a region of interest in left sensorimotor area, demonstrating cyclic change in signal intensity, which follows the periodicity of activation task. (From Jack et al.[73] By permission of the Radiological Society of North America.)

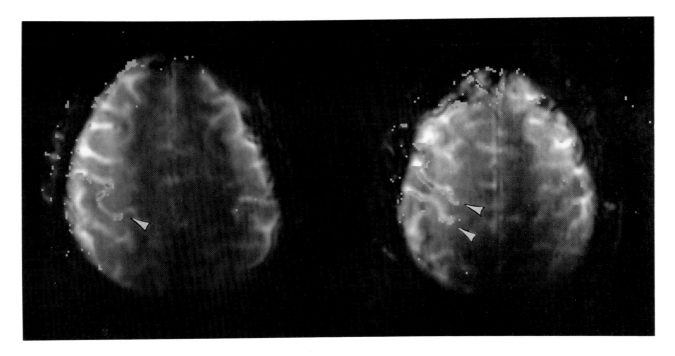

FIGURE 10-5. Intersubject variability in sensorimotor activation. Functional MRI (*f*MRI) studies in two different right-handed adult volunteers. Both performed an identical self-paced finger-to-thumb tapping task with the left hand. The method of *f*MRI acquisition (interleaved echo planar imaging single-slice acquisition at 1.5 T with phased array surface coil) was identical in the two studies. The method of processing *f*MRI data (cross-correlation with correlation coefficient of 0.48) was also identical, and cephalocaudal location of the anatomical slice was about the same in both volunteers. Note that in the volunteer on the left the activation is confined to a single sulcus (*arrowhead*) and activation in the volunteer on the right is in two adjacent sulci in the paracentral region (*arrowheads*).

precise concordance was demonstrated between the *f*MRI localization of the central sulcus and that obtained invasively.

Although the ability of *f*MRI to identify the functional sensorimotor area may appear to be a problem that has been entirely resolved, several key issues remain before this technique can be considered a clinically reliable test. First, we often find, in patients and volunteers, *f*MRI activation that meets statistical criteria for significance in more than one cortical sulcus (Figure 10-5). Furthermore, the method of processing the *f*MRI time series, which currently appears to be a fairly arbitrary choice made by individual investigators, can markedly influence the interpretation of the *f*MRI study (Figure 10-6). However, neurosurgeons need to know unequivocally which sulcus is the central sulcus. The second issue relates to the observation that some areas of the brain may be resected surgically with no apparent deficit but not others. If the primary motor strip is surgically violated, paresis results. Conversely, premotor cortical areas may be resected

without any apparent long-term adverse effects. In performing functional studies, the central sulcus region will routinely activate with a finger-tapping task but so will other "surgically insignificant" areas. Therefore, a distinction must be made between *f*MRI activation that is "surgically significant" and that which is "surgically insignificant." If *f*MRI is to become a useful routine procedure for preoperative planning, then criteria must be established to differentiate functionally active areas that can be surgically resected from those that cannot be resected.

In conclusion, preoperative surgical planning is a promising and potentially important application of *f*MRI in clinical practice. It also represents an ideal opportunity to correlate *f*MRI results with the established techniques of invasive electrical cortical mapping or, in the case of speech and language, amytal testing. Such correlative studies are necessary not only to establish the validity of the clinical usefulness of *f*MRI but to validate basic assumptions made about the neurophysiology underlying observed *f*MRI changes.

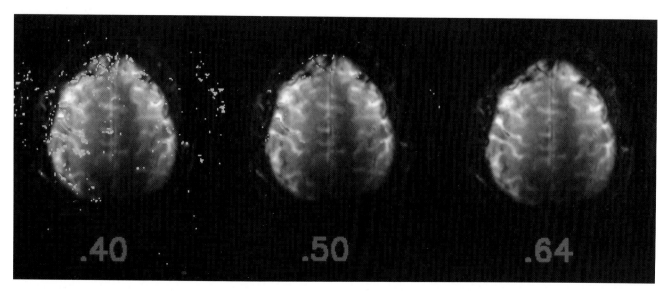

FIGURE 10-6. Effect of data processing on functional interpretation. Functional MRI (*f*MRI) of volunteer performing a unilateral (left hand) self-paced finger-to-thumb tapping task. Images were acquired using an interleaved echo planar imaging single-slice sequence with a homemade dual-phased array surface coil. The 96 time series images were processed using a cross-correlation algorithm. The image on the left is the result of a cross-correlation analysis with a correlation coefficient of 0.40; the middle image, with a correlation coefficient of 0.50; and the image on the right, with a correlation coefficient of 0.64. As the correlation coefficient is increased, the noise in the functional image is decreased. However, inspection of the image on the left (correlation coefficient of 0.40) would lead to the conclusion that the sensorimotor task produced significant activation in two adjacent sulci in the paracentral region. Conversely, the image on the right (correlation coefficient of 0.64) would lead to the conclusion that significant activation was located in a single sulcus in the paracentral region.

REFERENCES

1. Fox PT, Raichle ME, Mintun MA, et al. Nonoxidative glucose consumption during focal physiologic neural activity. Science 1988;241:462–4.

2. Fox PT, Mintun MA, Raichle ME, et al. Mapping human visual cortex with positron emission tomography. Nature 1986;323:806–9.

3. Fox PT, Raichle ME. Focal physiological uncoupling of cerebral blood flow and oxidative metabolism during somatosensory stimulation in human subjects. Proc Natl Acad Sci USA 1986;83:1140–4.

4. Prichard J, Rothman D, Novotny E, et al. Lactate rise detected by 1H NMR in human visual cortex during physiologic stimulation. Proc Natl Acad Sci USA 1991;88:5829–31.

5. Ogawa S, Lee TM, Nayak AS, et al. Oxygenation-sensitive contrast in magnetic resonance image of rodent brain at high magnetic fields. Magn Reson Med 1990;14:68–78.

6. Ogawa S, Lee TM, Kay AR, et al. Brain magnetic resonance imaging with contrast dependent on blood oxygenation. Proc Natl Acad Sci USA 1990;87:9868–72.

7. Ogawa S, Tank DW, Menon R, et al. Intrinsic signal changes accompanying sensory stimulation: functional brain mapping with magnetic resonance imaging. Proc Natl Acad Sci USA 1992;89:5951–5.

8. Brindle KM, Brown FF, Campbell ID, et al. Application of spin-echo nuclear magnetic resonance to whole-cell systems. Membrane transport. Biochem J 1979;180:37–44.

9. Thulborn KR, Waterton JC, Matthews PM, et al. Oxygenation dependence of the transverse relaxation time of water protons in whole blood at high field. Biochim Biophys Acta 1982;714:265–70.

10. Turner R, Le Bihan D, Moonen CT, et al. Echo-planar time course MRI of cat brain oxygenation changes. Magn Reson Med 1991;22:159–66.

11. Kwong KK, Belliveau JW, Chesler DA, et al. Dynamic magnetic resonance imaging of human brain activity during primary sensory stimulation. Proc Natl Acad Sci USA 1992;89:5675–9.

12. Bandettini PA, Wong EC, Hinks RS, et al. Time course EPI of human brain function during task activation. Magn Reson Med 1992;25:390–7.

13. Frostig RD, Lieke EE, Ts'o DY, et al. Cortical functional architecture and local coupling between neuronal activity and the microcirculation revealed by in vivo high-resolution optical imaging of intrinsic signals. Proc Natl Acad Sci USA 1990;87:6082–6.

14. Ernst T, Hennig J. Observation of a fast response in functional MR. Magn Reson Med 1994;32:146–9.

15. Belliveau JW, Kennedy DN Jr, McKinstry RC, et al. Functional mapping of the human visual cortex by magnetic resonance imaging. Science 1991;254:716–9.

16. Rosen BR, Belliveau JW, Vevea JM, et al. Perfusion imaging with NMR contrast agents. Magn Reson Med 1990;14:249–65.

17. Rosen BR, Belliveau JW, Buchbinder BR, et al. Contrast agents and cerebral hemodynamics. Magn Reson Med 1991;19:285–92.

18. Villringer A, Rosen BR, Belliveau JW, et al. Dynamic imaging with lanthanide chelates in normal brain: contrast due to magnetic susceptibility effects. Magn Reson Med 1988;6:164–74.

19. Detre JA, Leigh JS, Williams DS, et al. Perfusion imaging. Magn Reson Med 1992;23:37–45.

20. Williams DS, Detre JA, Leigh JS, et al. Magnetic resonance imaging of perfusion using spin inversion of arterial water. Proc Natl Acad Sci USA 1992;89:212–6.

21. Edelman RR, Siewert B, Darby DG, et al. Qualitative mapping of cerebral blood flow and functional localization with echo-planar MR imaging and signal targeting with alternating radio frequency. Radiology 1994;192:513–20.

22. Lai S, Hopkins AL, Haacke EM, et al. Identification of vascular structures as a major source of signal contrast in high resolution 2D and 3D functional activation imaging of the motor cortex at 1.5T: preliminary results. Magn Reson Med 1993;30:387–92.

23. Segebarth C, Belle V, Delon C, et al. Functional MRI of the human brain: predominance of signals from extracerebral veins. Neuroreport 1994;5:813–6.

24. Kim S-G, Hendrich K, Hu X, et al. Potential pitfalls of functional MRI using conventional gradient-recalled echo techniques. NMR Biomed 1994;7:69–74.

25. Duyn JH, Moonen CT, van Yperen GH, et al. Inflow versus deoxyhemoglobin effects in BOLD functional MRI using gradient echoes at 1.5 T. NMR Biomed 1994;7:83–8.

26. Haacke EM, Hopkins A, Lai S, et al. 2D and 3D high resolution gradient echo functional imaging of the brain: venous contributions to signal in motor cortex studies. NMR Biomed 1994;7:54–62.

27. Frahm J, Merboldt KD, Hanicke W, et al. Brain or vein—oxygenation or flow? On signal physiology in functional MRI of human brain activation. NMR Biomed 1994;7:45–53.

28. Connelly A, Jackson GD, Frackowiak RS, et al. Functional mapping of activated human primary cortex with a clinical MR imaging system. Radiology 1993;188:125–30.

29. Menon RS, Ogawa S, Kim SG, et al. Functional brain mapping using magnetic resonance imaging. Signal changes accompanying visual stimulation. Invest Radiol 1992;27 Suppl 2:S47–S53.

30. Frahm J, Bruhn H, Merboldt KD, et al. Dynamic MR imaging of human brain oxygenation during rest and photic stimulation. J Magn Reson Imaging 1992;2:501–5.

31. Belliveau JW, Kwong KK, Kennedy DN, et al. Magnetic resonance imaging mapping of brain function. Human visual cortex. Invest Radiol 1992;27 Suppl 2:S59–65.

32. Bandettini PA, Jesmanowicz A, Wong EC, et al. Processing strategies for time-course data sets in functional MRI of the human brain. Magn Reson Med 1993;30:161–73.

33. Binder JR, Rao SM, Hammeke TA, et al. Functional magnetic resonance imaging of human auditory cortex. Ann Neurol 1994;35:662–72.

34. Schad LR, Trost U, Knopp MV, et al. Motor cortex stimulation measured by magnetic resonance imaging on a standard 1.5 T clinical scanner. Magn Reson Imaging 1993;11:461–4.

35. Frahm J, Merboldt KD, Hanicke W. Functional MRI of human brain activation at high spatial resolution. Magn Reson Med 1993;29:139–44.

36. Blamire AM, Ogawa S, Ugurbil K, et al. Dynamic mapping of the human visual cortex by high-speed magnetic resonance imaging. Proc Natl Acad Sci USA 1992;89:11069–73.

37. Hajnal JV, Collins AG, White SJ, et al. Imaging of human brain activity at 0.15 T using fluid attenuated inversion recovery (FLAIR) pulse sequences. Magn Reson Med 1993; 30:650–3.

38. Constable RT, Kennan RP, Puce A, et al. Functional NMR imaging using fast spin echo at 1.5 T. Magn Reson Med 1994;31:686–90.

39. Duyn JH, Mattay VS, Sexton RH, et al. 3-dimensional functional imaging of human brain using echo-shifted FLASH MRI. Magn Reson Med 1994;32:150–5.

40. Cao Y, Towle VL, Levin DN, et al. Functional mapping of human motor cortical activation with conventional MR imaging at 1.5 T. J Magn Reson Imaging 1993;3:869–75.

41. Schneider W, Noll DC, Cohen JD. Functional topographic mapping of the cortical ribbon in human vision with conventional MRI scanners. Nature 1993;365:150–3.

42. Engel SA, Rumelhart DE, Wandell BA, et al. *f*MRI of human visual cortex (letter). Nature 1994;369:525.

43. Kim SG, Ashe J, Georgopoulos AP, et al. Functional imaging of human motor cortex at high magnetic field. J Neurophysiol 1993;69:297–302.

44. Rao SM, Binder JR, Bandettini PA, et al. Functional magnetic resonance imaging of complex human movements. Neurology 1993;43:2311–8.

45. Ellerman JM, Flament D, Kim SG, et al. Spatial patterns of functional activation of the cerebellum inves-

tigated using high field (4 T) MRI. NMR Biomed 1994;7:63–8.

46. Tyszka JM, Grafton ST, Chew W, et al. Parceling of mesial frontal motor areas during ideation and movement using functional magnetic resonance imaging at 1.5 tesla. Ann Neurol 1994;35:746–9.

47. Hathout GM, Kirlew KA, So GJ, et al. MR imaging signal response to sustained stimulation in human visual cortex. J Magn Reson Imaging 1994;4:537–43.

48. Schneider W, Casey BJ, Noll D. Functional MRI mapping of stimulus rate effects across visual processing stages. Hum Brain Mapping 1994;1:117–33.

49. McCarthy G, Blamire AM, Rothman DL, et al. Echo-planar magnetic resonance imaging studies of frontal cortex activation during word generation in humans. Proc Natl Acad Sci USA 1993;90:4952–6.

50. Cohen JD, Forman SD, Braver TS, et al. Activation of the prefrontal cortex in a nonspatial working memory task with functional MRI. Hum Brain Mapping 1994;1:293–304.

51. Saykin AJ, Weaver JB, Burr RB, et al. Functional magnetic resonance imaging in the evaluation of epilepsy surgery patients: a memory activation study. American Epilepsy Society Annual Meeting, Program Book, New Orleans, Louisiana, December 2 to 7, 1994:16.

52. Shaywitz BA, Shaywitz SE, Pugh KR, et al. Sex differences in the functional organization of the brain for language. Nature 1995;373:607–9.

53. Weisskoff RM, Zuo CS, Boxerman JL, et al. Microscopic susceptibility variation and transverse relaxation: theory and experiment. Magn Reson Med 1994;31:601–10.

54. Ogawa S, Menon RS, Tank DW, et al. Functional brain mapping by blood oxygenation level-dependent contrast magnetic resonance imaging. A comparison of signal characteristics with a biophysical model. Biophys J 1993;64:803–12.

55. Kennan RP, Zhong J, Gore JC. Intravascular susceptibility contrast mechanisms in tissues. Magn Reson Med 1994;31:9–21.

56. Fisel CR, Ackerman JL, Buxton RB, et al. MR contrast due to microscopically heterogeneous magnetic susceptibility: numerical simulations and applications to cerebral physiology. Magn Reson Med 1991;17:336–47.

57. Bandettini PA, Wong EC, Jesmanowicz A, et al. Spin-echo and gradient-echo EPI of human brain activation using BOLD contrast: a comparative study at 1.5T. NMR Biomed 1994;7:12–20.

58. Hoppel BE, Weisskoff RM, Thulborn KR, et al. Measurement of regional blood oxygenation and cerebral hemodynamics. Magn Reson Med 1993;30:715–23.

59. Turner R, Jezzard P, Wen H, et al. Functional mapping of the human visual cortex at 4 and 1.5 Tesla using deoxygenation contrast EPI. Magn Reson Med 1993;29:277–9.

60. Friston KJ, Jezzard P, Turner R. Analysis of functional MRI time-series. Hum Brain Mapping 1994;1:153–71.

61. Lee AT, Glover GH, Meyer CH. Discrimination of large venous vessels in spiral time-course blood-oxygen-level-dependent magnetic resonance functional neuroimaging (abstract). J Magn Reson Imaging 1994;Suppl 4P:62.

62. Jackson GD, Connelly A, Cross JH, et al. Functional magnetic resonance imaging of focal seizures. Neurology 1994;44:850–6.

63. Farzaneh F, Riederer SJ, Pelc NJ. Analysis of T2 limitations and off-resonance effects on spatial resolution and artifacts in echo-planar imaging. Magn Reson Med 1990;14:123–39.

64. Wong EC, Boskamp E, Hyde JS. Abstract 4015, 11th Annual Meeting, Society of Magnetic Resonance in Medicine, Berlin, 1992.

65. Butts K, Riederer SJ, Ehman RL, et al. Interleaved echo planar imaging on a standard MRI system. Magn Reson Med 1994;31:67–72.

66. Hajnal JV, Myers R, Oatridge A, et al. Artifacts due to stimulus correlated motion in functional imaging of the brain. Magn Reson Med 1994;31:283–91.

67. Noll DC, Schneider W, Cohen JD. Artifacts in functional MRI using conventional scanning (abstract). Proceedings of the Society of Magnetic Resonance in Medicine 1993;3:1407.

68. Simonson TM, Ehrhardt J, Lee HJ, et al. Evaluation of echo-planar and conventional MR imaging techniques for motion sensitivity (abstract). Radiology 1994;193(P):461.

69. Hu X, Kim SG. Reduction of signal fluctuation in functional MRI using navigator echoes. Magn Reson Med 1994;31:495–503.

70. Ehman RL, Felmlee JP. Adaptive technique for high-definition MR imaging of moving structures. Radiology 1989;173:255–63.

71. Woods RP, Cherry SR, Mazziotta JC. Rapid automated algorithm for aligning and reslicing PET images. J Comput Assist Tomogr 1992;16:620–33.

72. LeBihan D, Jezzard P, Turner R, et al. Analysis of functional MR images with Z maps: works in progress (abstract). J Magn Reson Imaging 1993;Suppl 3P:141.

73. Jack CR Jr, Thompson RM, Butts RK, et al. Sensory motor cortex: correlation of presurgical mapping with functional MR imaging and invasive cortical mapping. Radiology 1994;190:85–92.

74. Thompson RM, Jack CR Jr, Butts K, et al. Imaging of cerebral activation at 1.5 T: optimizing a technique for conventional hardware. Radiology 1994;190:873–7.

75. Penfield W, Rasmussen T. The cerebral cortex of man: a clinical study of localization of function. New York: Macmillan Company, 1950:57.

Positron Emission Tomography in the Evaluation of Epilepsy

William H. Theodore

POSITRON EMISSION TOMOGRAPHY: METHODOLOGIC ISSUES

To perform positron emission tomography (PET), a cyclotron must be available as part of the scanning facility. If 18-fluoro-2-deoxyglucose (FDG), with a half-life of 110 minutes, is the only isotope used, it can be shipped from a distant cyclotron. Because of the short half-lives of ^{15}O (2 minutes) and ^{11}C (20 minutes), cerebral blood flow studies that use the former and receptor or metabolic studies that use the latter require an on-site cyclotron.

Most PET studies of epilepsy have been performed with FDG. Measurements are made about 30 to 40 minutes after the isotope is injected to allow for its entry into the brain and for phosphorylation by hexokinase. The scan reflects the local cerebral metabolic rate for glucose (LCMRglc) during that 30- to 40-minute uptake period, weighted toward the beginning. A seizure occurring 3 minutes after injection would affect the results of the scan differently than an identical seizure that occurs 25 minutes after injection.

With the most recent scanners, sets of 30 to 50 images can be obtained and reconstructed in the coronal and sagittal planes as well as in the transverse plane. Three-dimensional imaging is also possible but requires greater computational complexity. Radial artery samples can be obtained to calculate absolute values of LCMRglc. It is uncertain how much information this adds if scans are to be used only for clinical localization. The spatial resolution of the best PET scanners is still slightly inferior to T_2 or volumetric magnetic resonance imaging (MRI) scans but superior to single-photon emission computed tomography (SPECT) or magnetic resonance spectroscopy (MRS).

REGISTRATION OF MULTIMODALITY IMAGES

Anatomical localization can be obtained with a high degree of accuracy with MRI, but this is more difficult to achieve with PET and is problematic with SPECT. Several strategies can be used to combine structural and functional imaging data or various functional modalities. Fox et al.[1] extrapolated the landmarks of a lateral skull radiograph performed with the patient in the PET scanner to a pneumoencephalographic atlas to obtain anatomical coordinates for cerebral blood flow measurements. Images can be obtained using a system of "fiducial" markers, such as a set of petrolatum-filled plastic tubes visible on MRI, attached to a thermoplastic face mask.[2] Both PET and MRI are performed with the mask and tube assembly in place, thus ensuring a common baseline. The zigzag pattern of the tubes can be used to identify the scanning level. MRI and PET can be performed with the patient in a common stereotactic frame that can also be used for depth electrode implantation.[3] Multimodality image registration can also be used for surgical planning, particularly for lesions difficult to approach by conventional methods.

Most recent approaches have used post hoc alignment procedures based on identification of a common feature visible on both PET and computed tomographic (CT) or MRI images, such as the contour of the scalp.[4-7] Dann et al.[8] matched the images by finding the center of mass of each independently and creating covariance matrices. Woods et al.[9] used a pixel-by-pixel alignment that had an alignment error of less than 3 mm in comparison with markers fixed in the skull (Figure 11-1).

PARTIAL SEIZURES

Cerebral Glucose Metabolism: Interictal Studies

By using FDG-PET, unilateral interictal hypometabolism, usually in the temporal lobe, is found in 70% to 80% of patients with complex partial seizures.[10-14] A decrease in the cerebral metabolic rate of glucose (CMRglc) is closely correlated with the presence of a histologic lesion (although not always one detectable with MRI) in resected temporal lobe specimens. However, it is not necessarily correlated with the degree of neuronal loss as measured by cell counts or with the degree of focal gliosis apparent on glial fibrillary acidic protein staining.[15-17] The amount of interindividual variation in hypometabolism is considerable, even in patients with seemingly similar electroencephalographic (EEG) seizure onset. However, the pattern seen in a patient seems to be stable from scan to scan as long as the time since the last seizure is controlled.[12,18]

When abnormalities are present on CT or MRI, the hypometabolism seen on PET is usually more extensive than the anatomical lesion.[10-14,19] This may be related to physiologic factors (the structural lesion causing more widespread dysfunction) and partial "voluming-smearing" of the visualized abnormality over an apparently wider area.

Technical factors may explain why the original studies reported that hypometabolism was more prominent in the lateral temporal lobe than in the mesial temporal lobe. The mesial temporal regions are subject more to difficulties such as partial volume effects in imaging studies. Moreover, the axial cuts usually used for PET studies may not be optimal for visualizing these regions (Figure 11-1). Using a scanner with an in-plane resolution of 9.5 mm, Sackellares et al.[20] reported that the

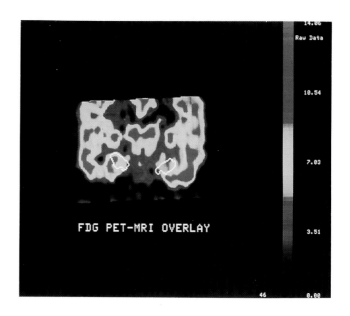

FIGURE 11-1. FDG-PET scan resliced in the coronal plane in a patient with a right temporal focus. Regions of interest were drawn on a coregistered MRI scan. No asymmetry was noted on the original axial images, but right mesial temporal hypometabolism is obvious on the resliced image. The patient had focal gliosis and neuronal loss.

mean asymmetry between the epileptogenic and contralateral side was 19.7% in the lateral temporal lobe and 10.8% in the mesial temporal lobe. Visualization of the mesial temporal cortex with PET is often poor, especially when low-resolution scanners are used. In our more recent studies with an advanced scanner with an in-plane resolution of 6.5 mm, we found no difference between the measured asymmetry in the lateral temporal cortex and the mesial temporal cortex. Hajek et al.[21] used PET to distinguish between complex partial seizures of mesial temporal origin and lateral temporal neocortical origin. The mean mesial LCMRglc was lower in patients with mesial temporal sclerosis than in those with lateral temporal lesions, but both groups showed a relatively larger decrease in metabolism in the mesial temporal lobe than in the lateral temporal lobe.

Detection of focal metabolism may be related to scanner resolution or the number of slices obtained. Engel et al.[22] reported that only 56% of patients studied with a single-slice scanner (in-plane resolution of 16 mm) showed focal hypometabolism, as opposed to 86% when a multislice instrument with 5-mm resolution was used.

A significant proportion of patients with complex partial seizures have frontal lobe as well as temporal lobe hypometabolism, even when EEG discharges appear well localized to the temporal lobe. In the latter, however, hypometabolism is usually more prominent in the temporal lobe than in the frontal lobe. In about 30% of patients, thalamic and parietal lobe hypometabolism is ipsilateral to temporal lobe EEG foci.[23-25] Thalamic hypometabolism, in particular, may be a valuable indicator of the lateralization of the epileptic focus.[26]

The finding of subcortical hypometabolism is particularly interesting because of the progressive recruitment of subcortical structures, including the substantia nigra and subthalamic and midline thalamic nuclei, during seizures in rodent and primate models.[27-29] Penicillin-induced kindling increases glucose utilization in the contralateral basal ganglia, nonspecific thalamic nuclei, and substantia nigra as well as in homotopic cortex, suggesting activation of crossed corticostriate pathways.[30,31] Lesions (usually bilateral) in the pontine or midbrain reticular formation or the injection of gamma-aminobutyric acid (GABA) into the substantia nigra retards seizure generalization; thus, these structures may serve as important gating points.[32-35] PET studies of cerebral blood flow in humans have shown prominent thalamic activation during seizures, which cannot always be explained by the motor components of the seizures.[25,36]

Well-localized hypometabolism may be less frequent when patients have extra-temporal EEG foci. [37-40] Swartz et al.[38] studied 22 patients with electroclinical features suggestive of frontal lobe epilepsy. The CT findings were abnormal in 32% of the patients, as were the MRI findings in 45% and the PET findings in 64%. The hypometabolic zones, although encompassing the region of probable seizure onset, tended to be regional or hemispheric, providing imprecise surgical-localizing data. However, in two patients, PET showed parietal lobe hypometabolism when electroclinical data suggested seizure onset in the frontal lobe. Both patients had abnormal MRI findings in the same region. Radtke et al.[40] found hypometabolism congruent with the EEG focus in 77% of their patients with temporal lobe ictal onset but in only 32% with frontal lobe ictal onset. Other investigators have stressed the difficulty of correlating the results of PET with clinical seizure phenomena thought to be indicative of the anatomical location of ictal onset.[37]

Patients with large structural lesions may have widespread associated metabolic defects not necessarily predicted by anatomical studies.[41] Also, these patients usually have diffuse or bilateral EEG discharges. PET may provide interesting physiologic information that may help to explain a patient's neuropsychologic dysfunction as well as the clinical features of seizures, but this information probably will not lead to specific changes in treatment.

Cerebral Glucose Metabolism: Ictal Studies

Ictal FDG studies usually occur by chance, because the half-life of FDG does not permit one to wait for a seizure to occur before injecting the isotope. Increased

metabolism at the site of interictal hypometabolism has been reported.[12,42,43] Because wider regions of the brain may be involved (related to the degree of clinical and electrographic seizure spread), ictal scans may not provide as accurate localizing data as interictal FDG studies. A complex partial seizure or even a generalized tonic-clonic seizure is usually much shorter than the 30- to 40-minute uptake period, which means that an "ictal" scan may include interictal, ictal, and postictal metabolic phases, depending on when the seizure occurs. Combinations of hypermetabolic and hypometabolic regions may be found. Ictal scans in particular, but interictal scans as well, should be performed with EEG and clinical monitoring to help in their interpretation.

Postictal depression of LCMRglc may be prolonged. Leiderman et al.[18] found that the metabolic rate in the inferior temporal lobe ipsilateral to a temporal lobe epileptic focus was relatively lower compared with the interictal rate in the 24- to 48-hour postictal period following simple partial seizures. In contrast, the relative regional increase in ipsilateral metabolism after a complex partial seizure persisted for 48 hours before decreasing. It may take the brain longer than 24 hours after a partial seizure to return to its metabolic baseline state.

COMPARISON WITH OTHER IMAGING MODALITIES

The rapid evolution of all neuroimaging techniques, particularly MRI, makes reports of intermodality comparisons difficult to evaluate. A particular group of investigators may not possess the most up-to-date hardware and software or have developed equivalent analytic models for each of the techniques they wish to compare. Their results are likely to favor the technique they have worked with most intensely.

Interictal FDG-PET reportedly reveals abnormalities in more patients than T_2-weighted MRI.[14,41,44] MRI may be more sensitive for detecting lesions such as small gliomas and hamartomas and PET more sensitive for regions of focal gliosis.[14,19,44,45] Initial studies have suggested that FDG-PET may also be more sensitive than volumetric MRI. Gaillard et al.[46] found that 87% of patients had decreased LCMRglc ipsilateral to the epileptic temporal lobe but only 60% had hippocampal atrophy. Garcia et al.[39] reported that MRS imaging showed an increase in pH on the side of the epileptic focus in five patients with frontal lobe epilepsy who had normal findings on FDG-PET and conventional MRI. Four of the patients had epilepsy surgery. Postoperatively, two had improvement, but none became seizure-free.

Interictal SPECT with either isopropyl-iodoamphetamine (IMP) or hexamethyl-propyleneamineoxime (HMPAO) was inferior to both FDG-PET and MRI for identifying epileptic foci.[47,48] However, ictal SPECT may be as sensitive and specific as either modality.[49]

POSITRON EMISSION TOMOGRAPHY ESTIMATION OF CEREBRAL BLOOD FLOW AND OXYGEN METABOLISM

Two methods have been used to measure cerebral blood flow with PET: injection of ^{15}O-labelled water and inhalation of ^{15}O-labelled gases (CO and CO_2), which can also provide information on cerebral oxygen metabolism ($CMRO_2$). Bolus injection of H_2^{15}O assumes homogeneous cerebral blood flow and tracer blood:tissue partition coefficient and shows a nearly linear relation of tissue counts to cerebral blood flow over physiologically encountered ranges. The 2-minute half-life of ^{15}O allows multiple doses to be administered without moving the patient from the scanner, making the technique useful for functional activation studies.

Steady state inhalation of ^{15}O-labelled gases is less appropriate for these applications, but it was used in a study that showed widespread decreases in mean cerebral blood flow and $CMRO_2$.[50] These findings, which could have been due partly to the effect of antiepileptic drugs, may suggest a more widespread effect of seizures on brain function. Decreased $CMRO_2$ and cerebral blood flow have been reported ipsilateral to EEG epileptic foci.[50–53] In some studies, a more widespread or bilateral dysfunction was found, although the temporal lobe ipsilateral to the EEG focus still had a relatively lower rate of cerebral blood flow and $CMRO_2$.[50]

Several investigators have suggested that interictal PET studies of cerebral blood flow may not be as specific as FDG-PET for delineating epileptic foci[51,53] (Figure 11-2). For technical reasons that include increased scatter and the higher energy of the ^{15}O photon, ^{15}O-PET scans usually have more background noise and somewhat less spatial resolution than FDG-PET. This may increase "partial voluming," making it more difficult to detect a region of hypoperfusion. However, it is also possible that mesial temporal lobe foci, especially if there is only a small region of focal gliosis and neuronal loss, may be hypometabolic but not hypoperfused.[53] There may be a mismatch between cerebral blood flow and CMRglc in epileptic foci, with a relatively greater depression of metabolism than of blood flow.[54,55] The implications of these studies, which need to be replicated, are unclear, but similar results have been obtained in patients with stroke.

Other physiologic derangements in epileptic foci have been described. In a patient with epilepsia partialis continua and a right frontocentral epileptic focus, cerebral blood flow was increased but $CMRO_2$ was decreased in the right parietal region, whereas CMRglc was symmetric.[56] On the basis of these findings, the authors suggested that aerobic glycolysis could occur in actively spiking human (as well as animal) epileptic tissue, but they noted that the conclusion had to be treated with caution because of possible seizure-induced alterations in the lumped constant, which describes the relation between the use of tracer (fluorodeoxyglucose) and physiologic substrate (glucose).

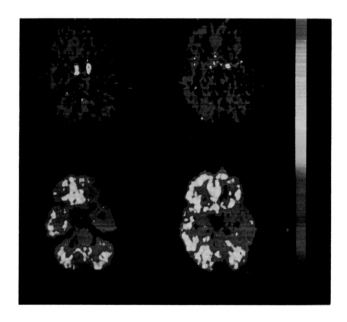

FIGURE 11-2. Comparison of blood flow and glucose metabolism in a patient with a right temporal lobe focus. The blood flow images show the asymmetry less clearly.

Because the half-life of ^{15}O is only 2 minutes, repeated scans can be performed during the same session under varying physiologic conditions. This eliminates the error introduced by comparing ictal and interictal scans on different days and by the patient being in a slightly different position in the scanner, as would have to be done with FDG.

Blood flow studies have a shorter time frame and may be more useful indicators of ictal function. Moreover, the bolus ^{15}O method is linear over the physiologic range of flow rates and, thus, is not subject to the methodologic problems associated with using FDG for ictal studies.[57] During complex partial seizures, cerebral blood flow increases bilaterally by 40% to 130% in temporal cortex, by 30% to 40% in the thalamus, and by 20% in frontal cortex[58–61] (Figure 11-3). The increased blood flow may be bitemporal even in patients with unilateral foci, although the increase is greater ipsilaterally. Cerebral blood flow changes accompanying secondarily generalized seizures may be asymmetric, with a greater increase in the region of presumed seizure origin.[61] Intracarotid injection of ^{77}Kr during a simple partial seizure showed that cerebral blood flow increased 30% to 130% contralaterally, with the greatest increase in the thalamus.[36]

Balish et al.[61] attempted to use ictal ^{15}O PET scans to show more specific alterations in cerebral blood flow.

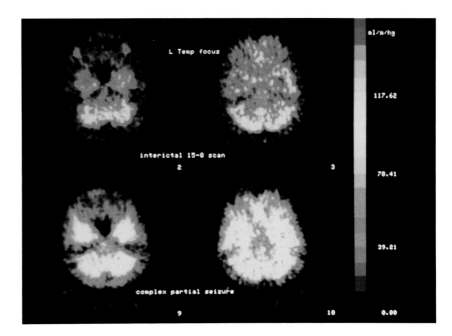

FIGURE 11-3. Interictal and ictal ^{15}O cerebral blood flow PET scan in a patient with a left temporal focus. During a complex partial seizure, cerebral blood flow increases bilaterally.

Serial injections of ^{15}O-labelled water were performed after activation of epileptic foci by pentylenetetrazol. However, the regions of increased cerebral blood flow were too widespread for accurate surgical localization, even when only partial seizures were induced.

In animal models, prolonged seizures (longer than 60 minutes) lead to mismatches between perfusion and metabolism, producing neuronal cell damage in certain brain regions such as the hippocampus.[62] Postictal increases in lactate are related to seizure duration.[63] Ictal alterations in cerebral blood flow and LCMRglc in animal models may depend on the convulsant used as well as on the experimental conditions, which usually bear little relation to seizures in humans. Bicuculline-induced seizures in rats may cause regional variations in increased perfusion of 150% to 500%.[64] ^{31}P magnetic resonance spectroscopy studies in children suggest that prolonged neonatal seizures lead to neuronal damage.[65]

FUNCTIONAL LOCALIZATION WITH POSITRON EMISSION TOMOGRAPHY

The correlation between alterations of cerebral blood flow or CMRglc and neuropsychologic function is broad. Imaging abnormalities may represent nonepileptic regions of cerebral dysfunction, even in patients with seizures. A relative decrease in glucose metabolism in the left temporal lobe is correlated with a lower verbal IQ score and impaired performance on verbal memory tasks.[66] It is important to remember that temporal lobe cortex that is not atrophied, even though epileptogenic,

may still have some functional reserve that can be evaluated with PET.

PET studies with ^{15}O-labelled water have mapped higher cortical function in normal human volunteers.[67,68] Control scans are subtracted from images obtained during task performance to obtain estimates of the associated increases in cerebral blood flow. The results of studies with echo-planar MRI are comparable to those of PET.[69]

Because specific language tasks cause alterations of cerebral blood flow and CMRglc, attempts have been made to use PET or SPECT as a substitute for Wada's test in establishing cerebral dominance for language and memory. However, choosing a stimulus that would provide a PET response that is sufficiently strong and clearly localized may be difficult.[70] In patients with left temporal EEG foci, hypometabolism of the left inferior temporal lobe was accentuated by a phonemic monitoring task (patients were asked to discriminate between the syllables "SA" and "AS").[71] Spontaneous speech during PET may be a less lateralizing task; greater relative hypometabolism was induced in patients with either left or right temporal foci.[72] The results of cerebral blood flow–PET studies in language localization have been compared with the results of subdural electrode stimulation in patients with uncontrolled epilepsy who were candidates for epilepsy surgery.[73] CT scans were performed with the subdural electrodes in place, and both the PET and CT scans were digitally coregistered with the MR images of each patient. Each point that showed language disruption with electrical stimulation was associated with increased cerebral blood flow. No change was found in cerebral blood flow at grid points that did not include language disruption.

POSITRON EMISSION TOMOGRAPHY IN PATIENTS WITH PARTIAL SEIZURES: SURGICAL LOCALIZATION

The predictive value of FDG-PET in patients undergoing temporal lobectomy has been evaluated.[74–76] The mean metabolic asymmetry in the lateral but not mesial temporal lobe on FDG-PET was significantly higher in patients who became seizure-free.[74] Patients with at least 15% hypometabolism are more likely to become seizure-free. False lateralization is rare.[77]

In contrast, PET studies of cerebral blood flow are not useful for surgical planning. There are no differences in the degree of hypoperfusion between patients who do and those who do not become seizure-free. Hypoperfusion may occur in up to 10% of temporal lobes contralateral to an epileptic focus.[78]

Focal hypometabolism is closely associated with the onset of a surface focal ictal seizure, and it is unclear what additional information PET can provide in this case.[74,79] Engel et al.[22] compared scalp-sphenoidal EEG, depth electrodes, and FDG-PET in identifying temporal lobe epileptic foci. Correct (agreeing with depth data or surgical results) lateralization/localization was found on scalp EEG in 47% of patients and false-positive results in 3%; about 50% of the studies were nondiagnostic. PET results were accurate in 60% to 64% of patients, wrong in 2% to 6%, and nondiagnostic in 34%. The results obtained with depth electrode studies were correct in 93% of patients, incorrect in 2%, and nondiagnostic in 5%. When the results of scalp-sphenoidal EEG and PET agreed (about one third of the patients), depth EEG studies never provided additional valuable information. The authors suggested that anterior temporal lobectomy could be performed without depth electrode studies in these patients if no contrary data (for example, from neuropsychologic studies or MRI) were found.

However, it has not been shown that epilepsy surgery can be performed successfully on the basis of PET (or other imaging data) alone if the surface EEG is nonlocalizing. Preliminary data suggest that FDG-PET hypometabolism predicts the results of seizure localization with subdural electrodes in about 50% of patients with a nonlocalizing surface EEG.[74] However, EEG abnormalities may mislocalize epileptic foci in the presence of structural abnormalities.[80] A clear mismatch between imaging and surface EEG findings is an indication for invasive electrode studies.

Modern imaging approaches have the advantage of viewing the whole brain simultaneously. This is important because bilateral abnormalities have been reported in 10% to 30% of patients with temporal lobe epilepsy. However, it is uncertain whether these abnormalities are related to the longer duration or greater severity of disease in cases that come to autopsy (for which both temporal lobes are available for pathologic study) than to the underlying pathophysiologic mechanism.[81]

POSITRON EMISSION TOMOGRAPHY IN PATIENTS WITH PRIMARY AND SECONDARY GENERALIZED EPILEPSIES

Patients with primary generalized absence seizures have a normal resting LCMRglc, but the LCMRglc increases markedly during seizures.[82,83] Using ^{15}O-labelled water, Prevett et al.[84,85] found thalamic activation in excess of global cerebral blood flow increases but no evidence for an alteration in benzodiazepine receptor binding. Interictal FDG metabolic patterns in Lennox-Gastaut syndrome include unilateral foci, bilateral multifocal, and diffuse hypometabolism.[86–88] The hypometabolic regions in some but not all of these patients are related to structural abnormalities.

In some patients with infantile spasms, PET demonstrates regions of hypometabolism, particularly the parieto-occipito-temporal region, associated with focal cortical dysgenesis not detected with MRI.[89,90] Symmetrical increases in metabolism in the lenticular nuclei have been reported, irrespective of whether there was focal cortical hypometabolism.[91] Cortical resection has led to encouraging early results. Pathologic examination revealed dysplastic or malformed cerebral cortex.[90]

Children with hemimegalencephaly may have diffuse cortical hypometabolism on the nonhemimegalencephalic side.[92] The prognosis after hemispherectomy may be worse in these patients than it is if the metabolism in the anatomically unaffected hemisphere is normal.

BLOOD FLOW, METABOLISM, AND BEHAVIOR IN EPILEPSY

PET has been used to study the relation between epilepsy and psychiatric disorders. The oxygen extraction ratio (cerebral metabolic rate for oxygen divided by cerebral blood flow) was lower in patients with epilepsy who had psychotic symptoms than in those who did not, suggesting that the decrease in metabolism was greater than in blood flow.[93] Patients with left temporal seizure onset and depression have bilateral inferior frontal hypometabolism, as compared with patients with seizures and no depression and with normal controls.[94] Hypometabolism in the left temporal lobe may be more common in patients with complex partial seizures and a history of a major depressive episode.[95]

Patients with schizophrenia may have relative decreases in the cerebral blood flow and LCMRglc of the frontal lobe.[96] Increased severity of the psychopathologic condition has been associated with increased cerebral blood flow in the left mesial temporal lobe.[97] Hypometabolism in the frontal lobe has been reported in patients with depression.[98]

NEUROIMAGING AND NEUROPHARMACOLOGY IN EPILEPSY

Baron et al.[99] used ^{11}C-labelled phenytoin to study antiepileptic drug concentration in patients with complex partial seizures. Because of the high lipophilicity and brain levels of the drug, the distribution of the tracer was uniform and binding was not increased in epileptic foci.

The effect of antiepileptic drugs on cerebral function has been studied with imaging techniques. The LCMRglc was decreased 37% by phenobarbital, 13% by phenytoin, 12% by carbamazepine, and 12% to 20% by valproic acid, depending on whether the drug was given to normal volunteers or to patients taking carbamazepine.[100–102] The effect of valproic acid on cerebral blood flow was particularly marked in the thalamus, which is of interest because of its value in the treatment of primary generalized absence seizures. Occipital levels of GABA, measured with MRS, were higher in patients taking vigabatrin, a GABA-transaminase inhibitor, than in control subjects.[103]

Endogenous opiates may be involved in regulation of cerebral blood flow in humans and possibly in maintenance of hypoperfusion in epileptic foci. Frost et al.[104] reported that the number of mu opiate receptors or binding affinity was increased in lateral temporal neocortex ipsilateral to epileptic foci but that mesial temporal cortex showed no differences in comparison with the contralateral homologous region. No abnormalities were found with diprenorphine, a ligand that binds to mu, delta, and kappa receptors, or with cyclofoxy, a mixed mu and kappa receptor ligand[105,106] (Figure 11-4). Possibly, only mu receptors are "increased" or mu receptors are increased and kappa (and perhaps delta) receptors are "decreased." Intravenous injection of naloxone (1 mg/kg) decreased blood flow but not glucose metabolism, and it also decreased the degree of asymmetry of cerebral blood flow in lateral temporal cortex in patients with hypoperfusion greater than 10% of baseline.[107]

The role of GABA in the pathophysiology of human epilepsy is complex. Increased GABAergic transmission in animal models of epilepsy has a clear anticonvulsant effect in a limited number of brain regions.[108] Moreover, direct stimulation of postsynaptic receptors by agents such as muscimol may have a different effect from a presynaptic increase in GABA. Human hippocampus resected from patients with complex partial seizures shows marked regional specificity: GABA and benzodiazepine receptor binding is decreased in CA1 and CA4 but not in the dentate gyrus.[109]

Although PET and SPECT do not have the sufficient resolution for distinguishing regional variations in

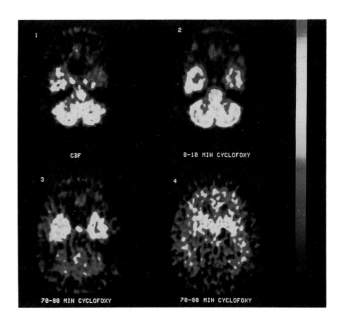

FIGURE 11-4. [15]Oxygen cerebral blood flow and cyclofoxy PET scans in a patient with a right temporal focus. The cerebral blood flow scan (1) shows right temporal hypoperfusion. Cyclofoxy scan in the early distribution phase (2) shows a pattern similar to the cerebral blood flow scan. The late phases (3 and 4) of cyclofoxy scan show receptor binding. Cerebellum (3) and occipital lobe (4) have little activity, which is high in temporal lobes, thalamus, and basal ganglia. There is relatively increased activity in the right lateral and mesial temporal cortex. At surgery, focal gliosis and neuronal loss were found.

receptor binding in the hippocampus, decreased benzodiazepine binding has been reported by investigators who used 11C-Ro 15-1788 (a central-type benzodiazepine receptor ligand) for PET studies and 123-I-iomazenil for SPECT studies.[110,111] The binding of 11C-Ro 15-1788 may be decreased in the mesial temporal cortex more than in the lateral temporal cortex.[112] In resected temporal lobe specimens from patients with mesial temporal sclerosis, central-type benzodiazepine receptors decreased and peripheral-type receptors increased in association with the degree of cell loss and focal gliosis in the hippocampus.[113] Savic et al.[114] suggested that 11C-Ro 15-1788 could be used as a marker for epileptic foci in patients being considered for temporal lobe resection.

Other neurotransmitter systems have also been studied. Increased monoamine oxidase β receptor binding measured with 11C-deprenyl probably reflects focal gliosis.[115]

CONCLUSIONS

Hypometabolism seen with FDG-PET is correlated with surface EEG ictal onset. FDG-PET may have a slight advantage in sensitivity over volumetric MRI, but technical improvements will probably eliminate this advantage. Temporal lobe resections could probably be performed on the basis of PET (or MRI) localization and consistent surface interictal EEG discharges, thus reducing the need for hospital admission, drug withdrawal, and ictal recording. It is uncertain whether improvements in resolution and data analysis will allow PET to be used to plan temporal lobe resections or to select patients for more limited operations such as amygdalohippocampectomy.

The role of FDG-PET for cases in which surface recording is nonlocalizing needs further prospective study in which imaging data would be collected and analyzed by investigators blinded to invasive electrode results. Children with infantile spasms and related syndromes who are identified as potential surgical candidates by PET studies could be randomized to surgical or experimental drug therapy, followed by cross-over if the initial therapy is unsuccessful. PET studies of cerebral blood flow with ^{15}O appear to be valuable for functional mapping but not useful for surgical localization.

Visualization of receptors in vivo may be the most important contribution of PET to understanding the pathophysiologic basis of human epilepsy.

REFERENCES

1. Fox PT, Perlmutter JS, Raichle ME. A stereotactic method of anatomical localization for positron emission tomography. J Comput Assist Tomogr 1985;9:141–53.

2. Meltzer CC, Bryan RN, Holcomb HH, et al. Anatomical localization for PET using MR imaging. J Comput Assist Tomogr 1990;14:418–26.

3. Henry TR, Engel J Jr, Mazziotta JC. PET studies of functional cerebral anatomy in human epilepsy. Curr Probl Epilepsy 1988;6:155–78.

4. Levin DN, Pelizzari CA, Chen GT, et al. Retrospective geometric correlation of MR, CT, and PET images. Radiology 1988;169:817–23.

5. Pelizzari CA, Chen GT, Spelbring DR, et al. Accurate three-dimensional registration of CT, PET, and/or MR images of the brain J Comput Assist Tomogr 1989;13:20–6.

6. Lemieux L, Lester S, Fish D. Multimodality imaging and intracranial EEG display for stereotactic surgery planning in epilepsy. Electroencephalogr Clin Neurophysiol 1992;82:399–407.

7. Grzeszczuk R, Tan KK, Levin DN, et al. Retrospective fusion of radiographic and MR data for localization of subdural electrodes. J Comput Assist Tomogr 1992;16:764–73.

8. Dann R, Hoford J, Kovacic S, et al. Evaluation of elastic matching system for anatomic (CT, MR) and functional (PET) cerebral images. J Comput Assist Tomogr 1989;13:603–11.

9. Woods RP, Mazziotta JC, Cherry SR. MRI-PET registration with automated algorithm. J Comput Assist Tomogr 1993;17:536–46.

10. Kuhl DE, Engel J Jr, Phelps ME, et al. Epileptic patterns of local cerebral metabolism and perfusion in humans determined by emission computed tomography of 18FDG and 13NH3. Ann Neurol 1980;8:348–60.

11. Engel J Jr, Kuhl DE, Phelps ME, et al. Interictal cerebral glucose metabolism in partial epilepsy and its relation to EEG changes. Ann Neurol 1982;12:510–7.

12. Theodore WH, Newmark ME, Sato S, et al. [18F]fluorodeoxyglucose positron emission tomography in refractory complex partial seizures. Ann Neurol 1983;14:429–37.

13. Franck G, Sadzot B, Salmon E, et al. Regional cerebral blood flow and metabolic rates in human focal epilepsy and status epilepticus. Adv Neurol 1986;44:935–48.

14. Abou-Khalil BW, Siegel GJ, Sackellares JC, et al. Positron emission tomography studies of cerebral glucose metabolism in chronic partial epilepsy. Ann Neurol 1987;22:480–6.

15. Engel J Jr, Brown WJ, Kuhl DE, et al. Pathological findings underlying focal temporal lobe hypometabolism in partial epilepsy. Ann Neurol 1982;12:518–28.

16. Henry TR, Babb TL, Engel J Jr, et al. Hippocampal neuronal loss and regional hypometabolism in temporal lobe epilepsy. Ann Neurol 1994;36:925–7.

17. Theodore WH, Katz D, Kufta C, et al. Pathology of temporal lobe foci: correlation with CT, MRI, and PET. Neurology 1990;40:797–803.

18. Leiderman DB, Albert P, Balish M, et al. The dynamics of metabolic change following seizures as measured by positron emission tomography with fludeoxyglucose F^{18}. Arch Neurol 1994;51:932–6.

19. Theodore WH, Dorwart R, Holmes M, et al. Neuroimaging in refractory partial seizures: comparison of PET, CT, and MRI. Neurology 1986;36:750–9.

20. Sackellares JC, Siegel GJ, Abou-Khalil BW, et al. Differences between lateral and mesial temporal metabolism interictally in epilepsy of mesial temporal origin. Neurology 1990;40:1420–6.

21. Hajek M, Antonini A, Leenders KL, et al. Mesiobasal versus lateral temporal lobe epilepsy: metabolic differences in the temporal lobe shown by interictal ^{18}F-FDG positron emission tomography. Neurology 1993;43:79–86.

22. Engel J Jr, Henry TR, Risinger MW, et al. Presurgical evaluation for partial epilepsy: relative contributions of chronic depth-electrode recordings versus FDG-PET and scalp-sphenoidal ictal EEG. Neurology 1990;40:1670–7.

23. Gur RC, Sussman NM, Gur RE, et al. Regional hypometabolism in focal epilepsy: a positron emission tomography study (abstract). Neurology 1987;37 Suppl 1:327.

24. Henry TR, Mazziotta JC, Engel J Jr. Interictal metabolic anatomy of mesial temporal lobe epilepsy. Arch Neurol 1993;50:582–9.

25. Balish M, Leiderman DB, Bromfield E, et al. Subcortical metabolism in partial epilepsy patients as measured by fluorodeoxyglucose positron emission tomography (abstract). Epilepsia 1989;30:707.

26. Henry TR, Mazziotta JC, Engel J Jr, et al. Quantifying interictal metabolic activity in human temporal lobe epilepsy. J Cereb Blood Flow Metab 1990;10:748–57.

27. Walker AE, Poggio GF, Andy OJ. Structural spread of cortically-induced epileptic discharges. Neurology 1956;6:616–26.

28. Collins RC, Kennedy C, Sokoloff L, et al. Metabolic anatomy of focal motor seizures. Arch Neurol 1976;33:536–42.

29. Caveness WF, Kato M, Malamut BL, et al. Propagation of focal motor seizures in the pubescent monkey. Ann Neurol 1980;7:213–21;232–5.

30. Collins RC. Kindling of neuroanatomic pathways during recurrent focal penicillin seizures. Brain Res 1978;150:503–17.

31. Engel J Jr, Wolfson L, Brown L. Anatomical correlates of electrical and behavioral events related to amygdaloid kindling. Ann Neurol 1978;3:538–44.

32. Iadarola MJ, Gale K. Substantia nigra: site of anticonvulsant activity mediated by gamma-aminobutyric acid. Science 1982;218:1237–40.

33. Garant DS, Gale K. Lesions of substantia nigra protect against experimentally induced seizures. Brain Res 1983;273:156–61.

34. McNamara JO, Galloway MT, Rigsbee LC, et al. Evidence implicating substantia nigra in regulation of kindled seizure threshold. J Neurosci 1984;4:2410–7.

35. Miller JW, McKeon AC, Ferrendelli JA. Functional anatomy of pentylenetetrazol and electroshock seizures in the rat brainstem. Ann Neurol 1987;22:615–21.

36. Feindel W, Gloor P, Yamamoto L, et al. Correlation of EEG and topographic cerebral blood flow in epilepsy by positron emission tomography. Adv Epileptol 1982;13:151–6.

37. Holmes MD, Kelly K, Theodore WH. Complex partial seizures. Correlation of clinical and metabolic features. Arch Neurol 1988;45:1191–3.

38. Swartz BE, Halgren E, Delgado-Escueta AV, et al. Neuroimaging in patients with seizures of probable frontal lobe origin. Epilepsia 1989;30:547–58.

39. Garcia PA, Laxer KD, van der Grond J, et al. Phosphorus magnetic resonance spectroscopic imaging in patients with frontal lobe epilepsy. Ann Neurol 1994;35:217–21.

40. Radtke RA, Hanson MW, Hoffman JM, et al. Positron emission tomography: comparison of clinical utility in temporal lobe and extratemporal epilepsy. J Epilepsy 1994;7:27–33.

41. Theodore WH, Holmes MD, Dorwart RH, et al. Complex partial seizures: cerebral structure and cerebral function. Epilepsia 1986;27:576–82.

42. Engel J Jr, Kuhl DE, Phelps ME. Patterns of human local cerebral glucose metabolism during epileptic seizures. Science 1982;218:64–6.

43. Engel J Jr, Kuhl DE, Phelps ME, et al. Local cerebral metabolism during partial seizures. Neurology 1983;33:400–13.

44. Sperling MR, Wilson G, Engel J Jr, et al. Magnetic resonance imaging in intractable partial epilepsy: correlative studies. Ann Neurol 1986;20:57–62.

45. Henry TR, Engel J Jr, Sutherling WW, et al. Correlation of structural and metabolic imaging with electrographic localization and histopathology in refractory complex partial epilepsy (abstract). Epilepsia 1987;28:601.

46. Gaillard WD, Bhatia S, Bookheimer SY, et al. FDG-PET and MRI volumetry in partial seizure focus localization (abstract). Neurology 1993;43 Suppl:A224.

47. Stefan H, Pawlik G, Bocher-Schwarz HG, et al. Functional and morphological abnormalities in temporal lobe epilepsy: a comparison of interictal and ictal EEG, CT, MRI, SPECT and PET. J Neurol 1987;234:377–84.

48. Ryvlin P, Philippon B, Cinotti L, et al. Functional neuroimaging strategy in temporal lobe epilepsy: a comparative study of ^{18}FDG-PET and ^{99m}Tc-HMPAO-SPECT. Ann Neurol 1992;31:650–6.

49. Ho SS, Berkovic SF, Berlangieri SU, et al. Comparison of ictal SPECT and interictal PET in the presurgical evaluation of temporal lobe epilepsy. Ann Neurol 1995;37:738–45.

50. Bernardi S, Trimble MR, Frackowiak RS, et al. An interictal study of partial epilepsy using positron emission tomography and the oxygen-15 inhalation technique. J Neurol Neurosurg Psychiatry 1983;46:473–7.

51. Ochs RF, Yamamoto L, Gloor P, et al. Correlation between the positron emission tomography measurement of glucose metabolism and oxygen utilization with focal epilepsy (abstract). Neurology 1984;34 Suppl 1:125.

52. Franck G, Salmon E, Sadzot B, et al. Epilepsy: the use of oxygen-15-labeled gases. Semin Neurol 1989;9:307–16.

53. Leiderman DB, Balish M, Sato S, et al. Comparison of PET measurements of cerebral blood flow and glucose metabolism for the localization of human epileptic foci. Epilepsy Res 1992;13:153–7.

54. Gaillard WD, White S, Reeves P, et al. Comparison of 18-FDG-PET with H$_2$O (O-15)-PET and Tc-99m HMPAO-SPECT in patients with intractable partial seizures (abstract). Neurology 1992;42 Suppl 3:298.

55. Pawlik G, Fink GR, Wienhard K, et al. Uncoupling of focal metabolism and hemodynamics in mesiolimbic temporal lobe epilepsy (abstract). Epilepsia 1993;34 Suppl 2:186.

56. Cowan JM, Rothwell JC, Wise RJ, et al. Electrophysiological and positron emission studies in a patient with cortical myoclonus, epilepsia partialis continua and motor epilepsy. J Neurol Neurosurg Psychiatry 1986;49:796–807.

57. Herscovitch P, Markham J, Raichle ME. Brain blood flow measured with intravenous H2(15)O. I. Theory and error analysis. J Nucl Med 1983;24:782–9.

58. Hougaard K, Oikawa T, Sveinsdottir E, et al. Regional cerebral blood flow in focal cortical epilepsy. Arch Neurol 1976;33:527–35.

59. Ingvar DH. rCBF in focal cortical epilepsy (abstract). Stroke 1973;4:359.

60. Herscovitch P, Raichle ME, Goldring S. Local blood flow increases dramatically in cerebral cortex and subcortical structures during focal seizures in humans (abstract). J Cereb Blood Flow Metab 1987;7 Suppl 1:S424.

61. Balish M, Leiderman D, Bromfield E, et al. The effect of seizures on cerebral blood flow measured with ^{15}O-H$_2$O (abstract). Neurology 1989;39 Suppl 1:299.

62. Ingvar M, Siesjo BK. Local blood flow and glucose consumption in the rat brain during sustained bicuculline-induced seizures. Acta Neurol Scand 1983;68:129–44.

63. Petroff OA, Prichard JW, Ogino T, et al. Combined ^{1}H and ^{31}P nuclear magnetic resonance spectroscopic studies of bicuculline-induced seizures in vivo. Ann Neurol 1986;20:185–93.

64. Siesjo BK, Abdul-Rahman A. A metabolic basis for the selective vulnerability of neurons in status epilepticus. Acta Physiol Scand 1979;106:377–8.

65. Younkin DP, Delivoria-Papadopoulos M, Maris J, et al. Cerebral metabolic effects of neonatal seizures measured with in vivo ^{31}P NMR spectroscopy. Ann Neurol 1986;20:513–9.

66. Rausch R, Henry TR, Ary CM, et al. Asymmetric interictal glucose hypometabolism and cognitive performance in epileptic patients. Arch Neurol 1994;51:139–44.

67. Petersen SE, Fox PT, Posner MI, et al. Positron emission tomographic studies of the cortical anatomy of single-word processing. Nature 1988;331:585–9.

68. Grasby PM, Frith CD, Friston KJ, et al. Functional mapping of brain areas implicated in auditory-verbal memory function. Brain 1993;116:1–20.

69. McCarthy G, Blamire AM, Rothman DL, et al. Echo-planar magnetic resonance imaging studies of frontal cortex activation during word generation in humans. Proc Natl Acad Sci USA 1993;90:4952–6.

70. Fox PT, Petersen S, Posner M, et al. PET assessment of hemispheric dominance for language (abstract). Neurology 1988;36 Suppl 1:365.

71. Bromfield EB, Ludlow CL, Sedory S, et al. Cerebral activation during speech discrimination in temporal lobe epilepsy. Epilepsy Res 1991;9:49–58.

72. Heiss W-D, Pawlik G, Hebold I, et al. Metabolic pattern of speech activation in healthy volunteers, aphasics, and focal epileptics (abstract). J Cereb Blood Flow Metab 1987;7 Suppl 1:S299.

73. Bookheimer SY, Zeffiro TA, Theodore W, et al. Multi-modal functional imaging for language localization in epilepsy (abstract). Neurology 1993;43 Suppl:A193.

74. Theodore WH, Sato S, Kufta C, et al. Temporal lobectomy for uncontrolled seizures: the role of positron emission tomography. Ann Neurol 1992;32:789–94.

75. Radtke RA, Hanson MW, Hoffman JM, et al. Temporal lobe hypometabolism on PET: predictor of seizure control after temporal lobectomy. Neurology 1993;43:1088–92.

76. Manno EM, Sperling MR, Ding X, et al. Predictors of outcome after anterior temporal lobectomy: positron emission tomography. Neurology 1994;44:2331–6.

77. Sperling MR, Alavi A, Reivich M, et al. False lateralization of temporal lobe epilepsy with FDG positron emission tomography. Epilepsia 1995;36:722–7.

78. Theodore WH, Gaillard WD, Sato S, et al. Positron emission tomographic measurement of cerebral blood flow and temporal lobectomy. Ann Neurol 1994;36:241–4.

79. Engel J Jr, Kuhl DE, Phelps ME, et al. Comparative localization of epileptic foci in partial epilepsy by PCT and EEG. Ann Neurol 1982;12:529–37.

80. Sammaritano M, de Lotbiniere A, Andermann F, et al. False lateralization by surface EEG of seizure onset in patients with temporal lobe epilepsy and gross focal cerebral lesions. Ann Neurol 1987;21:361–9.

81. Margerison JH, Corsellis JA. Epilepsy and the temporal lobes. A clinical, electroencephalographic and neuropathological study of the brain in epilepsy, with particular reference to the temporal lobes. Brain 1966;89:499–530.

82. Engel J Jr, Lubens P, Kuhl DE, et al. Local cerebral metabolic rate for glucose during petit mal absences. Ann Neurol 1985;17:121–8.

83. Theodore WH, Brooks R, Margolin R, et al. Positron emission tomography in generalized seizures. Neurology 1985;35:684–90.

84. Prevett MC, Lammertsma AA, Brooks DJ, et al. Benzodiazepine-GABA$_A$ receptor binding during absence seizures. Epilepsia 1995;36:592–9.

85. Prevett MC, Duncan JS, Jones T, et al. Demonstration of thalamic activation during typical absence seizures using H2(15)O and PET. Neurology 1995;45:1396–402.

86. Gur RC, Sussman NM, Alavi A, et al. Positron emission tomography in two cases of childhood epileptic encephalopathy (Lennox-Gastaut syndrome). Neurology 1982;32:1191–4.

87. Chugani HT, Mazziotta JC, Engel J Jr, et al. The Lennox-Gastaut syndrome: metabolic subtypes determined by 2-deoxy-2[^{18}F]fluoro-D-glucose positron emission tomography. Ann Neurol 1987;21:4–13.

88. Theodore WH, Rose D, Patronas N, et al. Cerebral glucose metabolism in the Lennox-Gastaut syndrome. Ann Neurol 1987;21:14–21.

89. Chugani HT, Shields WD, Shewmon DA, et al. Infantile spasms: I. PET identifies focal cortical dysgenesis in cryptogenic cases for surgical treatment. Ann Neurol 1990;27:406–13.

90. Chugani HT, Shewmon DA, Shields WD, et al. Surgery for intractable infantile spasms: neuroimaging perspectives. Epilepsia 1993;34:764–71.

91. Chugani HT, Shewmon DA, Sankar R, et al. Infantile spasms: II. Lenticular nuclei and brain stem activation on positron emission tomography. Ann Neurol 1992;31:212–9.

92. Rintahaka PJ, Chugani HT, Messa C, et al. Hemimegalencephaly: evaluation with positron emission tomography. Pediatr Neurol 1993;9:21–8.

93. Gallhofer B, Trimble MR, Frackowiak R, et al. A study of cerebral blood flow and metabolism in epileptic psychosis using positron emission tomography and oxygen. J Neurol Neurosurg Psychiatry 1985;48:201–6.

94. Bromfield EB, Altshuler L, Leiderman DB, et al. Cerebral metabolism and depression in patients with complex partial seizures. Arch Neurol 1992;49:617–23.

95. Victoroff JI, Benson F, Grafton ST, et al. Depression in complex partial seizures. Electroencephalography and cerebral metabolic correlates. Arch Neurol 1994;51:155–63.

96. Buchsbaum MS, Haier RJ, Potkin SG, et al. Frontostriatal disorder of cerebral metabolism in never-medicated schizophrenics. Arch Gen Psychiatry 1992;49:935–42.

97. Friston KJ, Liddle PF, Frith CD, et al. The left medial temporal region and schizophrenia. A PET study. Brain 1992;115:367–82.

98. Baxter LR Jr, Phelps ME, Mazziotta JC, et al. Cerebral metabolic rates for glucose in mood disorders. Studies with positron emission tomography and fluorodeoxyglucose F18. Arch Gen Psychiatry 1985;42:441–7.

99. Baron JC, Roeda D, Munari C, et al. Brain regional pharmacokinetics of 11C-labeled diphenylhydantoin: positron emission tomography in humans. Neurology 1983;33:580–5.

100. Theodore WH, Bromfield E, Onorati L. The effect of carbamazepine on cerebral glucose metabolism. Ann Neurol 1989;25:516–20.

101. Leiderman DB, Balish M, Bromfield EB, et al. Effect of valporate on human cerebral glucose metabolism. Epilepsia 1991;32:417–22.

102. Gaillard WD, White S, Fazilat S, et al. Effect of valproate on cerebral glucose metabolism and cerebral blood flow as determined by 18FDG and O-15 water PET (abstract). Epilepsia 1992;33 Suppl 3:54.

103. Petroff O, Rothman D, Behar K, et al. In vivo gamma-aminobutyric acid, glutamate, and glutamine levels in human brain (abstract). Ann Neurol 1993;34:262.

104. Frost JJ, Mayberg HS, Fisher RS, et al. Mu-opiate receptors measured by positron emission tomography are increased in temporal lobe epilepsy. Ann Neurol 1988;23:231–7.

105. Mayberg HS, Sadzot B, Meltzer CC, et al. Quantification of mu and non-mu opiate receptors in temporal lobe epilepsy using positron emission tomography. Ann Neurol 1991;30:3–11.

106. Theodore WH, Carson RE, Andreasen P, et al. PET imaging of opiate receptor binding in human epilepsy using [18F]cyclofoxy. Epilepsy Res 1992;13:129–39.

107. Theodore WH, Leiderman D, Gaillard W, et al. The effect of naloxone on cerebral blood flow and glucose metabolism in patients with complex partial seizures. Epilepsy Res 1993;16:51–4.

108. Gale K. GABA and epilepsy: basic concepts from preclinical research. Epilepsia 1992;33 Suppl 5:S3–12.

109. McDonald JW, Garofalo EA, Hood T, et al. Altered excitatory and inhibitory amino acid receptor binding in hippocampus of patients with temporal lobe epilepsy. Ann Neurol 1991;29:529–41.

110. Savic I, Persson A, Roland P, et al. In-vivo demonstration of reduced benzodiazepine receptor binding in human epileptic foci. Lancet 1988;2:863–6.

111. Cordes M, Henkes H, Ferstl F, et al. Evaluation of focal epilepsy: a SPECT scanning comparison of 123-I-iomazenil versus HM-PAO. AJNR Am J Neuroradiol 1992;13:249–53.

112. Henry TR, Frey KA, Sackellares JC, et al. In vivo cerebral metabolism and central benzodiazepine-receptor binding in temporal lobe epilepsy. Neurology 1993;43:1998–2006.

113. Johnson EW, de Lanerolle NC, Kim JH, et al. "Central" and "peripheral" benzodiazepine receptors: opposite changes in human epileptogenic tissue. Neurology 1992;42:811–5.

114. Savic I, Ingvar M, Stone-Elander S. Comparison of [11C]flumazenil and [18F]FDG as PET markers of epileptic foci. J Neurol Neurosurg Psychiatry 1993;56:615–21.

115. Kumlien E, Bergström M, Lilja A, et al. Positron emission tomography with [11C] deuterium-deprenyl in temporal lobe epilepsy. Epilepsia 1995;36:712–21.

CHAPTER

12

Interictal, Ictal, and Postictal Single-Photon Emission Computed Tomography

Mark R. Newton and Samuel F. Berkovic

BACKGROUND, METHODOLOGY, AND LIGANDS

Functional Imaging and Anatomical Imaging

Single-photon emission computed tomography (SPECT) is a functional imaging technique that allows relative cerebral blood flow to be determined at any point in time. This is in contrast with anatomical imaging methods, such as magnetic resonance imaging (MRI), which provide information on structure rather than on function. The investigation of refractory epilepsy requires data on both structure and function to guide epileptologists to the seizure focus; thus, SPECT and MRI should not be regarded as competing imaging methods but as complementary techniques. Whereas MRI-detected lesions in patients with intractable epilepsy are usually the cause of seizures, they are not always so. Therefore, measurement of function, such as regional cerebral blood flow, can provide essential information for localization of seizure focus that adds to the body of data derived from anatomical MRI, videoelectroencephalography (video-EEG), clinical observations, and neuropsychologic testing. Functional brain imaging is a rapidly developing investigational tool that is providing new clinical and scientific insights into epilepsy.

The origins of these techniques can be traced to Horsley's [1] observation a century ago of a local increase in blood flow during induced seizures. This observation was corroborated by Penfield[2] in the 1930s. Dymond and Crandall[3] described a similar phenomenon 40 years later with intracranial thermistors. The techniques used by these pioneer investigators required invasive procedures and gave information only on the regional perfusion changes; blood flow in other regions could not be recorded simultaneously. The development of functional imaging with radionuclides during the last 30 years has enabled the noninvasive measurement of relative blood flow changes throughout the brain. The evolution in radiotracers and detector technology has provided powerful functional imaging tools that can be applied clinically with simplicity and relatively low cost.

Nuclide Imaging

Nuclide imaging was the major step forward in the assessment of whole brain perfusion changes with seizures. Initially, xenon 133 was inhaled or injected, and data were collected by scintillation counters placed next to the patient's head.[4] Besides limited resolution, this dynamic SPECT method did not allow seizures to be captured whenever they happened to occur, so ictal study was a rare chance event when the patient happened to have a seizure during elective study.[5–7] Interictal study of patients with partial seizures sometimes revealed areas of focal hypoperfusion that corresponded to the epileptic focus.[6,8–10]

Positron emission tomography (PET) with ^{18}F-fluorodeoxyglucose showed hypometabolism in the epileptogenic zone,[11] with a sensitivity of about 80% in patients with temporal lobe epilepsy, in the interictal condition. PET is an expensive and elaborate technique. Also, it can be routinely applied only to interictal study because as with dynamic ^{133}X SPECT, ictal data are acquired purely by chance.[12,13]

The use of static SPECT in localizing seizure foci has become possible only in the last decade with the development of radioligands that are readily fixed in cerebral tissue during first-pass circulation. This has enabled ligands to be injected during seizures and scanning to be done shortly thereafter to produce a "snapshot" of cerebral blood flow very close to the time of injection. The combination of this technique with video-EEG telemetry has proved to be a powerful tool for investigating the pathophysiology of partial seizures.

Single-Photon Emission Computed Tomography Ligands

Perfusion Ligands

Iodinated Ligands. The ^{123}I-iodoamines isopropyl-iodoamphetamine (IMP) and trimethyl-(hydroxymethyl-^{123}I-iodobenzyl)-propanediamine (HIPDM) were the first ligands developed that were taken up rapidly by

cerebral tissues, thus reflecting the distribution of blood flow close to the time of injection.[14,15] In addition to studying the interictal condition, the stability of these compounds allows the ligand to be stored near the monitoring suite, enabling injection at the time of seizure. After the patient has recovered from the seizure and is cooperative, scanning can be performed at leisure. Hill et al.[16] reported the capture of a partial seizure using IMP, and Lee et al.[17–20] used HIPDM to study temporal lobe seizures. However, the ^{123}I-iodinated compounds are cyclotron products and, therefore, costly and of limited availability. Also, the long half-life of ^{123}I precludes study on sequential days.

Technetium Ligands. Exametazine, or hexamethyl-propyleneamineoxime (HMPAO), is a lipophilic compound that is rapidly fixed by cerebral tissues and has the advantage of binding to the relatively inexpensive and widely available isotope technetium^{99m} (^{99m}Tc).[21] The isotope has a much shorter half-life than ^{123}I and can be administered on sequential days if necessary. To date, the clinically valuable localizing data from SPECT has been derived with single-head rotating gamma cameras, yet the current generations of dual-head and triple-head cameras can produce superior resolution, allowing coregistration of the functional image with the anatomical data of magnetic resonance images.

The only disadvantage of ^{99m}Tc-HMPAO for peri-ictal studies is its instability, which requires mixing the isotope with the ligand immediately before use. This limitation has been overcome largely with a rapid mixing method that enables preparation of the compound within 30 seconds, thus allowing for capture of most seizures in the ictal or immediate postictal period.[22] Furthermore, ^{99m}Tc-HMPAO can be stabilized for the duration of the half-life of technetium by using cobalt chloride.[23] A new cerebral perfusion ligand, ethyl cysteinate dimer (ECD), that is stable when bound with technetium has been developed.[24,25]

Clearly, to make injections during the ictal and postictal periods, these ligands need to be stored next to the video monitoring suite. This is the arrangement in our unit, and all radioactive safety regulations are met. Such measures may not be possible in all medical centers, depending on the local regulations for storage of radioactive materials.

Receptor-Binding Ligands

Benzodiazepine Receptor-Binding Ligands. The recent development of two ^{123}I-binding compounds (the flumazenil analogue ^{123}I-iomazenil and the diazepam analogue 2'-iododiazepam) has allowed SPECT imaging of the distribution of central benzodiazepine receptors.[26–29] Currently, the few reports of the application of these ligands for the investigation of partial seizures[30–32] suggest that the technique can provide useful localizing data in the interictal period, similarly to the PET ligand ^{11}C-flumazenil.[33] Further studies with surgical outcome data in a larger number of patients will be needed to assess the place of this SPECT ligand in investigating epilepsy.

Cholinergic Receptor-Binding Ligand. The central distribution of muscarinic cholinergic receptors can also be imaged with SPECT using ^{123}I-iododexetimide.[34] Müller-Gartner et al.[34] reported decreased receptor binding in the epileptic temporal lobe in four patients with unilateral temporal lobe epilepsy. The differences in binding between patients and controls were much greater than the differences in perfusion shown by HMPAO SPECT in this pilot study. Boundy et al.[35] found decreased receptor binding using this ligand on the epileptic side in all nine patients with established unilateral temporal foci. These data were superior to those of interictal HMPAO SPECT, which were correctly localizing in six of the patients and falsely localizing in the three others.

The initial reports of SPECT using receptor-binding ligands suggested that valuable lateralizing information may be derived in the interictal condition, which offers the advantage of outpatient evaluation and technical simplicity. However, the principal disadvantage of these compounds is the necessity for access to a cyclotron for the generation of isotope. Further study with a greater number of patients and comparison with the perfusion ligands will be needed for comprehensive evaluation of these methods.

Methods for Single-Photon Emission Computed Tomography Study: Interictal, Ictal, and Postictal Conditions

Interictal Study

During the interictal period, ligand ideally is injected after the patient has been seizure-free for several hours, so that the cerebral perfusion image is most likely representative of the true interictal state. We attempt to perform interictal SPECT at least 24 hours after the last seizure, but in some cases, this long of a period is not possible because of the frequency of the seizures. Patients continue taking their antiepileptic medication, because this is the simplest and safest course for both outpatient and inpatient imaging. The ligand is injected with the patient supine, eyes closed, and silent, with a minimum of background noise. Data can be acquired very soon after the injection because of the rapid fixation of the ligand. SPECT images are derived from data collected by rotating gamma cameras that are found in virtually all nuclear medicine departments.

Ictal and Postictal Study

Ideally, the ligand kit (vial of freeze-dried HMPAO and syringe of technetium solution) is stored next to the monitoring suite, where trained personnel can rapidly mix the isotope and HMPAO after they have been alerted to the onset of a seizure and inject it into the patient through an in situ venous cannula. The methods for rapid deployment of this tracer have been described in detail elsewhere.[22] The essential requirements are prompt seizure alert, a rapid and safe mixing technique, and injection made during video-EEG monitoring. Personnel dedicated for this task would be ideal, although a luxury in most epilepsy programs; however, resident medical, nursing, or EEG staff can be easily trained. In the 6-year experience of the Austin Hospital (Melbourne), ligand was injected during the ictal period in more than 60% of cases, and as the number of available trained personnel increases, the ictal capture rate should increase accordingly.

We stress the importance of video-EEG surveillance, which provides exact timing of the injection relative to the onset and end of the seizure and correlation of the SPECT image with clinical and EEG data. Knowledge of the evolution of specific blood flow patterns, particularly in temporal lobe seizures, is essential for correct interpretation of SPECT data.[36,37] This can be achieved confidently only when the timing of ligand injection is established by video recording.

SINGLE-PHOTON EMISSION COMPUTED TOMOGRAPHY IN ADULT EPILEPSY

Temporal Lobe Epilepsy

Interictal Regional Cerebral Blood Flow

Regional hypoperfusion of the anterior temporal lobe on the side of the seizure focus was first reported using IMP,[16,38] but more rigorous and informative data on temporal lobe epilepsy came from Stefan et al.,[39] who used HMPAO, and later from Ryding et al.[40] and others [41–43] Although some authors claimed up to 80% incidence of focal hypoperfusion in the epileptic zone, few reports contained good critical methods of evaluation. Moreover, interictal focal hyperperfusion in the epileptic zone was described by Duncan et al.,[44] but this has yet to be confirmed in a large number of patients.

Interictal SPECT is not a sensitive test for identifying foci of temporal seizures. We examined the interictal SPECT scans of 119 patients with confirmed unilateral temporal lobe epilepsy by using readers blinded to clinical details and found the abnormality to be correct in 48% of cases, inconclusive in 42%, and incorrect in 10% (Table 12-1). Although the modest rate of correct lateralization may be helpful, the false-lateralization rate is of concern and mitigates the use of interictal SPECT in deciding the side of epileptic focus. Occasionally, the per-

Table 12-1.   Accuracy of Interictal, Postictal, and Ictal SPECT in Localizing Epileptic Foci in 119 Patients with Unilateral Temporal Lobe Epilepsy

SPECT lateralization*	Interictal, n = 119	Postictal,† n = 77	Ictal,‡ n = 51
Correct	48%	71%	97%
Inconclusive	42%	25%	3%
Incorrect	10%	4%	0%

*The first 46 cases were interpreted independently by two blinded reviewers, and the next 73 cases by three blinded reviewers. Values shown are the percentage means for the whole series.

†Seventy-seven studies in 77 patients, of whom 9 also had ictal studies.

‡Fifty-one studies in 51 patients. In 49 of the 51 patients, all three independent blinded reviewers correctly lateralized the foci. In one patient whose focus was not lateralized by any reviewer, a repeat ictal study showed the correct lateralization. In the other patient, the focus was not lateralized by only one of the three reviewers.

fusion defects are large and clear, but more often, they are subtle and subject to misinterpretation and, thus, should not be relied upon. The new generation of triple-headed scanners may improve the diagnostic yield of interictal SPECT, but extensive data are not available, and the incorrect lateralization rate will need to be significantly lower than 10% for the technique to be of major clinical value. However, interictal SPECT will still be necessary in many cases for comparison with the ictal and postictal studies in order to determine the extent of blood flow changes between conditions.

Ictal-Postictal Evolution of Blood Flow

Blood Flow Changes in the Temporal Lobe. Hyperperfusion of the temporal lobe was initially reported by Hill et al.[16] and Uren et al.[45] using IMP. Confirmatory findings in a larger series of patients with temporal lobe epilepsy were reported by Lee et al.[19] using HIPDM. The use of ^{123}I-iodinated compounds has been limited because their availability depends on having access to a cyclotron. In 1985, Biersack et al.[46] described ictal SPECT using ^{99m}Tc-HMPAO. Isolated reports followed from Andersen et al.[47] and Rowe et al.[48] These studies revealed the hyperperfusion of the anterior temporal lobe during temporal lobe seizures, but the extent and time frame of perfusion changes were not delineated until we reported the "postictal switch" of blood flow,[37] which elaborated on the novel observations of Rowe et al.[49] on postictal SPECT patterns in temporal lobe epilepsy.

The increased uptake of ^{99m}Tc-HMPAO in the anterior temporal lobe as seen in SPECT reflects the local increase in blood flow during the seizure (Figure 12-1).

The appearances are striking and unmistakable and provide powerful localizing data in patients being evaluated for temporal lobectomy. Side-to-side ratio analysis has shown a mean 30% increase in counts on the epileptic side compared with that of the interictal state. After the end of the seizure, this ictal hyperperfusion pattern persists into the immediate postictal period for about 60 seconds before there is a switch to a postictal pattern. This duration of ictal hyperperfusion was estimated from our observation that anterior temporal hyperperfusion was found after injections of ligand for up to 30 seconds after the end of the seizure. Allowing about 30 seconds for the cerebral distribution of the ligand, we calculated that this ictal increase in blood flow persists for the first minute of the postictal period.

The typical postictal pattern, which is found in about 70% of cases at our institution, consists of hypoperfusion of the lateral temporal cortex on the side of the focus, often with persisting perfusion in the mesial temporal cortex (see Figure 12-1). This was originally described by Rowe et al.,[43,48-50] whose injections were given at a mean 6.3 minutes after seizure onset (about 5 minutes after the end of the seizure), and confirmed by Duncan et al.[36] in a similar group of patients. The postictal changes may be subtle and often require comparison with the interictal study.

Perfusion Changes Distant from the Temporal Lobe.   SPECT allows examination of the relative blood flow changes in all cerebral regions, thus providing unique insight into the pathophysiology of temporal lobe seizures.   A qualitative and semiquantitative analysis of 72 ictal and postictal SPECT studies compared with the interictal condition in patients with established temporal lobe epilepsy has revealed that the peri-ictal perfusion changes evolve at different rates in different cortical and subcortical regions.[48] Although perfusion declines in the lateral temporal lobe earlier than in the mesial temporal lobe in the immediate postictal period, perfusion in the lateral frontal, central, and parietal cortical areas decreases abruptly from interictal levels at the end of the seizure. The combination of lateral temporal lobe hypoperfusion with these extratemporal cortical changes establishes a pattern of extensive hypoperfusion throughout the hemisphere on the side of seizure origin. This appearance, confirmed by Duncan et al.,[36] is useful for lateralization of temporal lobe seizures.

Peri-ictal blood flow in subcortical gray matter can also be analyzed. Ictal hyperperfusion of the basal ganglia ipsilateral to the epileptic temporal lobe is associated with dystonic posturing of the contralateral upper limb[51] (Figure 12-2). This observation supports the hypothesis that the spread of the seizure from the temporal lobe to the ipsilateral basal ganglia is responsible for the dystonia[52] rather than spread to the supplementary motor area.[53]

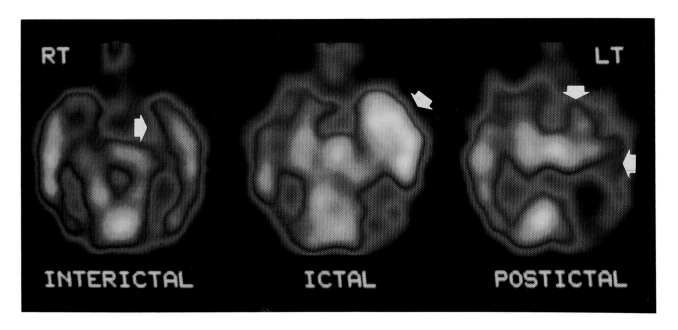

FIGURE 12-1. Transaxial slices showing sequential changes in temporal lobe perfusion before, during, and after complex partial seizure. Interictal condition. Reduced perfusion in the mesial temporal region (*arrow*). Ictal condition. Marked increase in perfusion in the anterior temporal lobe during seizure (*arrow*). Postictal condition (1.5 minutes after seizure end). Reduced lateral temporal perfusion (*horizontal arrow*) with relative hyperperfusion in the mesial temporal region (*vertical arrow*). (*LT*) left, (*RT*) right. (From Newton et al.[37] By permission of *Journal of Neurology, Neurosurgery, and Psychiatry*.)

Thalamic hyperperfusion is also seen ipsilateral to the seizure focus during the seizure and, similarly to basal ganglia hyperperfusion, decreases rapidly to interictal levels during the initial 90 seconds of the postictal period. Perfusion in the cerebellar hemispheres, however, remains symmetrical throughout the ictal and postictal periods in complex partial seizures of temporal lobe origin.[54]

Clinical Value

The striking and unambiguous changes seen with ictal SPECT provide powerful lateralizing data. In a review of 119 cases of established unilateral temporal lobe epilepsy from the Austin Hospital in Melbourne, Australia, 97% of 51 ictal SPECT studies were correctly lateralized by two blinded observers, with no incorrect lateralizations. Only one case was inconclusive. Second best are the postictal changes that allowed correct lateralization in 71% of 77 studies but were incorrect in 4%. Interictal SPECT, by contrast, allowed only 48% correct lateralizations in the 119 cases, with an unacceptable 10% being incorrectly lateralized.[54] Similar results have been reported by other authors in comparable groups of patients. Markand et al.[55] found ictal hyperperfusion in 91% of 38 patients who underwent temporal lobectomy. Duncan et al.[36] reported an interictal lateralization rate of 54% in 28 patients and

ictal/postictal changes in 93% that were congruent with other localizing data.

It is of interest that the ictal hyperperfusion found during temporal lobe seizures is usually limited to the ipsilateral temporal region, in contrast to the electrical activity that frequently spreads to the contralateral hippocampus. Why the topography of perfusion changes does not match the electrographic spread in complex partial seizures is not clear. However, in complex partial events that hemigeneralize, hyperperfusion can be seen along the motor strip ipsilateral to the epileptic focus, an observation initially reported by Lee et al.[18] using HIPDM SPECT.

We have seen two cases in which ictal EEG showed seizure origin in one temporal lobe that then activated the contralateral temporal lobe, and because the ligand was injected late in the seizure, the hyperperfusion was seen in the temporal lobe contralateral to the focus. Although this has been found in only 2 of more than 100 ictal SPECT studies performed at our institution, it emphasizes that SPECT is complementary to the clinical and electrographic data and cannot be interpreted independently of them.

It should be noted that the above ictal SPECT results were found in complex partial seizures. In our experience, injections of ligand during simple partial seizures have rarely yielded diagnostic information.

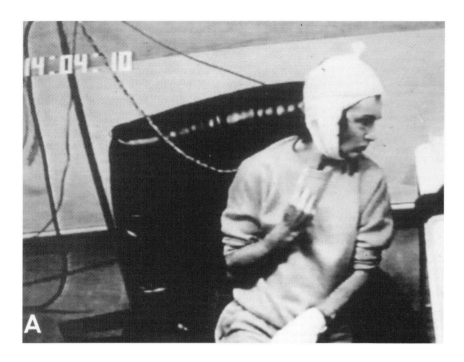

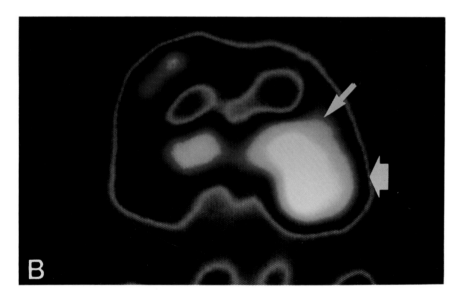

FIGURE 12-2. Ictal dystonia associated with increased perfusion of basal ganglia. A. Dystonic posturing of patient's right arm during complex partial seizure. B. Coronal slice of SPECT obtained after ligand injection during the seizure. Hyperperfusion is seen in both the left temporal lobe (*lower arrow*) and adjacent basal ganglia (*upper arrow*). (A from Newton et al.[51] By permission of Little, Brown and Company.)

However, partial status epilepticus has been reported to show hyperperfusion congruent with the EEG focus in seven patients.[56] One of these patients showed focal hyperperfusion that resolved over 6 days. There is some experimental evidence that the cerebral hypermetabolism associated with partial status epilepticus persists for up to 7 days after the cessation of seizure activity.[57]

Pathology, Single-Photon Emission Computed Tomography, and Surgical Outcome

Pathology and Ictal Perfusion Subtypes. In a study of 30 operated on patients, Ho et al.[58] found that different patterns of ictal temporal hyperperfusion were associated with different underlying pathologic conditions. Patients with hippocampal sclerosis (n = 10) or those with foreign tissue lesions in the mesial temporal lobe (n = 8) had typical ictal SPECT patterns of ipsilateral mesial and lateral temporal lobe hyperperfusion. Five patients with good surgical outcome but no demonstrable lesion showed ictal hyperperfusion similarly restricted to the ipsilateral anterior temporal lobe region. In contrast, patients with foreign tissue lesions in the lateral temporal lobe (n = 7) had hyperperfusion bilaterally, with predominant changes in the region of the lesion. No differences were seen in the seizure symptoms of these four groups. These observations suggest that the location of the lesion determines the ictal blood flow pattern, which probably follows the anatomical pathways of seizure spread.

Single-Photon Emission Computed Tomography and Surgical Outcome.   The relatively low lateralizing power of interictal SPECT, as described above, was confirmed in a series of patients with temporal lobe epilepsy whose SPECT findings were related to surgical outcome.[59] These data suggested that the interictal perfusion patterns were not a sensitive index of cortical dysfunction in the temporal lobe. The experience at our hospital is similar, as would be expected from the interictal SPECT data shown in Table 12-1. Because ictal SPECT has significantly greater lateralizing power, surgical outcome should be closely related to the ictal perfusion pattern. Review of the ictal SPECT and surgical outcome data by Ho et al. (Ho SS, Berkovic SF, Newton MR, et al., unpublished data) showed that typical ictal SPECT patterns predicted good outcome, in contrast to atypical ictal SPECT scans.

Extratemporal Focal Epilepsies

Interictal Study

The localization of foci in seizures of extratemporal origin has long been a major diagnostic challenge. In the absence of structural lesions, little information is often derived from the EEG and clinical data. Therefore, the advent of functional imaging provided hope for more effective localization in this difficult group of epilepsies. Interictal SPECT has been of limited localizing value in extratemporal partial seizures. Marks et al.[60] obtained interictal SPECT in 8 of 11 patients evaluated for extratemporal partial seizures and found widespread areas of hypoperfusion not seen in the ictal scans in only 2 of them. Four other patients had hypoperfusion defects that corresponded to known lesions. Our experience is similar.[61]

The parietal epilepsy series reported by Ho et al.[62] contained interictal SPECT data on all 14 patients, but only 4 showed perfusion defects, and these were related to known structural defects. It would appear, then, that the current role of interictal SPECT in extratemporal partial seizures is for comparison with ictal and postictal studies of cerebral perfusion. The role of interictal SPECT using receptor ligands has yet to be defined. Interictal PET with ^{18}F-fluorodeoxyglucose is probably more useful than interictal perfusion SPECT studies; we have identified a few cases in which PET showed hypometabolic areas despite normal MRI findings.

Ictal Study

Seizures of extratemporal origin are a challenge to ictal perfusion SPECT studies because they commonly are brief, shorter than temporal lobe seizures and, therefore, allow little time for the preparation and injection of ^{99m}Tc-HMPAO, which in our hands takes 30 seconds. Despite these obstacles, injection of ligand in the ictal period has been achieved in many patients in different medical centers. To date, the results indicate that ictal SPECT is of much greater value in localizing extratemporal seizure foci than interictal SPECT studies. Focal hyperperfusion at the site of seizure origin has been reported by several investigators.[46,60,63] Marks et al.[60] found ictal SPECT of value in localizing foci in 10 of 12 studies in 11 patients with extratemporal foci.

At our institution, Ho et al.[62] studied the clinical and ictal SPECT features of 14 patients with parietal lobe epilepsy. The images showed focal hyperperfusion in all patients and corresponded with the structural lesions that were present in nine. Semiquantitative analysis of side-to-side ratios in the parietal regions of interest revealed increases of 11% to 51% (mean, 25.5%) compared with interictal scans. In addition, two main clinical seizure patterns were recognized in association with the SPECT patterns: (1) seizures with sensorimotor manifestations characterized by hyperperfusion in the anterior parietal area and (2) complex partial seizures of the psychoparetic type associated with hyperperfusion in the posterior parietal region (Figure 12-3). These two clinical seizure patterns may reflect seizure propagation via association fibers that connect the anterior parietal region with the primary motor, premotor, and supplementary motor areas. The posterior parietal region, however, is connected with the cingulate gyrus, insula, and parahippocampal gyrus so that seizure propagation to these structures may well imitate the psychoparetic seizures of temporal lobe epilepsy.

The presence of abnormality on MRI does not appear to influence the ictal perfusion pattern in parietal lobe epilepsy. Five of the 14 patients with parietal seizure foci reported by Ho et al.[62] had no lesion seen on MRI, and the SPECT appearances were not different from those of cases with abnormal MRI findings (Figure 12-3 C and D). Normal MRI findings, of course, do not exclude pathologic conditions such as cortical microdysgenesis, which may be epileptogenic.

Postictal Study

Examination of our postictal injections in the extratemporal cases has been of limited localizing value.[61] Postictal SPECT suggested localization in 10 of 26 patients with no other diagnostic data, in contrast to ictal SPECT that suggested a seizure focus in 8 of 9 patients whose seizure was captured with ligand. Furthermore, in 12 patients with established parietal, frontal, or occipital foci, ictal SPECT was congruent in all 9 patients in

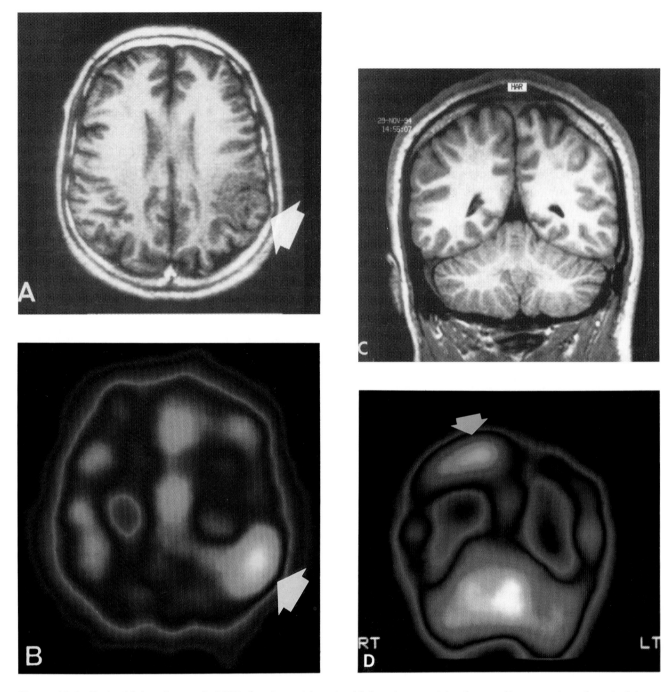

Figure 12-3. Parietal lobe seizures. A. MRI of patient with parietal lobe seizures arising from a discrete region of cortical dysgenesis (*arrow*). B. Transverse slice of ictal SPECT study showing focal hyperperfusion (*arrow*) in an area corresponding to region of cortical dysgenesis. C. In this patient with parietal lobe seizures, MRI does not reveal any lesion, but ictal SPECT (D) shows parietal hyperperfusion (*arrow*) in coronal slice through brain. (*LT*) left, (*RT*) right.

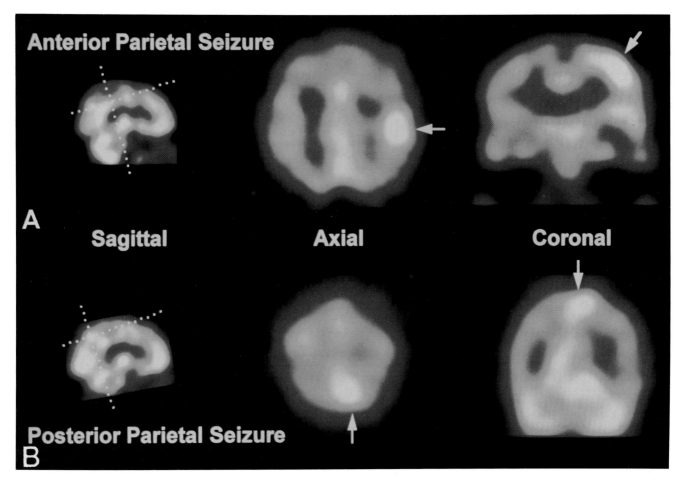

FIGURE 12-4. A. Anterior parietal hyperperfusion (*arrows*) in patient with complex partial seizures. B. Posterior parietal hyperperfusion (*arrows*) in another patient with sensorimotor seizures. (From Ho et al.[62] By permission of Little, Brown and Company.)

whom injection was achieved during the ictal period (Figure 12-4). However, postictal studies in this group revealed changes in only two of five patients studied in that condition. These data make the ictal injection of ligand during the ictal period even a greater priority than in the case of temporal lobe seizures.

SINGLE-PHOTON EMISSION COMPUTED TOMOGRAPHY IN PEDIATRIC EPILEPSY

Physiologic Considerations

Brain development is associated with changes in regional cerebral blood flow so that knowledge of these changes becomes essential for the interpretation of pathologic situations in children. The most critical development occurs in the first years of life, when the values of cerebral blood flow exceed those of adults and the regional patterns of blood flow differ.[64–68]

At birth, the mean regional cerebral blood flow is the same as in adults (50 mg/100 g per minute), but it increases rapidly to 60 mg/100 g per minute by age 1 year and to 70 mg/100 g per minute by age 3. Mean cerebral blood flow gradually decreases after the age of 10 years to reach adult values by age 20. These changes in cerebral blood flow parallel most markers of synaptogenesis,[69–72] which is most prolific during the first few years of life and stabilizes after the first decade.

The regional changes in cerebral blood flow are characterized by intermittent increases that mirror an anteroposterior gradient of cortical maturation. Increases in cerebral blood flow in the sensorimotor and posterior cortices are found at birth and are followed by increases in the primary visual cortex by age 3 months and in the posterior associative cortex by age 6 months.[64,73,74] Regional cerebral blood flow in the frontal cortex gradually increases after the first year of life,[64] in contrast to the specific spurts of increased flow seen in the posterior cortex, which have stabilized by that age. This evolution of regional cerebral blood flow corresponds with the sequence of cognitive development, that is, visual and auditory faculties develop in the first year of life and are followed by the development of frontal lobe functions in succeeding years.

Evolution of Cerebral Blood Flow in Childhood and Epilepsy

Clinical observations of childhood epilepsy parallel the age-related changes in regional cerebral blood flow. Rolandic and occipital epilepsy are relatively common in infants, whereas frontal epilepsy rarely occurs. Preexisting epileptogenic areas may become symptomatic at different ages, depending on their location. In tuberous sclerosis, for example, tubers at different sites may produce seizures at different times of life. West's syndrome, which has a peak onset by age 6 months, can be associated with lesions in the occipital and associated posterior areas,[75,76] 6 months being the age at which cerebral blood flow normally increases in those regions. In addition, the severe mental regression usually seen in West's syndrome at the 6-month mark is due to the lack of visual function, the main faculty for communicating at this age.

Temporal Lobe Epilepsy

The patterns of regional cerebral blood flow associated with temporal lobe epilepsy in children, as shown by SPECT, are similar to those seen in adults in the interictal, ictal, and postictal periods. Lateralization rates up to 80% or more[77,78] have been found with ictal studies, as compared with the interictal SPECT perfusion defects that are seen in 40% to 60% of cases.[79–82] The high proportion of correct localizations has been supported by congruence with other investigative data and postoperative pathologic findings. This makes ictal SPECT a very useful tool in the preoperative work-up of children with temporal lobe epilepsy.[77,83]

Extratemporal Focal Epilepsies

Seizures arising in sites other than the temporal lobe are difficult to localize. If localizing data from clinical observations and EEG studies are sparse, few options remain for further investigation. However, ictal SPECT can demonstrate the epileptic region in frontal lobe epilepsy, as reported by Harvey et al.,[84] who studied 22 children with this condition (Figure 12-5). Focal frontal hyperperfusion was seen in 20 of 22 cases (91%), the distribution being lobar in one child and restricted to focal frontal regions in the others. Semiquantitative measurement using side-to-side ratios of counts revealed a mean 20% increase in counts at the

epileptic focus, as compared with the interictal state. The ictal studies frequently showed hyperperfusion of the ipsilateral basal ganglia and contralateral cerebellum, presumably reflecting regions of subcortical activation via corticostriatopontocerebellar connections. Occipital and parietal seizure foci have been localized with ictal SPECT by the same authors (Harvey AS, personal communication).

The experience with interictal SPECT in pediatric extratemporal seizures disorders has been similar to that in adults with extratemporal foci. Harvey et al.[84] found interictal focal hypoperfusion in only 2 of 22 children with frontal lobe epilepsy. Uvebrant et al.[82] reported an 83% abnormality rate in children with focal seizures, but the hypoperfusion defects were often widespread and in multiple sites. Other authors have reported a spectrum of abnormalities, including multifocal perfusion defects, regions of hyperperfusion, and bilateral abnormalities, in addition to focal hypoperfusion.[79,85–87]

Infantile spasms (West's syndrome) have been studied with 133X SPECT by Chiron et al.,[88] who found foci of hyperperfusion in the frontal cortex and hypoperfusion in posterior cerebral cortex. The hyperperfused areas decreased with spasm control with corticosteroid treatment. Similarly, areas of hypometabolism in children with infantile spasms, as demonstrated by PET,[75,89] were distributed predominantly in the parietal region. These areas were found in the absence of MRI abnormalities in 14 of 23 children, and pathologic examination showed dysplastic cortex in nearly all the subjects. These data show strong concordance between SPECT and PET in locating the epileptogenic regions in children with infantile spasms.

LIMITATIONS OF SINGLE-PHOTON EMISSION COMPUTED TOMOGRAPHY

This review has highlighted the diagnostic power of ictal SPECT studies in focal seizure disorders of adults and children. Current data suggest (1) that postictal SPECT has more value in temporal lobe epilepsies than in extratemporal seizure disorders and (2) that interictal SPECT is limited by relatively lower sensitivity in both types of epilepsy, and the false localization rate in the interictal condition is unacceptably high for temporal lobe epilepsy. Having determined that the ictal condition is optimal for SPECT study, we consider below the factors that currently limit its application.

Seizures of very brief duration (for example, less than 30 seconds) are likely to be associated with short-lived hyperperfusion of small magnitude. This factor militates against seizure capture with ^{99m}Tc-HMPAO SPECT, because of the minimum 30 seconds required to prepare the ligand. However, the new stabilized ligands

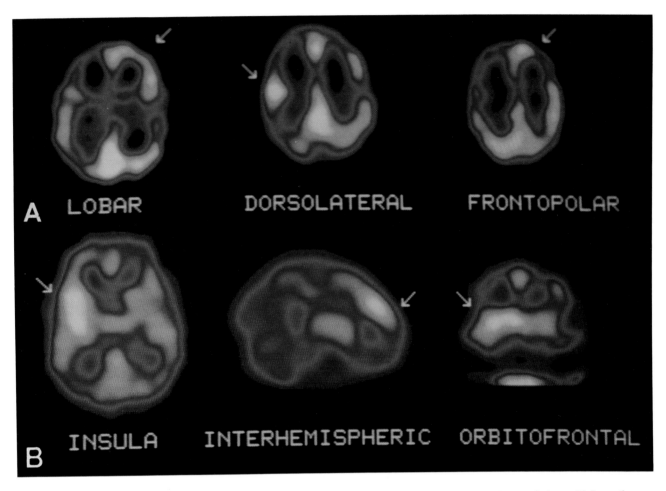

FIGURE 12-5. SPECT patterns of frontal lobe seizures in children. Ictal SPECT studies in six children with frontal lobe epilepsy. A. Regional hyperperfusion (*arrow*) in left lobar distribution, focal hyperperfusion (*arrow*) in right dorsolateral region, and frontopolar hyperperfusion (*arrow*). B. A seizure arising from right insula is associated with regional hyperperfusion (*arrow*). Interhemispheric focus (*arrow*) is shown on sagittal slice and orbitofrontal hyperperfusion (*arrow*) on coronal slice. (From Harvey et al.[84] By permission of Little, Brown and Company.)

may enable the study of shorter seizures. Also, the current limits of SPECT resolution may prevent the detection of ictal hyperperfusion in extratemporal seizures that affect a small cortical region. Furthermore, seizures that spread rapidly to a distant cortical focus or that secondarily generalize may not show a restricted hyperperfused focus with ligand injection during the ictal period at least 30 seconds after seizure onset. The ictal-postictal evolution of regional cerebral blood flow appears to be quite different in temporal and extratemporal seizures. The prolonged postictal hypoperfusion often present in SPECT studies of temporal lobe seizures is not found in postictal SPECT of the extratemporal seizures that we have studied so far, which limits the value of ligand injection during the postictal period in the latter. However, these circumstances are relatively uncommon in the spectrum of refractory partial seizures.

CURRENT ROLE OF SINGLE-PHOTON EMISSION COMPUTED TOMOGRAPHY IN COMPREHENSIVE EPILEPSY EVALUATION

The tools of investigation currently available to epileptologists provide a wide range of data on cerebral structure and function in patients with refractory partial seizures. There is now enough information on the usefulness of these tools to choose the most efficient localization protocol in selected patient groups.

In most cases of temporal lobe tumors, video-EEG and congruent neuropsychologic data are sufficient for operation. However, if the EEG data are not useful, functional imaging with ictal SPECT or interictal PET is necessary to confirm the suspected seizure focus and to exclude any other foci.

When video-EEG and neuropsychologic data are congruent for patients with a clinical picture of temporal lobe epilepsy and mesial temporal sclerosis on MRI, we confirm the site of the epileptogenic focus with either interictal PET (an outpatient procedure) or ictal SPECT (an inpatient procedure). When the PET findings are normal or equivocal, we consider it mandatory to use ictal SPECT to confirm the localization of the seizure focus. Therefore, initial functioning imaging is most simply done with PET, if available. However, ictal SPECT will become increasingly easy to acquire as the use of stable technetium isotopes becomes widespread.

When the MRI findings are normal in a patient with complex partial seizures, it is essential to confirm any localizing video-EEG data with functional imaging. Ideally, we obtain both ictal SPECT and interictal PET with ^{18}F-fluorodeoxyglucose. These imaging techniques have a high chance of indicating a temporal focus, and for extratemporal seizures, in which EEG may not be clearly and consistently localizing, ictal SPECT may reveal the primary focus, as can interictal PET (although less often).

Frequently, EEG localizing data are not good in patients with extratemporal lesions and partial seizures. In these cases, ictal SPECT study can provide the functional evidence that complements the anatomical MRI data to confirm seizure localization. Although interictal PET might show a metabolic abnormality in the region of the lesion, it would not provide the dynamic changes revealed by SPECT in the ictal condition. When seizures arise from an extratemporal focus in the absence of a lesion, ictal SPECT may provide the only definite clue to seizure focus; therefore, it is an invaluable guide to planning intracranial EEG study.

FUTURE DIRECTIONS

In the decade since the development of cerebral blood flow ligands, SPECT has become a valuable adjunct in the preoperative assessment of patients with refractory focal epilepsy. However, more clinical and scientific information probably will be obtained with refinement of ligand delivery and SPECT resolution.

Stabilization of the ^{99m}Tc-HMPAO complex has been achieved with cobalt chloride,[23] and another technetium binding ligand, ECD, has been evaluated in normal human subjects.[24,25] Both compounds can be injected immediately without the preparation time delay currently required with ^{99m}Tc-HMPAO. Grünwald et al.[90] have recently confirmed this with ECD. This improvement will lead to capture of short-lived seizures and markedly simplify the training required for the personnel injecting the ligand. SPECT resolution provided by current generation triple-headed gamma cameras is between 9 and 12 mm; future developments should improve on this to detect more subtle perfusion changes

during seizures. Receptor ligands may provide localizing data in patients with the very brief seizures that are often found in frontal and parietal lobe epilepsies.

CONCLUSIONS

Ictal SPECT is a reliable and highly accurate method of identifying the lateralization of temporal lobe seizures.[91,92] Injection of ligand during the seizure or immediately afterward produces striking and obvious changes that are readily and precisely interpretable. Such studies can be undertaken securely only in the context of video-EEG monitoring, which enables the precise timing of injection relative to the end of the seizure. Knowledge of the postictal switch in blood flow in temporal lobe seizures is essential for the proper interpretation of SPECT images. Postictal SPECT studies provide less powerful but still clinically useful lateralizing data and are more reliable than interictal SPECT data. Although ictal SPECT has not been as rigorously validated in children as in adults, it appears to provide almost identical lateralizing data.

Initial experience with ictal SPECT in extratemporal seizures promises that this method will be extremely valuable for those epilepsies that often defy localization. This has also been the case in children with frontal lobe epilepsies, in which SPECT demonstrated frontal foci in more than 90% of cases in one series.[62]

SPECT, when deployed in the ictal condition, has developed into a powerful tool for the localization of refractory partial seizures in adults and children. In addition, it provides novel scientific insights into the pathophysiology of focal epilepsies. The widespread availability of SPECT, its ease of use, and relative economy make it a very powerful method that can be universally exploited. In addition, the development of stable technetium perfusion ligands promises to enhance the usefulness of this unique functional imaging method.

Acknowledgments

The authors gratefully acknowledge the contributions of Drs. C.C. Rowe and S.S. Ho and the staff of the Department of Nuclear Medicine, Austin Hospital, Melbourne, Australia.

REFERENCES

1. Horsley V. An address on the origin and seat of epileptic disturbance. Br Med J 1892;1:693–6.
2. Penfield W. The circulation of the epileptic brain. Assoc Res Nerv Dis Proc 1938;18:605–37.
3. Dymond AM, Crandall PH. Oxygen availability and blood flow in the temporal lobes during spontaneous epileptic seizures in man. Brain Res 1976;102:191–6.
4. Ingvar DH, Lassen NA. Quantitative determination of regional cerebral blood-flow in man (letter to the editor). Lancet 1961;2:806–7.

5. Hougaard K, Oikawa T, Sveinsdottir E, et al. Regional cerebral blood flow in focal cortical epilepsy. Arch Neurol 1976;33:527–35.

6. Ingvar DH. rCBF in focal cortical epilepsy (abstract). Stroke 1973;4:359.

7. Ingvar DH. rCBF in focal cortical epilepsy. In: Langfitt TW, McHenry LC Jr, Reivich M, et al., eds. Cerebral circulation and metabolism. New York: Springer-Verlag, 1975:361–4.

8. Lavy S, Melamed E, Portnoy Z, et al. Interictal regional cerebral blood flow in patients with partial seizures. Neurology 1976;26:418–22.

9. Touchon J, Valmier J, Baldy-Moulinier M. Regional cerebral blood flow in temporal lobe epilepsy: inter-ictal studies. In: Baldy-Moulinier M, Ingvar DH, Meldrum BS, eds. Cerebral blood flow, metabolism and epilepsy. London: John Libbey, 1983:33–8.

10. Valmier J, Touchon J, Daures P, et al. Correlations between cerebral blood flow variations and clinical parameters in temporal lobe epilepsy: an interictal study. J Neurol Neurosurg Psychiatry 1987;50:1306–11.

11. Engel J Jr, Henry TR, Risinger MW, et al. Presurgical evaluation for partial epilepsy: relative contributions of chronic depth-electrode recordings versus FDG-PET and scalp-sphenoidal ictal EEG. Neurology 1990;40:1670–7.

12. Engel J Jr, Kuhl DE, Phelps ME. Patterns of human local cerebral glucose metabolism during epileptic seizures. Science 1982;218:64–6.

13. Theodore WH, Newmark ME, Sato S, et al. [18F]Fluorodeoxyglucose positron emission tomography in refractory complex partial seizures. Ann Neurol 1983;14:429–37.

14. Kung HF, Tramposch KM, Blau M. A new brain perfusion imaging agent: [I-123]HIPDM:N,N,N'-trimethyl-N'-[2-hydroxy-3-methyl-5-iodobenzyl]-1,3-propanediamine. J Nucl Med 1983;24:66–72.

15. Winchell HS, Baldwin RM, Lin TH. Development of I-123-labeled amines for brain studies: localization of I-123 iodophenylalkyl amines in rat brain. J Nucl Med 1980;21:940–6.

16. Hill TC, Holman BL, Lovett R, et al. Initial experience with SPECT (single-photon computerized tomography) of the brain using N-isopropyl I-123 p-iodoamphetamine: concise communication. J Nucl Med 1982;23:191–5.

17. Lee BI, Markand ON, Siddiqui AR, et al. Single photon emission computed tomography (SPECT) brain imaging using N,N,N'-trimethyl-N'-(2 hydroxy-3-methyl-5-123I-iodobenzyl)-1,3-propanediamine 2 HCl (HIPDM): intractable complex partial seizures. Neurology 1986;36:1471–7.

18. Lee BI, Park HM, Siddiqui AR, et al. Interictal HIPDM-SPECT in patients with complex partial seizures (abstract). Neurology 1988;38 Suppl 1:406.

19. Lee BI, Markand ON, Wellman HN, et al. HIPDM single photon emission computed tomography brain imaging in partial onset secondarily generalized tonic-clonic seizures. Epilepsia 1987;28:305–11.

20. Lee BI, Markand ON, Wellman HN, et al. HIPDM-SPECT in patients with medically intractable complex partial seizures. Ictal study. Arch Neurol 1988;45:397–402.

21. Neirinckx RD, Canning LR, Piper IM, et al. Technetium^{99m} d,l-HM-PAO: a new radiopharmaceutical for SPECT imaging of regional cerebral blood perfusion. J Nucl Med 1987;28:191–202.

22. Newton MR, Austin MC, Chan JG, et al. Ictal SPECT using technetium-^{99m}-HMPAO: methods for rapid preparation and optimal deployment of tracer during spontaneous seizures. J Nucl Med 1993;34:666–70.

23. Weisner PS, Bower GR, Dollimore LA, et al. A method for stabilising technetium^{99m} exametazime prepared from a commercial kit. Eur J Nucl Med 1993; 20:661–6.

24. Vallabhajosula S, Zimmerman RE, Picard M, et al. Technetium^{99m} ECD: a new brain imaging agent: in vivo kinetics and biodistribution studies in normal human subjects. J Nucl Med 1989;30:599–604.

25. Léveillé J, Demonceau G, De Roo M, et al. Characterization of technetium-^{99m}-L,L-ECD for brain perfusion imaging. Part 2: Biodistribution and brain imaging in humans. J Nucl Med 1989;30:1902–10.

26. Beer H-F, Blauenstein PA, Hasler PH, et al. In vitro and in vivo evaluation of iodine-123-Ro 16-0154: a new imaging agent for SPECT investigations of benzodiazepine receptors. J Nucl Med 1990;31:1007–14.

27. Schubiger PA, Hasler PH, Beer-Wohlfahrt H, et al. Evaluation of a multicentre study with Iomazenil—a benzodiazepine receptor ligand. Nucl Med Commun 1991;12:569–82.

28. Verhoeff NP, Erbas B, Kapucu O, et al. Quantification of central benzodiazepine receptor binding potential in the brain with 123I-iomazenil SPECT: technical and interobserver variability. Nucl Med Commun 1993;14:634–43.

29. Saji H, Iida Y, Nakatsuka I, et al. Radioiodinated 2'-iododiazepam: a potential imaging agent for SPECT investigations of benzodiazepine receptors. J Nucl Med 1993;34:932–7.

30. van Huffelen AC, van Isselt JW, van Veelen CW, et al. Identification of the side of epileptic focus with ^{123}I-Iomazenil SPECT. A comparison with ^{18}FDG-PET and ictal EEG findings in patients with medically intractable complex partial seizures. Acta Neurochir Suppl (Wien) 1990;50:95–9.

31. Bartenstein P, Ludolph A, Schober O, et al. Benzodiazepine receptors and cerebral blood flow in partial epilepsy. Eur J Nucl Med 1991;18:111–8.

32. Cordes M, Henkes H, Ferstl F, et al. Evaluation of focal epilepsy: a SPECT scanning comparison of ^{123}I-

iomazenil versus HM-PAO. AJNR Am J Neuroradiol 1992;13:249–53.

33. Savic I, Persson A, Roland P, et al. In-vivo demonstration of reduced benzodiazepine receptor binding in human epileptic foci. Lancet 1988;2:863–6.

34. Müller-Gartner HW, Mayberg HS, Fisher RS, et al. Decreased hippocampal muscarinic cholinergic receptor binding measured by 123I-iododexetimide and single-photon emission computed tomography in epilepsy. Ann Neurol 1993;34:235–8.

35. Boundy KL, Rowe CC, Black A, et al. Cholinergic neuroreceptor imaging with I[123] iododexetimide (IDEX) SPECT in temporal lobe epilepsy (abstract). Aust NZ J Med 1994;24:613.

36. Duncan R, Patterson J, Roberts R, et al. Ictal/postictal SPECT in the pre-surgical localisation of complex partial seizures. J Neurol Neurosurg Psychiatry 1993;56:141–8.

37. Newton MR, Berkovic SF, Austin MC, et al. Postictal switch in blood flow distribution and temporal lobe seizures. J Neurol Neurosurg Psychiatry 1992;55:891–4.

38. Sanabria E, Chauvel P, Askienazy S, et al. Single photon emission computed tomography (SPECT) using 123I-isopropyl-iodo-amphetamine (IAMP) in partial epilepsy. In: Baldy-Moulinier M, Ingvar D, Meldrum BS, eds. Cerebral blood flow, metabolism and epilepsy. London: John Libbey, 1983:82–7.

39. Stefan H, Pawlik G, Bocher-Schwarz HG, et al. Functional and morphological abnormalities in temporal lobe epilepsy: a comparison of interictal and ictal EEG, CT, MRI, SPECT and PET. J Neurol 1987;234:377–84.

40. Ryding E, Rosen I, Elmqvist D, et al. SPECT measurements with 99mTc-HM-PAO in focal epilepsy. J Cereb Blood Flow Metab 1988;8:S95–100.

41. Andersen AR, Gram L, Kjaer L, et al. SPECT in partial epilepsy: identifying side of the focus. Acta Neurol Scand Suppl 1988;117:90–5.

42. Bluestone DL, Engelstad BL, Barbaro NM, et al. Tc-HMPAO SPECT imaging for intractable compex partial seizures of temporal lobe origin (abstract). Epilepsia 1989;30:690.

43. Rowe CC, Berkovic SF, Austin MC, et al. Visual and quantitative analysis of interictal SPECT with technetium-99m-HMPAO in temporal lobe epilepsy. J Nucl Med 1991;32:1688–94.

44. Duncan R, Patterson J, Hadley DM, et al. CT, MR and SPECT imaging in temporal lobe epilepsy. J Neurol Neurosurg Psychiatry 1990;53:11–5.

45. Uren RF, Magistretti PL, Royal HD, et al. Single-photon emission computed tomography. A method of measuring cerebral blood flow in three dimensions (preliminary results of studies in patients with epilepsy and stroke). Med J Aust 1983;1:411–3.

46. Biersack HJ, Reichmann K, Winkler C, et al. 99mTc-labelled hexamethylpropyleneamine oxime photon emission scans in epilepsy (letter). Lancet 1985;2:1436–7.

47. Andersen AR, Waldemar G, Dam M, et al. SPECT in the presurgical evaluation of patients with temporal lobe epilepsy—a preliminary report. Acta Neurochir Suppl (Wien) 1990;50:80–3.

48. Rowe CC, Berkovic SF, Sia ST, et al. Localization of epileptic foci with postictal single photon emission computed tomography. Ann Neurol 1989;26:660–8.

49. Rowe CC, Berkovic SF, Austin MC, et al. Patterns of postictal cerebral blood flow in temporal lobe epilepsy: qualitative and quantitative analysis. Neurology 1991;41:1096–103.

50. Rowe CC, Berkovic SF, Austin MC, et al. Interictal and postictal cerebral blood flow in temporal lobe epilepsy. Curr Probl Epilepsy 1990;7:143–50.

51. Newton MR, Berkovic SF, Austin MC, et al. Dystonia, clinical lateralization, and regional blood flow changes in temporal lobe seizures. Neurology 1992;42:371–7.

52. Kotagal P, Luders H, Morris HH, et al. Dystonic posturing in complex partial seizures of temporal lobe onset: a new lateralizing sign. Neurology 1989;39:196–201.

53. Bennett DA, Ristanovic RK, Morrell F, et al. Dystonic posturing in temporal lobe seizures (letter). Neurology 1989;39:1270–2.

54. Newton MR, Berkovic SF, Austin MC, et al. Time course and distribution of cerebral blood flow in temporal lobe seizures using technetium-99m-HMPAO SPECT (abstract). J Nucl Med 1994;35 Suppl:208P.

55. Markand ON, Shen W, Park HM, et al. Single photon imaging computed tomography (SPECT) for localization of epileptogenic focus in patients with intractable complex partial seizures. Epilepsy Res Suppl 1992;5:121–6.

56. Tatum WO, Alavi A, Stecker MM. Technetium-99m-HMPAO SPECT in partial status epilepticus. J Nucl Med 1994;35:1087–94.

57. VanLandingham KE, Lothman EW. Self-sustaining limbic status epilepticus. I. Acute and chronic cerebral metabolic studies: limbic hypermetabolism and neocortical hypometabolism. Neurology 1991;41:1942–9.

58. Ho SS, Berkovic SF, McKay WJ, et al. Ictal SPECT shows different perfusion patterns in subtypes of temporal lobe epilepsy (abstract). Epilepsia 1994;35 Suppl 8:20.

59. Jack CR Jr, Mullan BP, Sharbrough FW, et al. Intractable nonlesional epilepsy of temporal lobe origin: lateralization by interictal SPECT versus MRI. Neurology 1994;44:829–36.

60. Marks DA, Katz A, Hoffer P, et al. Localization of extratemporal epileptic foci during ictal single photon emission computed tomography. Ann Neurol 1992;31:250–5.

61. Newton MR, Berkovic SF, Austin MC, et al. SPECT in the localisation of extratemporal and temporal seizure foci. J Neurol Neurosurg Psychiatry 1995;59:26–30.

62. Ho SS, Berkovic SF, Newton MR, et al. Parietal lobe epilepsy: clinical features and seizure localization by ictal SPECT. Neurology 1994;44:2277–84.

63. Stefan H, Bauer J, Feistel H, et al. Regional cerebral blood flow during focal seizures of temporal and frontocentral onset. Ann Neurol 1990;27:162–6.

64. Chiron C, Raynaud C, Maziere B, et al. Changes in regional cerebral blood flow during brain maturation in children and adolescents. J Nucl Med 1992;33:696–703.

65. Chugani HT, Phelps ME. Maturational changes in cerebral function in infants determined by ^{18}FDG positron emission tomography. Science 1986;231:840–3.

66. Chugani HT, Phelps ME, Mazziotta JC. Positron emission tomography study of human brain functional development. Ann Neurol 1987;22:487–97.

67. Kennedy C, Grave GD, Jehle JW, et al. Blood flow to white matter during maturation of the brain. Neurology 1970;20:613–8.

68. Kennedy C, Sokoloff L. An adaptation of the nitrous oxide method to the study of the cerebral circulation in children: normal values for cerebral blood flow and cerebral metabolic rate in childhood. J Clin Invest 1957;36:1130–7.

69. Farkas-Bargeton E, Diebler MF, Rosenberg B, et al. Histochemical changes of the developing human cerebral neocortex. Studies on two enzymes of energy metabolism in three cortical areas. Neuropediatrics 1984;15:82–91.

70. Huttenlocher PR. Synaptic density in human frontal cortex—developmental changes and effects of aging. Brain Res 1979;163:195–205.

71. McDonald JW, Johnston MV. Physiological and pathophysiological roles of excitatory amino acids during central nervous system development. Brain Res Brain Res Rev 1990;15:41–70.

72. Seeman P, Bzowej NH, Guan HC, et al. Human brain dopamine receptors in children and aging adults. Synapse 1987;1:399–404.

73. Denays R, Ham H, Tondeur M, et al. Detection of bilateral and symmetrical anomalies in technetium-^{99m}-HMPAO brain SPECT studies. J Nucl Med 1992;33:485–90.

74. Rubinstein M, Denays R, Ham HR, et al. Functional imaging of brain maturation in humans using iodine-123 iodoamphetamine and SPECT. J Nucl Med 1989;30:1982–5.

75. Chugani HT, Shields WD, Shewmon DA, et al. Infantile spasms: I. PET identifies focal cortical dysgenesis in cryptogenic cases for surgical treatment. Ann Neurol 1990;27:406–13.

76. Dulac O, Chiron C, Jambaqué I, et al. Infantile spasms. Prog Clin Neurosci 1987;2:97–109.

77. Harvey AS, Bowe JM, Hopkins IJ, et al. Ictal ^{99m}Tc-HMPAO single photon emission computed tomog-raphy in children with temporal lobe epilepsy. Epilepsia 1993;34:869–77.

78. Hwang PA, Gilday DL, Ash JM, et al. Perturbations in regional cerebral blood flow detected by SPECT scanning with ^{99m}Tc-HmPAO correlate with EEG abnormalities in children with epilepsy (abstract). J Cereb Blood Flow Metab 1987;7 Suppl 1:S573.

79. Chiron C, Raynaud C, Dulac O, et al. Study of the cerebral blood flow in partial epilepsy of childhood using the SPECT method. J Neuroradiol 1989;16:317–24.

80. Denays R, Rubinstein M, Ham H, et al. Single photon emission computed tomography in seizure disorders. Arch Dis Child 1988;63:1184–8.

81. Hwang P, Adams C, Gilday DL, et al. SPECT studies in epilepsy: applications to epilepsy surgery in children. J Epilepsy 1990;3 Suppl:83–92.

82. Uvebrant P, Bjure J, Hedstrom A, et al. Brain single photon emission computed tomography (SPECT) in neuropediatrics. Neuropediatrics 1991;22:3–9.

83. Harvey AS, Berkovic SF. Functional neuroimaging with SPECT in children with partial epilepsy. J Child Neurol 1994;9 Suppl 1:S71–81.

84. Harvey AS, Hopkins IJ, Bowe JM, et al. Frontal lobe epilepsy: clinical seizure characteristics and localization with ictal ^{99m}Tc-HMPAO SPECT. Neurology 1993;43:1966–80.

85. Adams C, Hwang PA, Gilday DL, et al. Comparison of SPECT, EEG, CT, MRI, and pathology in partial epilepsy. Pediatr Neurol 1992;8:97–103.

86. Iivanainen M, Launes J, Pihko H, et al. Single-photon emission computed tomography of brain perfusion: analysis of 60 paediatric cases. Dev Med Child Neurol 1990;32:63–8.

87. Vles JS, Demandt E, Ceulemans B, et al. Single photon emission computed tomography (SPECT) in seizure disorders in childhood. Brain Dev 1990;12:385–9.

88. Chiron C, Dulac O, Bulteau C, et al. Study of regional cerebral blood flow in West syndrome. Epilepsia 1993;34:707–15.

89. Chugani HT, Shewmon DA, Shields WD, et al. Surgery for intractable infantile spasms: neuroimaging perspectives. Epilepsia 1993;34:764–71.

90. Grünwald F, Menzel C, Pavics L, et al. Ictal and interictal brain SPECT imaging in epilepsy using technetium-^{99m}-ECD. J Nucl Med 1994;35:1896–901.

91. Berkovic SF, Newton MR, Rowe CC. Localization of epileptic foci using SPECT. In: Lüders HO, ed. Epilepsy surgery. New York: Raven Press, 1992:251–6.

92. Berkovic SF, Newton MR, Chiron C, et al. Single photon emission tomography. In: Engel J Jr, ed. Surgical treatment of the epilepsies. 2nd ed. New York: Raven Press, 1993:233–43.

Magnetoencephalography: Functional Imaging in Epilepsy

Jeffrey David Lewine, William W. Orrison, Jr., Andrea Halliday, Frank Morrell, Sylvester Chuang, Paul Hwang, and John A. Sanders

Successful neurosurgical treatment of epilepsy requires identifying the epileptic focus and using a surgical approach that minimizes postoperative deficits. Therefore, it is imperative that the precise spatial relationship between the lesion and functional areas of the brain be determined, especially when the intended region of resection is suspected to be near functionally essential cortex, such as the sensorimotor strip. Years of invasive and noninvasive studies have yielded some guidelines about the relationship between brain function and structure (for example, the central sulcus is the boundary between the motor area and somatosensory area). However, because of variability in brain structure and function, this information often is of limited use in neurosurgical planning. For example, even with magnetic resonance imaging (MRI) (which is the best available noninvasive neuroanatomical technique), it is sometimes difficult to identify the left and right central sulci in normal brains.[1] This invariably is more difficult when the normal structure has been severely distorted by a neoplasm or vascular malformation.

The standard neurosurgical procedures for functional localization of sensorimotor cortex involve electrical stimulation of the cortex either intraoperatively or extraoperatively after subdural grid implantation[2] or electrocorticographic monitoring of somatosensory evoked responses at the cortical surface[3,4] (or both).

However, these methods have limitations.[5] For example, electrocorticographic data are not always easily interpreted, especially when the surgical exposure of the relevant cortical regions is limited.[6] The greatest limitation is that critical data are not obtained until after craniotomy and after commitment to a particular neurosurgical approach. Clearly, if detailed knowledge of the location of sensorimotor cortex were available preoperatively, it would facilitate risk assessment, craniotomy site selection, and decisions about how aggressively to resect pathologic tissue. This can be especially important in cases without life-threatening lesions in which the possibility of significant postoperative motor deficit may be an unacceptable surgical risk.

Several techniques offer promise in the area of noninvasive localization of epileptic foci and noninvasive presurgical functional mapping. These include metabolic and hemodynamic techniques such as positron emission tomography (PET), single-photon emission computed tomography (SPECT), and functional magnetic resonance imaging (*f*MRI) and neurophysiologic techniques such as electroencephalography (EEG), magnetoencephalography (MEG), and transcranial magnetic stimulation (TMS). As described below, MEG is perhaps the most powerful single technique because its high resolution of brain electrophysiology in both spatial and temporal domains allows rapid identification of pathophysiologic regions and nearby areas of essential cortex.

TECHNICAL ASPECTS OF MAGNETOENCEPHALOGRAPHY

MEG is a technique whereby weak magnetic fields generated by intracellular neuronal currents are measured external to the skull surface.[7–9] Just as current flow in a wire produces a surrounding magnetic field, current flow in neurons produces a surrounding neuromagnetic field. Because of biophysical considerations, postsynaptic currents in the dendrites of pyramidal cells oriented parallel to the skull are the most significant contributors to the extracranial neuromagnetic field. The magnetic field produced by a single neuron is negligible, but when the activity of tens of thousands of neurons is in synchrony, the summated field can be detected by specialized sensors. This type of synchrony is usually present in primary sensory and motor cortical areas during response to a sensory stimulus or generation of a motor event; it is also present during the generation of an epileptic spike.

The device used for measuring neuromagnetic signals is known as a "biomagnetometer." The simplest biomagnetic detection coil consists of an induction loop of niobium titanium wire maintained in a superconducting state by immersion in liquid helium, at a temperature of 4.2°K. Superconductivity is a property whereby a material loses its electric resistivity when it is brought below its transition temperature. When a time-varying neuromagnetic field passes perpendicular to the plane of the wire loop, it induces a change in the amount of current flowing in the wire. In modern biomagnetometers, the detection coil is inductively coupled to a superconducting quantum interference device (SQUID) that acts as a high-gain current-to-voltage converter (Figure 13-1).

The largest of neuromagnetic signals (that is, those associated with epileptic spikes) are more than a million times weaker than the magnetic signals generated by nearby hospital equipment, so it is essential that the system be able to isolate neuromagnetic signals from extensive background noise. To reduce the amount of external noise reaching the detector, the biomagnetometer is operated in a magnetically shielded room made of high-permeability materials such as mu-metal. Rather than passing into the shielded room, impinging magnetic fields flow through the walls of the chamber, around and away from the sensor system in the room.

The shielded room provides significant attenuation of external magnetic signals, but the strength of the noise that reaches the biomagnetometer is still several orders of magnitude larger than the neuromagnetic signals of interest. To increase the signal-to-noise ratio, the sensors of clinical biomagnetometers are configured as gradiometers, consisting of oppositely wound induction coils connected in series. Most systems use an axial first-

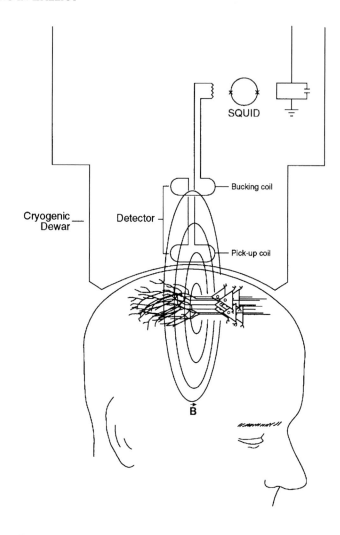

FIGURE 13-1. Basic concepts in magnetoelectroencephalography: Current flow in dendrites of neurons produces a surrounding magnetic field (*B*) that induces currents in the superconducting coils of the detection system. The detection circuit is inductively coupled to a superconducting quantum interference device (*SQUID*), which acts as a high-gain current-to-voltage converter.

order configuration. The lower "pickup" coil and the upper "bucking" coil are separated by a few centimeters (see Figure 13-1). The sensing unit, as a whole, measures the spatial gradient rather than the magnitude of the field. Near a magnetic source, the gradient of the magnetic field is steep. For example, as one moves from 2 cm to 4 cm from a source, the field strength decreases by more than 75%. Far from a source, the gradient is shallow. For example, as one moves from 1002 cm to 1004 cm, the field changes by less than 1%. When a source is far from the sensor, the pickup and bucking coils measure nearly equivalent magnetic signals from the source, so the net output of the sensor is small. In contrast, when the sensor is positioned over the cranium, the neuromagnetic signal measured by the bucking coil is significantly smaller than that detected by the pickup coil, so the sensor output is large. In this fashion, the biomagnetometer is made sensitive to nearby neural sources and insensitive to distant ones.

The magnetic field that a current element produces at a particular sensor location outside the head can be specified exactly with Maxwell's equations and the Biot-Savart law. The inverse problem of specifying the currents that generate a particular measured magnetic field pattern is much more inexact because many configurations of current produce the same external magnetic field pattern. Indeed, without the use of simplifying assumptions, the inverse problem has no unique solution. However, by making certain assumptions about the shape of the head and the nature of the underlying current configuration, the problem can be made mathematically tractable, and computer algorithms can be used to infer the location of the neuronal activity that generates a recorded magnetic field pattern.

The most common model used in the analysis of neuromagnetic data is that of a dipole-in-a-sphere. This model makes two fundamental assumptions. First, it is assumed that the head can be treated as a spherically symmetrical volume conductor. Whereas this is correct only as a first-order approximation, it greatly simplifies the mathematics of inverse modeling. Experimental data suggest that real-world deviations from sphericity have only a minor impact on the types of studies described herein. Second, it is assumed that the magnetic field recorded at each instant in time can be modeled as though it were produced by a single current dipole embedded within the conducting volume. This dipole provides a simplified biophysical representation of the actual currents that generate the recorded signal—currents postulated to be associated with the focal activation of a small cortical region. Given these assumptions, it is possible to identify the location, orientation, and strength of the dipole that best accounts for the measured magnetic field pattern.

Briefly, the relevant computer algorithms work as follows. First, a dipole of particular position, orientation, and strength is hypothesized. Second, the Biot-Savart law is used to forward calculate the magnetic signal that this hypothetical dipole would generate at each of the sensors. The magnitude of this forward calculated field is compared with the signal actually measured and a mismatch term is calculated. Mismatch terms at each sensor are squared and summated across all sensors to generate an overall error term. A new dipole is then postulated at a different position, and its error term calculated. By using iterative minimization procedures, the computer algorithm continues to hypothesize dipoles until it determines the position, orientation, and strength of the dipole that provides the smallest error term. That is, the algorithm specifies the best-fitting dipole. The position, ori-

entation, and strength of this dipole are taken as indicative of the position, orientation, and strength of the relevant neuronal currents. By identifying common physical landmarks for both MEG and MRI data, it is possible to align coordinate axes so that MEG sources can be plotted directly on the relevant anatomical images. The resulting magnetic source localization images thereby provide surgeons with pictographic details about the spatial relationships between brain structure, function, and pathology (Figure 13-2).

In considering the usefulness of the dipole model, it is important not to confuse the model (a dipole) with what is being modeled (a complex pattern of neuronal currents). Provided that the external neuromagnetic field mostly reflects activation of a single cortical region and provided that the spatial extent of the active region is small relative to the distance to the pickup coil, localization of the best-fitting dipole provides for excellent localization of the activated region. However, if multiple, separated cortical regions simultaneously make significant contributions to the field pattern and a single dipole model is used erroneously, the dipole solution will fail to accurately characterize the neuronal activity. Therefore, investigators must be careful in determining those circumstances under which the dipole model may be validly applied. As described below, the dipole model is generally valid for localizing the generators of certain components of the neuromagnetic signal found (1) before the onset of movement and (2) after somatosensory stimulation. The model is also valid for the characterization of some epileptic spikes, sharp waves, and paroxysmal slow waves.

MAGNETOENCEPHALOGRAPHY AND EPILEPSY: CHARACTERIZATION OF EPILEPTIC SPIKES

Effective surgical intervention in epilepsy requires accurate knowledge of the location of the relevant pathologic tissue, and this is one of the oldest and most important clinical applications of MEG. Monitoring of a seizure with depth probes is the standard method for localizing an epileptic focus before surgical resection,[10] but the implantation of electrodes is a risky and expensive surgical procedure that is not tolerated by all patients. Relatively few hospitals have the appropriate facilities and expertise for depth monitoring; thus, the development of noninvasive alternatives is a high priority.

During the 1980s, several major centers of MEG epilepsy research emerged. Efforts at these institutions focused on characterizing epileptic spikes, but the investigations were partly hampered by the small size (seven or fewer sensors) of available sensor arrays. Accurate dipole modeling depends on adequate spatial sampling of the instantaneous neuromagnetic field pattern. This was not possible with a single placement of a small array

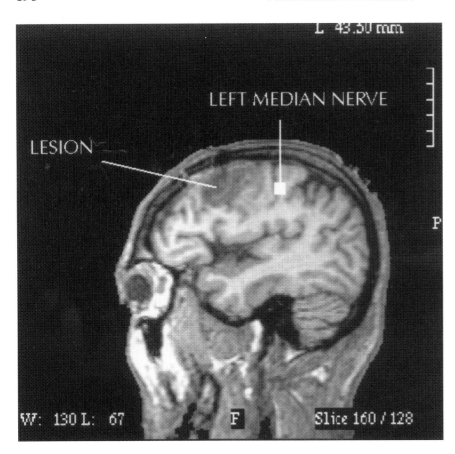

FIGURE 13-2. Magnetic source localization image of a 41-year-old man with a high-grade astrocytoma in left frontal cortex. The image shows the relationship between the neoplasm and the primary somatosensory cortex activated by median nerve stimulation.

instrument. Therefore, investigators were forced to develop special triggering, relative covariance, and signal averaging techniques that allowed for combination of data sets obtained during sequential samplings of the magnetic field pattern. Several excellent reviews of these innovative methods and the early results are available.[11–14] During the last few years, large-array systems with 37 or more sensors have become available (Figure 13-3). Single placements of these sensor arrays often provide adequate sampling of the spatial pattern of the magnetic field generated by individual epileptic events,[15–18] thus allowing for efficient localization of epileptic activity.

In evaluating data from epileptic patients, care must be used in applying the single dipole model. Some epileptic spikes clearly reflect activation of a focal brain region, as evidenced by the good quality ($r > 0.97$) and positional stability of sequential single dipole fits calculated every few milliseconds during the duration of the spike. However, for other spikes, individual dipole fits are poor ($r < 0.80$) and the dipole position is temporally unstable. This latter situation implies that multiple sources contribute to the generation of the spike. Because multiple dipole modeling is a far more complex and time-consuming procedure than single dipole modeling, the tendency is to focus only on dipolar events. Although this strategy can provide a clear indication of one pathophysiologic region, clinicians must not ignore the presence of more complex source configurations for some epileptic events.

Clinicians also need to be aware that the magnetic field generated by activation of a spatially extended (but contiguous) cortical region is indistinguishable from that generated by a deeper dipole source. Thus, when application of a dipole model to a particular field pattern localizes the source to be deep in the white matter, it is almost certainly the case that the data really reflect neuronal activation of a large (> 1 cm) region of the overlying cortical mantle.

One of the dominant uses of MEG in epilepsy is in the characterization of temporal lobe foci in cases in which decisions must be made about which portions of the temporal lobe are to be resected. Work by Ebersole and colleagues[19,20] has shown that certain epileptiform events can occur in the MEG without obvious EEG correlates and vice versa. In many cases, it is easier to model MEG data than simultaneously obtained EEG data, and MEG source localizations are generally more consistent with data from depth probes. Sample MEG data obtained from a patient with a known right temporal lobe focus is shown in Figure 13-4.

In extratemporal epilepsy, MEG can provide very important information, especially in cases of frontal lobe epilepsy in which traditional neuroimaging techniques often fail to reveal focal changes (Figure 13-5). Bihemi-

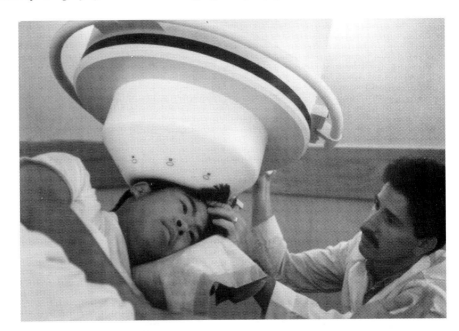

FIGURE 13-3. The large-array Magnes system (Biomagnetic Technologies Incorporated) is used at several clinical facilities in the United States. The cryogenic dewar contains 37 first-order axial gradiometers. The unit is easily positioned over regions of interest.

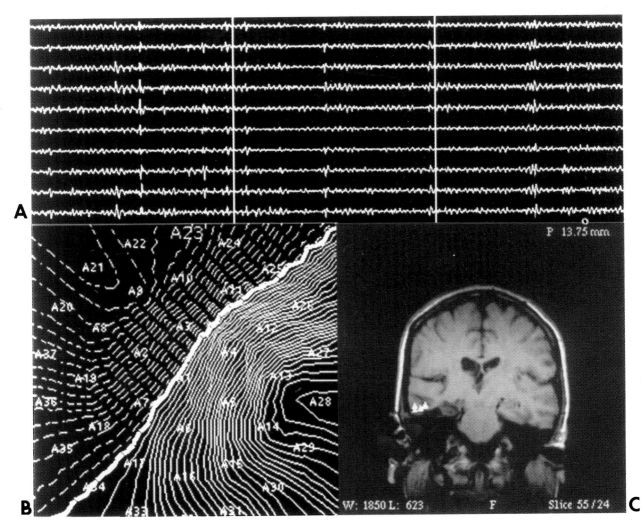

FIGURE 13-4. Neuromagnetic data from a 36-year-old woman with epilepsy. A. Magnetoencephalographic waveforms with multiple epileptic events. B. Dipolar isofield contour map for one of the spikes. C. Magnetic source localization image showing the right temporal location of dipolar sources (*white triangles*) that account for individual epileptic events (spikes).

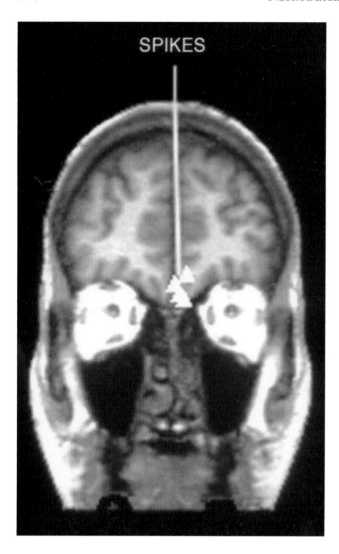

FIGURE 13-5. Magnetic source localization images from a 50-year-old man with intractable epilepsy. Data show localization of interictal spike sources (*triangles*) to mesial surface of right frontal cortex.

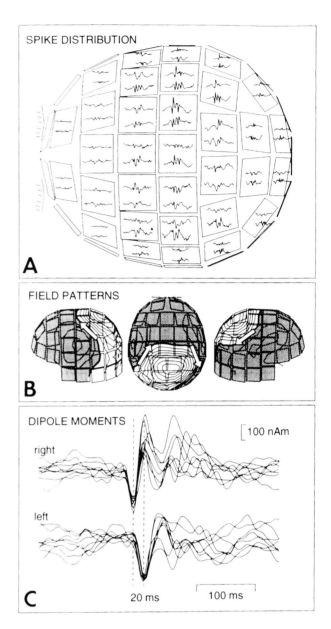

FIGURE 13-6. Whole-head neuromagnetic data from an 18-year-old woman with uncontrolled epilepsy. A. Spatial distribution of one spike displayed on the sensor array. B. Isofield pattern at peak latency of spike, showing contributions from both right and left hemispheres. C. Time course of activation for right versus left neuronal populations. Data show that left hemisphere activity lags that of the right hemisphere by 20 ms. (From Hari et al.[21] By permission of Rapid Communications of Oxford.)

spheric MEG examinations using new whole head and dual-probe systems are especially useful in cases of epilepsy in which it is necessary to determine whether the two hemispheres show independent spiking versus correlated spiking, with one side leading the other[21] (Figure 13-6).

Children often fail to tolerate depth monitoring, so noninvasive assessment is especially important. However, traditional neuroimaging studies often produce inconclusive or contradictory results. For example, PET and SPECT generally show very diffuse abnormalities, even in patients subsequently shown to have focal seizures, and conventional EEG often mislocalizes the epileptic zone or fails to reveal important characteristics about the focus.

This latter limitation of EEG studies is illustrated in the case of a 5-year-old left-handed boy who was eval-

uated at the Albuquerque Magnetic Source Imaging Facility. The patient was diagnosed to have Landau-Kleffner syndrome, a condition in which rapid reduction in language skills occurs around age 4 and frequent spiking is found at left posterior temporal EEG leads. This condition can be ameliorated by multiple subpial transections through Wernicke's area. The challenge to the surgical team was to decide whether additional transections along the upper bank of the superior temporal gyrus were needed. The danger in proceeding medially is that branches of the middle cerebral artery that emerge from the sylvian fissure can be damaged. Therefore, clear evidence of a medial epileptic focus is desired before extending the surgical approach. Preoperative scalp EEG is generally inadequate to address the issue because the apical dendrites of the pyramidal neurons in the floor of the sylvian fissure are oriented in a superior-inferior direction that is unfavorable for EEG assessment. In contrast, this orientation, that is, parallel to the lateral skull surface, is ideal for preoperative MEG evaluation.

In the 5-year-old boy, MEG data were recorded sequentially over each hemisphere with a 37-channel biomagnetometer. Three regions were identified as generating epileptic spikes (Figure 13-7). The most intense focus was in the vicinity of Wernicke's area. The spike generation zone extended 3 cm medial along the upper bank of the superior temporal gyrus, with a very intense focus about 2 cm medial to Wernicke's area. A second focus was found just deep to an inferior left frontal site that was believed to correspond to Broca's area. Spike generators were also found somewhat diffusely throughout the auditory association areas of the right hemisphere. By analyzing the timing of the MEG spikes with respect to spikes observed in simultaneous EEG records, it became apparent that the MEG spikes generated in the left sylvian area were coincident with the lead-edge of EEG spikes. Spikes in Broca's area and on the right side trailed the lead-edge of EEG spikes by 20 and 25 milliseconds, respectively. That is, the timing data suggested that the left sylvian area was the triggering focus, with the activity in the other two areas reflecting propagation along known anatomical pathways.

Originally, a series of subpial transections along only the lateral surface of Wernicke's area had been planned, but the MEG data clearly indicated the need for more aggressive intervention extending into the sylvian fissure. The magnetic source localization images for this patient were used to guide the procedure medially along the upper bank of the superior temporal sulcus, where electrocorticography confirmed MEG-inferred zones of epileptiform activity. The surgical treatment was successful, and the child is recovering several lost language skills.

MAGNETOENCEPHALOGRAPHY AND EPILEPSY: CHARACTERIZATION OF ABNORMAL LOW-FREQUENCY MAGNETIC ACTIVITY

Although the first MEG study of epilepsy focused on hyperventilation-induced changes in slow activity,[22] most of the subsequent work has focused on characterization

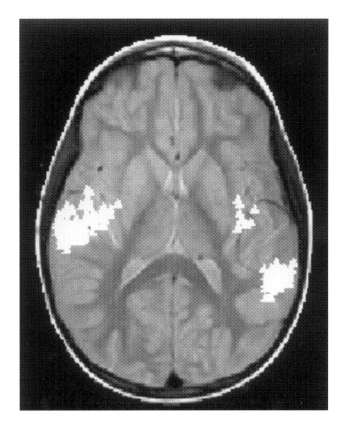

FIGURE 13-7. Magnetic source localization image from a 5-year-old boy with Landau-Kleffner syndrome. Each triangle shows the dipole source location associated with an individual epileptic spike. Dipolar sources were found to extend medially from Wernicke's area along the floor of the sylvian fissure, at Broca's area, and at auditory association areas on the right side. The activity in Broca's area and on the right side appears to reflect propagation from a triggering zone in Wernicke's area.

of epileptic spikes. A limitation of this approach is that it is useful only for patients who have fairly frequent interictal spikes. Recent work at several MEG sites[22–25] indicates that MEG analysis of paroxysmal slowing, sometimes referred to as "abnormal low-frequency magnetic activity" (ALFMA) is an alternative approach, because focal slowing is generally seen even in patients without interictal spiking. The spontaneous EEG and MEG of normal healthy subjects is dominated by signals of 8 Hz or higher, but in cases of abnormality there is often an increase in the amount of delta and theta power in the 1- to 4-Hz and 4- to 6-Hz bandwidths, respectively. In many forms of abnormality, this slowing of the spontaneous record is diffuse across recording sites (especially in the EEG), but in some patients (for example, those with focal epilepsy), the slowing can be quite focal, especially in the MEG[23–25] (Lewine JD, Orrison WW, Davis JT, unpublished data).

Different laboratories have slightly different approaches to the analysis of ALFMA, but the basic strategies are similar. Briefly, spontaneous MEG signals are band-pass filtered from 1 to 4 or 1 to 6 Hz. Slow wave events are then identified visually or with automatic processing routines that search for high-amplitude signals (> 200 fT). After a slow wave event is identified, standard dipole modeling strategies are applied to the signal. At most instants in time, several brain regions contribute nearly equally to the spontaneous neuromagnetic signal, and a dipole model of this situation is wholly inappropriate. However, at certain instants, the neuromagnetic field generated by a region of focal abnormality may be so large (> 200 fT) that it dominates the recorded signal, with the dipole model proving to be appropriate and accurate for localizing the physiologically abnormal area. Even in the most severely pathologic cases, less than 1% of the spontaneous data record can be characterized by a dipole model. Yet, this 1% of data can provide important clinical information in epilepsy. It would be of interest to characterize more fully the more prevalent nondipolar signals, but currently, this cannot be done routinely.

The false-positive rate for identification of ALFMA in neurologically normal adults is low (< 15%), but it is quite high for normal children (around 40%). This is because high-amplitude alpha and theta activity (that is prevalent in normal children) is not suppressed fully by standard 1- to 4-Hz digital filtering, so automatic data processing routines of the type described above occasionally misidentify these signals as ALFMA. Before automated dipole processing, avoidance of this type of false-positive result required inefficient "by-hand" identification of delta bursts.

In a study of 50 unselected adult patients with epilepsy, Lewine and colleagues (Lewine JD, Orrison WW, Davis JT, unpublished data) found significant ALFMA in 80% of them, whereas significant interictal spiking was found in only 30%. Similar percentages have been observed in other studies. [24] When single ALFMA foci were observed, the implied physiologically abnormal area was in agreement with that indicated by other methods (intracranial monitoring or video EEG or both) in 90% of cases (Figure 13-8). Multiple ALFMA foci were observed in more than 50% of patients. In 80% of these cases, the location of the most intense focus correctly identified the side and lobe of the lesion as independently indicated by depth probes or video EEG monitoring (or both). Identification of ALFMA has correctly identified the location of seizure onset (when confirmed by invasive ictal EEG recording) in cases in which traditional noninvasive structural (MRI and CT) and functional (PET and SPECT) methods were unrevealing.[24] In several patients, electrocorticography has confirmed the validity of source localizations of ALFMA and their relevance to epileptic pathology (Oommen KJ, Galen C,

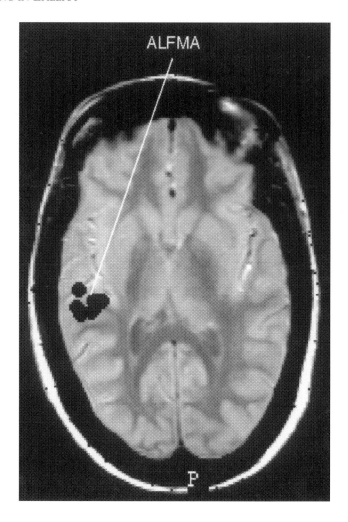

FIGURE 13-8. Magnetic source localization image from a 32-year-old woman with right temporal lobe epilepsy. She did not show any interictal spikes during the examination, but significant abnormal low-frequency magnetic activity (ALFMA) was observed (*small circles*).

Hirschkoff E, et al., presented at meeting of the American Electroencephalographic Society, New Orleans, Louisiana, October 10–15, 1993).

MAGNETOENCEPHALOGRAPHY AND EPILEPSY: FUNCTIONAL MAPPING

Identification of the epileptogenic zone is only the first step in planning a successful surgical intervention in epilepsy. It is equally critical that functional regions be identified. In all cases, the experiments take advantage of standard signal-averaging techniques. A stimulus is presented multiple times and data epochs spanning the stimulus are averaged to extract time-locked neuromagnetic signals from the background noise. Functional mapping of sensorimotor cortex is easily performed with MEG

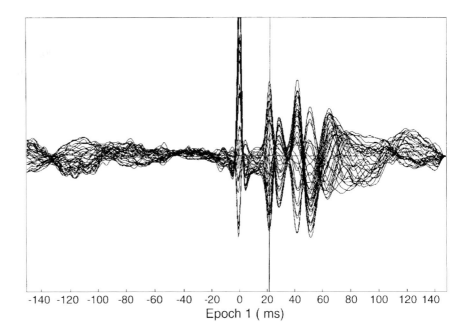

FIGURE 13-9. Neuromagnetic signals evoked by electrical stimulation of the left median nerve. Data were recorded with a 37-channel biomagnetometer, and waveforms from all channels were overlaid. There is a large electrical artifact at time zero, followed by a sequence of neuromagnetic oscillations.

technology and is part of the routine clinical practice of several MEG facilities.[26–28] Mapping of auditory cortex is also performed frequently, although its clinical usefulness is generally less than that for sensorimotor mapping. For each of these modalities, it is possible to identify time points in the evoked neuromagnetic signal where the field is generated by a focal neuronal population. Studies of the visual system are less frequent because visual evoked fields generally have complex morphologies indicative of concurrent activation of multiple visual cortical regions. Several MEG facilities are trying to develop strategies for preoperative mapping of language function, but definitive successes in this area are elusive. In this chapter, the discussion is confined to the most significant neurosurgical situation of mapping sensorimotor cortices.

Mapping of somatosensory cortex is generally considered the easiest and most reliable of the MEG mapping procedures. Electrical stimulation of the median nerve allows rapid identification of the postcentral gyrus. An example set of neuromagnetic waveforms evoked by stimulation of the left median nerve is shown in Figure 13-9. The waveforms are characterized by a stimulus artifact associated with the applied electrical current and a sequence of subsequent neuromagnetic oscillations. The instantaneous magnetic field pattern at the peak latency for each of the early neuromagnetic components (at about 20, 30, and 40 ms) is highly dipolar (Figure 13-10), and a single dipole model provides an excellent account of the empirical data ($r > 0.97$). Source locations for each peak invariably fall within a few millimeters of each other, and in normal subjects, the sources consistently localize to the primary somatosensory cortex of the postcentral gyrus, as identified by structural methods

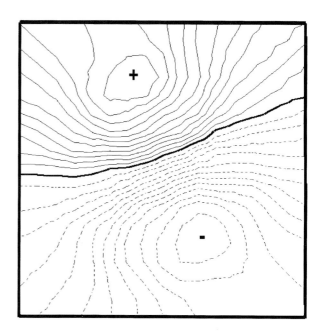

FIGURE 13-10. Isofield contour map associated with a 22-ms response. *Solid lines* indicate emerging flux, and *dashed lines* indicate entering flux. The step size is 20 fT. The field is highly dipolar, characterized by single regions of emerging and entering flux.

(Figure 13-11). Later components of the waveform (at latencies > 70 ms) usually are not adequately characterized by single dipole models. Multiple dipole modeling of these data indicates that these components reflect concurrent activation of primary somatosensory cortex and

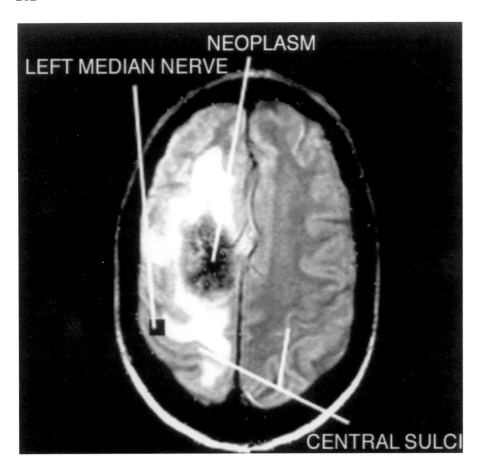

FIGURE 13-11. Magnetic source localization image for the median nerve data in Figure 13-10. The patient was a 63-year-old man with a right medial frontal adenocarcinoma. The data show that the median nerve response is lateral and posterior to the lesion but within the zone of edema.

secondary somatosensory cortex (which is located along the inferior parietal lobule).

The accuracy of MEG localizations of the postcentral gyrus of patients has been confirmed by electrocorticography.[5,28,29] In all instances, MEG has correctly identified sensorimotor cortex, even in cases in which the structure has been severely distorted by a space-occupying lesion (Figure 13-12). It is noteworthy that the entire MEG examination for localizing the median nerve response (including data analysis) takes less than 15 minutes to perform.

In addition to mapping the cortical representation of the median nerve, it is sometimes useful to characterize activation after stimulation of other areas of the body. Mapping of the face representation is generally done with tactile or vibratory stimulation of the lower lip or tongue. Detailed information on the hand area can be assessed by tactile, vibratory, or electrical stimulation of the digits. Electrical stimulation of the tibial nerve is used to locate the foot representation in somatosensory cortex. The exact latencies at which activation of primary somatosensory cortex dominates the neuromagnetic signal depend on the site and type of stimulation, but in all cases, evoked signal components earlier than 50 ms mostly reflect primary cortical activation.

Direct MEG studies of motor function are somewhat more difficult to perform because they require the patient to make smooth, well-controlled movements of the hand. Even in patients with significantly compromised motor function, median nerve somatosensory responses usually are strong and can be used to provide the critical information about the location of the central sulcus.

In a typical motor experiment, subjects flex or extend one or more digits of the hand in a self-paced or visually cued fashion. Signals are back-averaged with respect to movement onset to identify the primary motor field. Figure 13-13 is an example of motor waveforms recorded with a 37-channel first-order axial gradiometer system. Beginning a few hundred ms before movement onset, a slow dipolar shift in the magnetic signal peaks at 20 to 50 ms prior to movement onset. This is followed by a large dipolar signal that reflects feedforward and feedback activation of somatosensory cortex, whereas the signal peaking at 20 to 50 ms before movement onset reflects activation of primary motor cortex. The motor field is generally dipolar, and its source localizes to the anterior bank of the central sulcus (Figure 13-14). A motor MEG examination takes approximately 20 to 25 minutes to complete.

As illustrated below in the case study, the ability of MEG to localize precisely both functionally essential

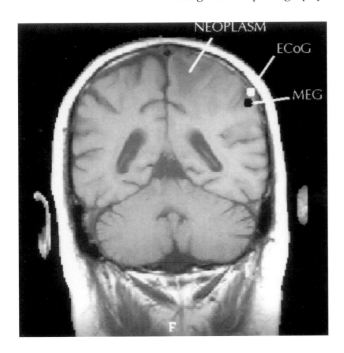

FIGURE 13-12. Somatosensory cortex identified by magnetoencephalography (*MEG*) and stereotaxic intraoperative electrocorticographic (*ECoG*) monitoring of the somatosensory evoked potential. The data show excellent agreement between the noninvasive and invasive methods, with ECoG by necessity identifying a superficial cortical site.

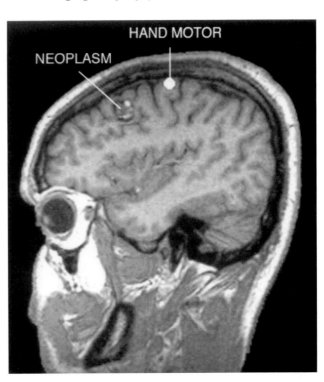

FIGURE 13-14. Magnetic source localization image of a 30-year-old man with a right frontal lesion. The source of activity associated with thumb movement is in the precentral gyrus (*hand motor*), posterior to the lesion.

FIGURE 13-13. Neuromagnetic signals evoked by movement of the left thumb. Data were recorded with a 37-channel biomagnetometer and waveforms from all channels were overlaid. The primary motor field response begins about 300 ms before movement (time 0) and peaks at about −40 ms. A large somatosensory cortex response begins immediately after the movement and peaks at about 85 ms.

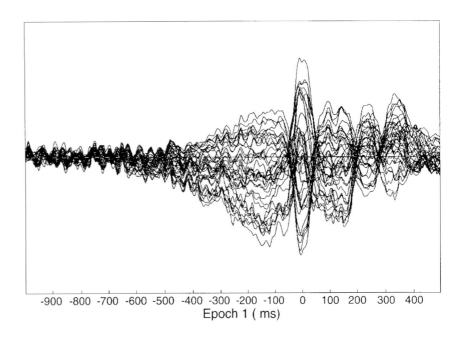

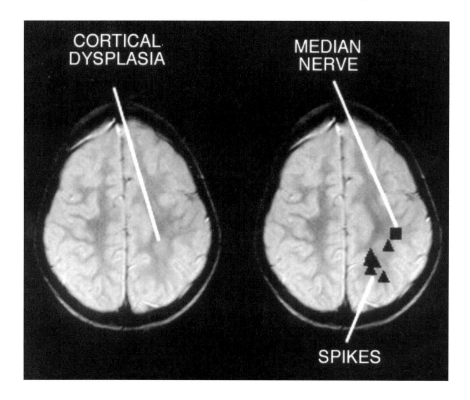

FIGURE 13-15. Magnetic source imaging data from a 5-year-old boy with intractable seizures. The data show the relationship between a region of cortical dysplasia and sources for epileptic spikes (*triangles*) and median nerve evoked responses (*square*). The data indicate spike clustering around the structural lesion, just posterior to primary somatosensory cortex.

regions and regions of epileptic dysfunction makes it an important noninvasive diagnostic procedure for the evaluation of epilepsy.

The patient was a 5-year-old boy with a history of uncontrolled partial complex and tonic-clonic seizures. MRI studies were interpreted differently. One study indicated thickening of the cortical mantle at left parietal locations and a region of left parietal dysplasia (Figure 13-15), and the other study, in which there was a problem with artifact, indicated a more diffuse hemispheric abnormality. EEG showed frequent interictal spikes maximal at left frontocentral sites. PET showed abnormal metabolism of the left parietal lobe, and SPECT showed decreased blood flow throughout the left hemisphere. The initial surgical recommendation was for restricted resection near the structural lesion, but physicians at another institution recommended complete hemispherectomy. The patient was referred to the Albuquerque Magnetic Source Imaging Facility for examination of sensorimotor function and epileptiform activity. MEG revealed frequent dipolar interictal spiking at the suspect left parietal region without any evidence of spikes originating from temporal or frontal locations. The dipole sources were oriented in an anterior-posterior direction, pointing toward F3 and F7. ALFMA analyses showed a dominant left parietal focus at the lesion site, with some extension inferiorly. Median nerve stimulation showed that somatosensory cortex was anterior to the lesion and spike focus. Thus, the MEG data supported the

original recommendation for restricted resection. The patient has not yet had surgical treatment, but if he does, a restricted resection is planned.

COMPARISON WITH OTHER TECHNIQUES

A major drawback of the neuromagnetic method is the high capital equipment cost (> $2 million) of a large-array biomagnetometer system. It often is suggested that less expensive and more readily available techniques can provide preoperative functional mapping as accurately and efficiently as MEG. To address this issue, researchers at the Albuquerque Magnetic Source Imaging Facility have initiated a series of studies to compare alternative electromagnetic techniques for functional localization of the central sulcus in control subjects and neurosurgical patients.[30] Techniques that are being evaluated include MEG, EEG, *f*MRI, and TMS. MEG, EEG, and *f*MRI evaluations have focused on both somatosensory and motor source localizations, and TMS experiments have focused solely on localization of motor cortex. For normal subjects, each of the techniques provides good localization of the central sulcus (as identified by structural MRI evaluation).

MEG data are generally the easiest to analyze, with single dipole models proving adequate for characterizing the relevant components of somatosensory and motor evoked fields. EEG analyses are somewhat more difficult because two or more distinct sources generally contribute to each component of the evoked signal, and failure to take all the sources into the model results in mislocalization of activity. EEG data generally reflect more sources than MEG does, because EEG is more sensitive to thalamic and brain stem activity, and it is sensitive to current flow in neurons with both tangential and radial orientations (MEG is sensitive to tangential currents only).

Readily available 1.5-T clinical magnetic resonance scanners are sufficient for identifying the central sulcus with *f*MRI. However, many normal subjects show multiple areas of activation during motor tasks, and anatomical knowledge must be used to distinguish primary motor cortex aligning the central sulcus from supplementary motor areas (Figure 13-16). This usually can be accomplished for normal subjects with undistorted anatomy, but it may be a problem in patients with space-occupying neoplasms.

TMS data are somewhat problematic to interpret because the exact relationship between the surface position of the stimulation coil and the region of induced neuronal activation is not well understood. In each of five patients tested, the Albuquerque group has found that this projection line passes through motor cortex, as identified by structural MRI methods and MEG (Figure 13-17).

Results of a comparative mapping study with a normal control subject are shown in Figure 13-18. MEG data were obtained with a 37-channel biomagnetometer and analyzed with a single dipole model. EEG data were obtained with 32 electrodes distributed over the head surface, and analyses were performed with a commercially available multiple dipole algorithm (BESA).[31] Only the dominant cortical source is shown in Figure 13-18. Functional MRI data were obtained with a clinical 1.5-T scanner (Siemens). Only the region of statistically significant change between rest and movement conditions is shown in Figure 13-18. TMS was effected by using a Cadwell magnetic stimulation unit, with the projection point through the cortical surface displayed.

Although the different methods identify slightly different locations for functional regions, all lead to correct identification of the central sulcus in control subjects. Evaluation of the techniques with patients is complicated because each technique places different demands on the patient. For example, motor mapping with MEG and EEG requires that the patient be able to make reasonably smooth and well-controlled movements, because of the requirement for time-locked signal averaging. On the one hand, the patients most in need of motor cortex mapping generally have some compromise of motor function. On the other hand, somatosensory mapping usually can be performed even in patients with severe compromise of motor function. Another consideration in MEG and EEG experiments is possible distortion of the magnetic and electric activity patterns by anomalous electric conductivity barriers at the margins of neoplasms and vascular

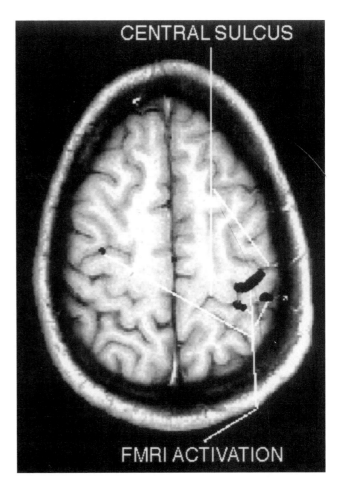

FIGURE 13-16. Functional MRI (*FMRI*) data set showing movement-related changes in hemodynamics. The data were obtained with a 1.5-T clinical imager without special hardware. During the experiment, images were acquired during rest periods and periods in which the right hand was moved repeatedly. The presented statistical difference image (superimposed on a standard T_1-weighted image) shows multiple regions of significant activation (*in black*). The largest focus of activity aligns the central sulcus (as determined by anatomical methods).

malformations. Available data suggest that such distortions can cause very significant mislocalizations in neuroelectric experiments, and whereas the distortion of neuromagnetic signals by unusual conductivity barriers is generally less, mislocalizations of several millimeters may still occur.[32]

Very few studies have been conducted with TMS in patients, and some of the above concerns about electrical conductivity barriers may apply to TMS, where "hot spots" of induced current theoretically could develop around lesions. Another concern in TMS experiments is the remote possibility of inducing an epileptic seizure in a seizure-prone patient.

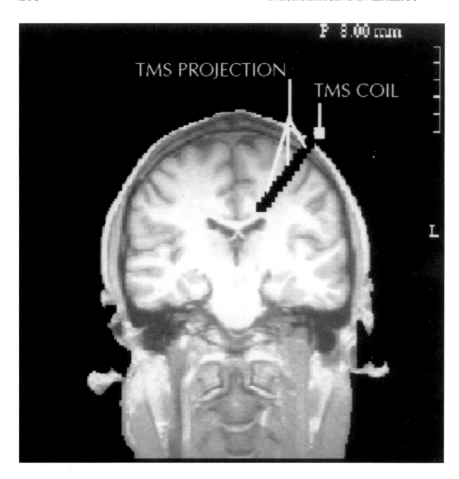

FIGURE 13-17. Integration of transcranial magnetic stimulation (*TMS*) and magnetic resonance imaging is achieved by plotting the center position of the coil and calculating the projection line through the center of the sphere that best describes the local curvature of the head underneath the coil. The projection line passes through primary motor cortex.

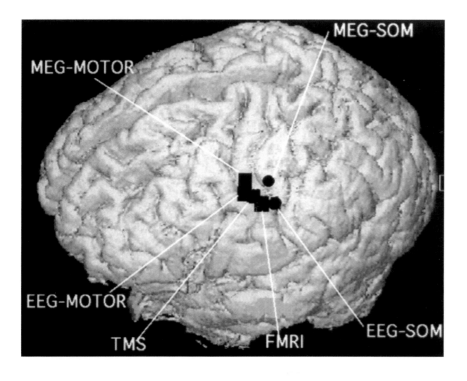

FIGURE 13-18. Multimodal imaging data from a control subject showing both somatosensory (*SOM*) and motor functional mappings. (*EEG*) electroencephalography, (*FMRI*) functional magnetic resonance imaging, (*MEG*) magnetoencephalography, (*TMS*) transcranial magnetic stimulation.

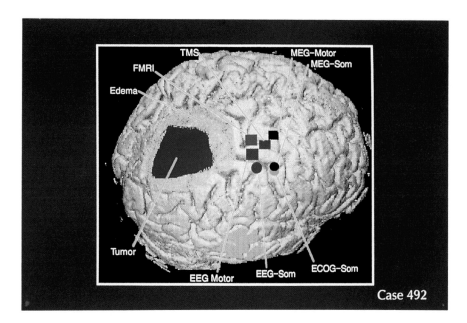

FIGURE 13-19. Multimodal imaging data for a patient with a right parietal neoplasm. Electrocorticographic (*ECoG*) data were obtained intraoperatively with a 32-contact electrode grid. The positions of the contacts were determined stereotaxically. Electroencephalographic (*EEG*) data led to erroneous localization of the central sulcus. (*FMRI*) functional magnetic resonance imaging, (*MEG*) magnetoencephalography, (*SOM*) somatosensory, (*TMS*) transcranial magnetic stimulation.

Currently, the quality of motor movement required for good *f*MRI responses is unknown, and too few studies of somatosensory mapping by median nerve stimulation or hand brushing have assessed the reliability of this method. Another complication in *f*MRI is that the extent to which a lesion disrupts local hemodynamic mechanisms is not well characterized, although some studies with patients[33] suggest that good data can be obtained even from those with lesions near the motor cortex.

Figure 13-19 shows data from a comparative mapping study of a neurosurgical patient. The method used was identical to that described above. The patient was a 57-year-old man with a metastatic lesion of the right parietal lobe. Notice the scatter in functional localization across techniques, although MEG, *f*MRI, and TMS all led to correct identification of the central sulcus, as confirmed intraoperatively by corticographic monitoring of the median nerve somatosensory evoked potential. It is important to note that EEG source localizations led to incorrect identification of the central sulcus because the electrical conductivity barrier at the anterior margin of the lesion causes unmodeled distortions in the electric potential pattern. (This distortion did not affect the corticographic data because cortical surface electrodes perform only very local sampling of the electric potential pattern and the corticographic grid was several centimeters distant from the lesion.)

SUMMARY AND CONCLUSIONS

In summary, MEG is an extremely powerful tool for localizing functional and dysfunctional brain regions. Given the relative simplicity of MEG data collection and analysis procedures and the high reliability of functional mapping results, as repeatedly confirmed by intraoperative methods, MEG is quickly becoming the method

of choice for preoperative functional mapping at medical centers where a choice can be made between noninvasive methods. By integrating MEG and MRI data into magnetic source localization images, neurosurgeons can be provided with precise preoperative information on the spatial relationships between lesions, zones of epileptiform activity, and regions of cortex supporting normal sensory and motor functions. The MEG approach to the evaluation of epilepsy has already been shown to have a positive impact on patient care, and as the relevant equipment becomes more readily available, MEG is certain to be increasingly important in the preoperative assessment of neurosurgical patients.

Acknowledgments

The authors are grateful to S. Conviser, J. M. Cottrell, J. Meyer, and K. Paulson for their technical assistance in collection of some of the data presented herein.

Portions of the work were supported by funds from the Department of Veterans Affairs, the University of New Mexico, the McDonnell-Pew Program in Cognitive Neuroscience, and Biomagnetic Technologies Inc.

REFERENCES

1. Sobel DF, Gallen CC, Schwartz BJ, et al. Locating the central sulcus: comparison of MRI anatomic and magnetoencephalographic functional methods. AJNR Am J Neuroradiol 1993;14:915–25.

2. Penfield W, Boldrey E. Somatic motor and sensory representation in the cerebral cortex of man as studied by electrical stimulation. Brain 1937;60:389–443.

3. Black PM, Ronner SF. Cortical mapping for defining the limits of tumor resection. Neurosurgery 1987;20:914–9.

4. Berger MS, Kincaid J, Ojemann GA, et al. Brain mapping techniques to maximize resection, safety, and seizure control in children with brain tumors. Neurosurgery 1989;25:786–92.

5. Sutherling WW, Crandall PH, Darcey TM, et al. The magnetic and electric fields agree with intracranial localizations of somatosensory cortex. Neurology 1988;38:1705–14.

6. Suzuki A, Yasui N. Intraoperative localization of the central sulcus by cortical somatosensory evoked potentials in brain tumor. Case report. J Neurosurg 1992;76:867–70.

7. Hari R, Ilmoniemi RJ. Cerebral magnetic fields. Crit Rev Biomed Eng 1986;14:93–126.

8. Williamson SJ, Kaufman L. Analysis of neuromagnetic signals. In: Gevins AS, Rémond A, eds. Handbook of electroencephalography and clinical neurophysiology. Vol 1: Methods of analysis of brain electrical and magnetic signals. Amsterdam: Elsevier Science Publishers, 1987:405–48.

9. Lewine JD. Neuromagnetic techniques for the noninvasive analysis of brain function. In: Freeman SE, Fukushima E, Greene ER, eds. Noninvasive techniques in biology and medicine. San Francisco: San Francisco Press, 1990:33–74.

10. Engel J Jr, Ojemann GA. The next step. In: Engel J Jr, ed. Surgical treatment of the epilepsies. 2nd ed. New York: Raven Press, 1993:319–29.

11. Rose DF, Smith PD, Sato S. Magnetoencephalography and epilepsy research. Science 1987;238:329–35.

12. Sato S. Epilepsy research: NIH experience. Adv Neurol 1990;54:223–30.

13. Sutherling WW, Barth DS. Magnetoencephalography in clinical epilepsy studies: the UCLA experience. Adv Neurol 1990;54:231–45.

14. Ricci GB. Italian contributions to magnetoencephalographic studies of the epilepsies. Adv Neurol 1990;54:247–60.

15. Stefan H, Schneider S, Abraham-Fuchs K, et al. Magnetic source localization in focal epilepsy. Multichannel magnetoencephalography correlated with magnetic resonance brain imaging. Brain 1990;113:1347–59.

16. Stefan H, Schneider S, Abraham-Fuchs K, et al. The neocortico to mesio-basal limbic propagation of focal epileptic activity during the spike-wave complex. Electroencephalogr Clin Neurophysiol 1991;79:1–10.

17. Paetau R, Kajola M, Korkman M, et al. Landau-Kleffner syndrome: epileptic activity in the auditory cortex. Neuroreport 1991;2:201–4.

18. Paetau R, Kajola M, Karhu J, et al. Magnetoencephalographic localization of epileptic cortex—impact on surgical treatment. Ann Neurol 1992;32:106–9.

19. Ebersole JS, Squires K, Gamelin J, et al. Simultaneous MEG and EEG provide complementary dipole models of temporal lobe spikes (abstract). Epilepsia 1993;34:143.

20. Ebersole JS, Squires K, Gamelin J, et al. Dipole models of temporal lobe spikes from simultaneous MEG and EEG. In: Deecke L, Baumgartner C, Stroink G, et al., eds. Advances in biomagnetism, abstracts. Vienna, 1993: 6–7.

21. Hari R, Ahonen A, Forss N, et al. Parietal epileptic mirror focus detected with a whole-head neuromagnetometer. Neuroreport 1993;5:45–8.

22. Cohen D. Magnetoencephalography: detection of the brain's electrical activity with a superconducting magnetometer. Science 1972;175:664–6.

23. Vieth JB, Sack G, Schueler P, et al. Ischemic and epileptic lesions measured by AC- and DC-MEG. In: Williamson SJ, Hoke M, Kotani M, et al., eds. Advances in biomagnetism. New York: Plenum Press, 1990:307–10.

24. Gallen CC, Iragi V, Tecoma E, et al. Identification of epileptic regions via MEG focal slow wave localizations: comparison with EEG monitoring. In: Deecke L, Baumgartner C, Stroink G, et al., eds. Advances in biomagnetism, abstracts. Vienna, 1993:36–7.

25. Lewine JD, Orrison WW, Astur RS, et al. Explorations of pathophysiological spontaneous activity by magnetic source imaging. In: Deecke L, Baumgartner C, Stroink G, et al., eds. Advances in biomagnetism, 1993. New York: Plenum Press (in press).

26. Lewine JD, Benzel EC, Baldwin NG, et al. Magnetoencephalography. In: Wilkins R, Rengachary S, eds. Neurosurgery. 2nd ed. New York: McGraw-Hill (in press).

27. Benzel EC, Lewine JD, Bucholz RD, et al. Magnetic source imaging: a review of the Magnes System of Biomagnetic Technologies Incorporated. Neurosurgery 1993;33:252–9.

28. Galen CC, Sobel DF, Waltz T, et al. Noninvasive presurgical neuromagnetic mapping of somatosensory cortex. Neurosurgery 1993;33:260–8.

29. Lewine JD, Orrison WW, Maclin EL, et al. Event-related magnetic fields and neurosurgical practice. In: Deecke L, Baumgartner C, Stroink G, et al., eds. Advances in biomagnetism, 1993. New York: Plenum Press (in press).

30. Lewine JD, Sanders JA, George JS, et al. Analysis of motor function by MEG, fMRI and TMS. Abstracts Soc Neurosci 1993;19:1209.

31. Scherg M, Vajsar J, Picton TW. A source analysis of the late human auditory evoked potentials. J Cognitive Neurosci 1989;1:336–55.

32. Lewine JD, Edgar JC, Repa K, et al. A physical phantom for simulating the impact of pathology on magnetic source imaging. In: Deecke L, Baumgartner C, Stroink G, et al., eds. Advances in biomagnetism, 1993. New York: Plenum Press (in press).

33. Jack CR, Thompson RM, Butts RK, et al. Sensory motor cortex—correlation of presurgical mapping with functional MR imaging and invasive cortical mapping. Radiology 1994;190:85–92.

Selection of Candidates for Surgical Treatment of Epilepsy

Gregory D. Cascino

Surgery is a potential alternative treatment for a patient with epilepsy who has medically refractory seizures that are socially or physically disabling (or both).[1–3,4a,5,6] Most patients who undergo epilepsy surgery have intractable partial or focal seizures.[3,4b,6] A significant percentage of patients with partial epilepsy do not have remission with pharmacotherapy alone.[7] Medically resistant seizures develop in about 45% of patients with partial epilepsy.[3] The initial response to antiepileptic drug medication may be highly predictive of the responsiveness of the seizure disorder to medical therapy.[7] Patients are unlikely to enter a seizure remission if they have not done so within 5 years after diagnosis.[7] The presence of a space-occupying mass lesion, developmental delay, and a remote symptomatic cause are factors predictive of an unfavorable response to medical treatment.[7] The most commonly performed and successful surgical procedure for partial epilepsy is focal resection of epileptogenic cortex.[4b,8–12] Other operative procedures that are beneficial in the management of intractable partial epilepsy include lesionectomy and hemispherectomy.[13–17] Recently, multiple subpial transections have been introduced as an alternative to cortical resection in selected patients.[18] Corpus callosotomy may be efficacious for seizures associated with drop attacks in patients with symptomatic generalized epilepsy.[19,20]

THEORETICAL CONCEPTS FOR PARTIAL EPILEPSY

Several important theoretical concepts need to be considered in patients with partial epilepsy.[21] The term "epileptic focus" is an inaccurate description of the *region or regions of epileptogenesis* in partial seizure disorders. The "epileptogenic lesion," or "lesional zone," refers to a structural abnormality identified with neuroimaging studies or pathologic examination (or both) that is intimately associated with the development of partial seizure activity.[21] The "irritative zone" is the region of cerebral cortex identified by interictal electroencephalographic (EEG) epileptiform alterations.[21] Electrocorticography (ECoG) may be used to define further the region of the interictal spiking. The "functional deficit zone" represents the region of nonepileptic brain dysfunction as demonstrated by the neurologic examination, postictal deficits, neuropsychologic studies, the sodium amobarbital test, or interictal EEG nonepileptiform changes.[21] Positron emission tomography (PET) and single-photon emission computed tomography

(SPECT) may also identify functional abnormalities that coexist with the region of seizure onset.[21–24]

The "symptomatogenic zone" is the region of the brain that gives rise to the characteristic ictal behavior or symptoms.[21] This zone may be in proximity with or quite remote from the epileptic brain tissue. The "pacemaker zone" refers to the site of seizure initiation as determined with EEG recordings.[21] Most seizures "confined" to the pacemaker zone do not produce a clinical seizure until there is secondary propagation to the symptomatogenic zone. Finally, the "epileptogenic zone" should be considered the epileptic brain tissue that is critical for seizure onset and that must be resected to render the patient seizure-free.[21] Ictal extracranial or intracranial EEG recordings are used to delineate the limits of the epileptogenic zone before consideration of epilepsy surgery. In most patients with partial epilepsy, the operative strategy is to completely resect the epileptogenic zone.

TERMINOLOGY FOR PARTIAL OR FOCAL SEIZURES

The current terminology for classifying partial seizures is largely based on the presence or absence of an impairment in consciousness during the ictus.[25] "Complex partial seizures" are defined as ictal events associated with a localization-related electrographic abnormality and incomplete or complete loss of consciousness.[25] Variably, patients may exhibit auras and automatisms during complex partial seizure activity. The localization of the epileptogenic zone and specific ictal behavior are not considered in classifying seizure type.[25] Commonly, it is impossible, even with inpatient ictal EEG monitoring, to determine whether a patient has had an impairment in alertness during an ictus, for example, frontal lobe complex partial seizure. The term "partial seizure" has also proved troublesome because some physicians and patients perceive that it implies an *incomplete* event or a seizure involving only *part* of the body.

Another point of confusion in dealing with the currently accepted classification is the differentiation between aura and simple partial seizure. "Aura" is a useful term for indicating the specific ictal behavior before impairment in consciousness. Currently, focal motor seizure activity lasting for several years in an awake patient with Rasmussen's encephalitis and an abdominal discomfort lasting a few seconds in a patient with hippocampal epilepsy would be labeled identically as "simple partial seizure activity." Also, the currently used classification is not of predictive value for patients undergoing surgical treatment and provides no information about the likely pathologic process underlying the epileptogenic zone. An alternative classification has been proposed that emphasizes the specific ictal semiology and is more informative and operational for patient care[26] (Lüders HO, personal communication, 1994). *Focal* is substituted for *partial* because of the potential ambiguity associated with the lat-

ter term. Wieser[27] has indicated his preference for retaining the term "psychomotor seizure" to describe focal seizures with confusion that are predominantly although not exclusively of temporal lobe origin. The Cleveland Clinic group reports the patient's symptoms as the seizure progresses, for example, abdominal aura → confusion with automatisms → right upper extremity dystonic posturing[26] (Lüders HO, personal communication, 1994). The ictal behavior provided in this example would indicate the likely medial temporal onset of seizure activity, with lateralization of the epileptogenic zone to the left cerebral hemisphere. Statistically, this patient probably would have mesial temporal sclerosis as the underlying lesion and be a favorable candidate for epilepsy surgery. In this chapter, whenever possible, the alternative classification is substituted for the conventional terminology.

WHO SHOULD BE REFERRED FOR SURGICAL TREATMENT?

Patients with medically refractory partial epilepsy may be candidates for epilepsy surgery if there is an impairment in the quality of life related to the seizures or to medical therapy (or both) and if the epileptic brain tissue can be resected without neurologic morbidity.[1,3,4a,5,10,12,27–33] The age of the patient, the duration of epilepsy, and the age at seizure onset may affect operative outcome but seldom should be used as exclusionary criteria. Younger patients (for example, younger than 30 years) may be preferred because of the putative beneficial effect of successful surgical treatment on the ability of the person to be employed or to return to school.[1] There is now consensus that epilepsy surgery may be an important treatment option for pediatric patients, even in the first months of life, because of the profound detrimental effect of poorly controlled seizures on development.[32,34,35] Older persons may also be good candidates for surgical treatment. Finally, the specific epileptic syndrome (see below) may affect the referral of a patient with intractable partial epilepsy for surgical evaluation.

How Bad Do the Seizures Have to Be for Surgical Treatment to be Considered?

Patients should be considered surgical candidates when the seizure disorder or medical treatment (or both) is associated with significant problems in daily living.[3,4b,5,28,30,33] The psychosocially disabling effects of intractable partial epilepsy (for example, the inability to drive a motor vehicle or to work) often motivate patients to consider surgical treatment.[28] Seizures associated with impairment of consciousness, loss of postural tone, or recurrent episodes of status epilepticus may be particularly disabling physically and, thus, prompt earlier referral to an epilepsy center for surgical consideration. Importantly, even seizures that appear relatively "minor" may be socially disabling if the patient cannot legally operate a motor vehicle. Patients with auras only are not usually considered appropriate candidates for surgical treatment.

Another important issue is the required frequency of seizure activity before surgical treatment is considered. Most patients with medically refractory psychomotor seizures of temporal lobe origin experience several seizures (for example, two to four) per month. All too often, physicians are satisfied with occasional psychomotor seizures if the generalized tonic-clonic seizures are medically controlled. Even less than one seizure per month may affect a person's quality of life. The presence of psychomotor seizure activity may not be only socially or physically disabling but may also expose the patient to chronic antiepileptic drug toxicity.[3]

When Should the Patient Be Referred?

Patients with partial epilepsy who have not had remission with initial medical therapy should be referred to an appropriate neurologic specialist within several months after the diagnosis.[4b] The first-line antiepileptic drugs for partial epilepsy are carbamazepine and phenytoin. If treatment with the initial antiepileptic drug is unsuccessful, then the likelihood that the seizures will be well controlled is about 10%.[36] Medication with antiepileptic drugs should be increased as needed until the patient is seizure-free or toxic effects related to the medication develop.[36] The plasma levels of antiepileptic drugs are of secondary importance in deciding drug dosing. Monotherapy with high doses of a drug is preferred, and polypharmacy should be discouraged in the initial management of partial epilepsy because of problems with compliance, cost of medication, pharmacokinetic interactions, and limited efficacy.[36] Unnecessary medication trials with barbiturates or benzodiazepines should be discouraged because of neurotoxicity and lack of efficacy relative to first-line antiepileptic drugs.[36] If the seizures prove refractory to the first-line antiepileptic drugs, the patient should be referred to an appropriate epilepsy center that can consider several alternative treatment options, for example, epilepsy surgery, investigational drugs, combination drugs, and conventional medications that have not been used previously.[36] The specific ictal behavior also affects the timing of epilepsy surgery. Patients with psychomotor or tonic-clonic seizures are evaluated earlier than those with auras only or with seizures that are not associated with an impairment of consciousness. The issue of timing is perhaps most important in pediatric patients (see Chapter 17).

SURGICALLY REMEDIABLE PARTIAL EPILEPTIC SYNDROMES

Syndromes associated with partial epilepsy that are amenable to focal cortical resection have been identified. Surgically remediable epileptic syndromes include medi-

al temporal lobe epilepsy, lesional epilepsy, neocortical (extrahippocampal) epilepsy, and certain childhood seizure disorders. Surgical treatment for pediatric epilepsy is discussed in Chapter 17.

Nonlesional Medial Temporal Lobe Epilepsy

Patients with medial temporal lobe epilepsy are favorable candidates for operative management.[29,37,38] In one study at the Mayo Clinic, about 80% of patients with presumed medial temporal lobe epilepsy were seizure-free postoperatively.[38] The region of seizure onset is in the temporal lobe in nearly 80% of patients with partial epilepsy.[4a] The most epileptogenic region of the temporal lobe involves the limbic "detonator structures," that is, the amygdala and hippocampus.[4a,26,27] Depth EEG studies have shown that about 90% of seizures in patients with nonlesional temporal lobe epilepsy emanate from the hippocampus.[39] The most common lesion underlying medial temporal lobe epilepsy is mesial temporal sclerosis[40–42] (see Chapter 4). Mesial temporal sclerosis is characterized by differential neuronal loss with a gliotic response.[41,43] Typically, the neuronal loss is maximal in the prosubiculum, CA1, and CA3 and is less prominent in CA2, the dentate gyrus, and the subiculum.[43] The most consistent finding in patients with nonlesional medial temporal lobe epilepsy is hilar neuronal loss.[43] Variable pathologic features associated with mesial temporal sclerosis include neuronal loss in the amygdala and entorhinal cortex. Currently, the consensus is that hippocampal neuronal loss is the cause of the focal seizures in patients with medial temporal lobe epilepsy.[43] Secondary effects associated with seizures may contribute to the neuronal loss and the gliosis.[43]

The medical history of patients with medial temporal lobe epilepsy is often positive for an acute symptomatic neurologic disease in childhood. Complex or prolonged febrile seizures, bacterial meningitis, and seizures associated with a diphtheria-pertussis-tetanus (DPT) vaccination in the first several years of life are important risk factors for the development of unprovoked partial seizures and medial temporal lobe epilepsy.[41] The importance of childhood febrile seizures in the pathogenesis of mesial temporal sclerosis has been emphasized.[41]

Typically, the early life insult produces generalized tonic-clonic seizures, with a latency of several years (maybe even decades) before the emergence of aura and psychomotor seizures.[26] Initially, the psychomotor seizures may be responsive to antiepileptic drugs, but ultimately the presence of medial temporal lobe epilepsy is an unfavorable predictor for medical treatment. The ictal behavior often includes an aura followed by a brief psychomotor seizure with gestural, mimetic, or oroalimentary automatisms.[26,27,44] The common auras include abdominal discomfort (for example, "butterflies in the stomach"), a nonspecific cephalic sensation, an unpleasant taste or odor, and an experiential phenomenon (for example, déjà vu or jamais vu).[26] The auras may occur in isolation or variably precede the psychomotor seizure.[26]

The psychomotor seizure for each patient with medial temporal lobe epilepsy is usually quite stereotypic in character and duration. Most patients experience several psychomotor seizures per month. Postictally the patient may be confused and appear drowsy. The psychomotor seizure may last 1 to 2 minutes, but the postictal state may be more prolonged, from several minutes to 1 hour. Secondarily generalized tonic-clonic seizures are usually infrequent and medically responsive. The ictal semiology may suggest the lateralization or localization (or both) of the epileptogenic zone.[26,27] The psychomotor seizure may be associated with contralateral dystonic posturing in the upper extremity, reflecting seizure propagation to the basal ganglia.[44] Aphasia is intimately involved with partial seizures that arise from the language-dominant hemisphere. This is demonstrated best by language testing in the immediate postictal period.

The interictal EEG reveals unilateral or bilateral anterior-mid temporal lobe spike or sharp wave discharges in most patients with medial temporal lobe epilepsy.[27] Monitoring with sphenoidal electrodes may be useful in identifying the mesial temporal origin of interictal discharges. Recording during drowsiness or light sleep may be necessary to identify epileptiform alterations. The topography of the interictal epileptiform discharges may suggest a regional distribution, for example, frontotemporal spiking. Bitemporal spike activity during sleep is not uncommon and should not necessarily be considered to indicate bitemporal seizures. During the aura, the EEG may reveal only nonspecific localized or generalized attenuation. Extracranial ictal EEG may show a lateralized ictal theta discharge that is maximal in the frontotemporal region. Supplementary scalp or sphenoidal electrodes may indicate the anterior temporal topography of the ictal epileptiform abnormality. Other scalp-recorded changes that occur during a partial seizure in patients with medial temporal lobe epilepsy include a bisynchronous alteration or a discharge that is contralateral to the epileptic temporal lobe.

Neuroimaging alterations in the mesial temporal lobe may be useful in identifying the epileptogenic lesion and in indicating the epileptic temporal lobe[22,24,38,40,45] (see Chapters 5, 6, 11, and 12). The introduction of structural and functional neuroimaging procedures has resulted in decreased use of chronic intracranial EEG monitoring in preoperative evaluations. Magnetic resonance imaging (MRI) in patients with medial temporal lobe epilepsy associated with mesial temporal sclerosis has been shown to be a reliable indicator of the hippocampal origin of the partial seizures (Figure 14-1) (see Chapter 5). The high sensitivity and specificity of MRI in patients with mesial temporal sclerosis have been con-

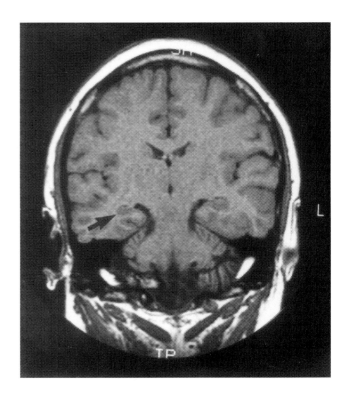

FIGURE 14-1. T_1-weighted MRI study in the oblique-coronal plane revealing atrophy of the right hippocampal formation (*arrow*). Mesial temporal sclerosis was verified pathologically at the time of resection of right anterior temporal lobe cortex.

firmed.[40] MRI provides excellent resolution of the anatomical details of the medial temporal lobe and, thus, demonstrates the hippocampal lesions in mesial temporal sclerosis. Common MRI findings in patients with mesial temporal sclerosis include atrophy of the hippocampal formation, increased alteration of T_2 signal intensity, and loss of internal structure.[45] The methodology for an MRI study is critical for demonstrating changes related to mesial temporal sclerosis. A coronal T_1-weighted sequence is optimal for identifying atrophy because of the ability to differentiate gray and white matter.[38] A coronal T_2-weighted sequence may be useful in determining the presence of increased signal intensity. Interictal PET usually reveals regional hypometabolism in patients with medial temporal lobe epilepsy[23,24] (see Chapter 11). Ictal SPECT has been shown to indicate reliably the epileptic temporal lobe[22] (see Chapter 12). Interictal SPECT studies have a relatively low sensitivity and specificity and are less useful than the ictal images.

Lesional Epileptic Syndromes

Intractable partial epilepsy is related to foreign-tissue lesions (tumor, vascular malformation, or neuronal migrational disorder) in about 30% of patients who have surgical treatment.[14–16,42,46–50] There is a high coherence between the site of the lesional pathology and the localization of the epileptogenic zone.[14] MRI has been shown to be highly sensitive and specific in patients with lesional epileptic syndromes[46] (see Chapters 2 and 3). The neurologic history, physical examination findings, and EEG are unable to identify patients with a lesion as the underlying abnormality. Neuroimaging studies, especially MRI, are of critical importance in establishing the likely nature of the epileptogenic lesion (see Chapters 2 and 3). The rationale for the preoperative evaluation in these patients is to confirm the epileptogenic nature of the imaged alteration. Rarely, the site of seizure onset may be remote from the lesional pathology.[21]

There is consensus that the most effective operative strategy in patients with lesional epileptic syndromes includes extirpation of the foreign-tissue lesion.[14,15,48] The reasons for surgical failure include inadequate resection of the lesion or inadequate resection of the epileptogenic zone (or both). Inadequate resection of the lesion has been shown to be of greatest prognostic importance.[49] Selective resection of the foreign-tissue lesion with incomplete excision of the epileptogenic zone may be effective in some patients with intractable partial epilepsy.[16] Comparative studies have suggested that complete excision of the epileptic brain tissue is more effective than lesionectomy in rendering patients with lesional epilepsy seizure-free.[14] The nature of the lesion has also been shown to have predictive value. Patients with neoplasms and vascular malformations are more likely to be rendered seizure-free than patients with neuronal migrational disorders.[14–16,49]

Neoplasms commonly associated with medically refractory seizure disorders include low-grade gliomas, gangliogliomas, and dysembryoplastic neuroepithelial tumors (Figure 14-2).[42,50] Commonly, patients present with a seizure disorder of several years' duration.[47] Potential causes of the partial seizures in these patients include denervation hypersensitivity and a direct cortical "irritating" effect of the tumor.[51] Morphological alterations that are potentially epileptogenic have been shown in the cerebral cortex adjacent to a neoplasm. Long-term follow-up studies have indicated that most patients with tumoral epilepsy are rendered seizure-free or experience a significant decrease in seizure tendency after epilepsy surgery.[52] Selected series have indicated that nearly 90% of patients with tumoral epilepsy may be rendered seizure-free if the lesion and epileptogenic cortex are excised.[52]

The common vascular malformations associated with chronic epilepsy include cavernous hemangiomas and arteriovenous malformations (Figure 14-3).[53] The latter lesions characteristically are angiographically occult.[53] The relatively low epileptogenic potential of venous angiomas has been confirmed. Epilepsy surgery in patients with vascular malforma-

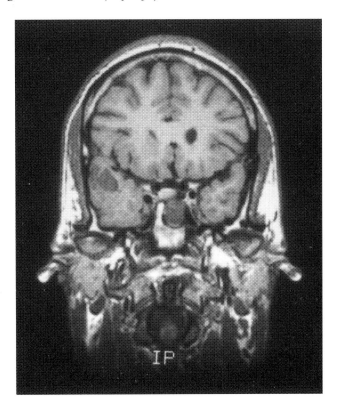

FIGURE 14-2. T_1-weighted MRI study in the oblique-coronal plane showing a mass lesion in right anterior temporal lobe. At the time of surgical extirpation, the lesion was shown to be a grade II oligodendroglioma.

tions has a favorable outcome.[53] The cause of seizure activity in patients with vascular malformations is not clear. One reason may be the presence of bleeding at the site of the lesion. Invariably, there is evidence of remote hemorrhage on pathologic examination.[53] Yeh et al.[54] showed that 16 of 18 patients (89%) who had resection of an arteriovenous malformation with a focal corticectomy were seizure-free. A recent study at the Mayo Clinic found that nearly 80% of patients with lesional epilepsy related to a vascular malformation were seizure-free after resection of the lesion and that most of the other 20% had some decrease in seizure activity.[53]

Neuronal migrational disorders (Figure 14-4) include a large group of developmental abnormalities that are outlined in Chapter 3.[49] The outcome of epilepsy surgery in these patients depends on the specific type of lesion. The most common abnormality underlying the epileptogenic zone is focal cortical dysplasia.[49] The pathologic feature of focal cortical dysplasia is disorganization of the cortical architecture, with aberrant giant neurons and glial cells scattered throughout the cortical layers. In one study, only 2 of 26 patients were rendered seizure-free after surgical treatment for focal cortical

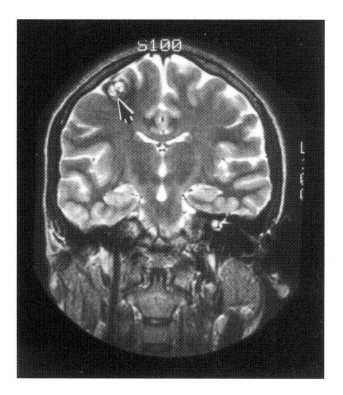

FIGURE 14-3. T$_2$-weighted MRI study in the oblique-coronal plane revealing a cavernous hemangioma *(arrow)* in the right posterior frontal lobe, with evidence of remote hemorrhage. The lesion was shown to involve the precentral gyrus. The vascular malformation was resected in its entirety without neurologic morbidity.

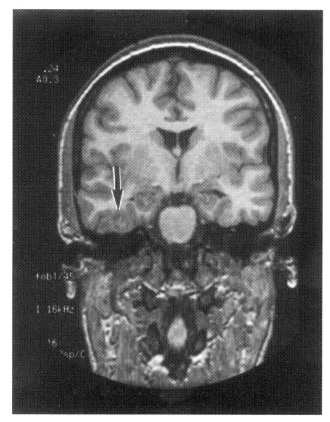

FIGURE 14-4. T$_1$-weighted MRI study in the oblique-coronal plane showing a neuronal migrational abnormality *(arrow)* in the inferior aspect of the right temporal lobe, with evidence of polymicrogyria.

dysplasia, but 59% of the patients experienced greater than a 50% decrease in seizures.[49]

Nonlesional Neocortical, Extrahippocampal Epilepsy

The operative results in patients undergoing a neocortical, extrahippocampal resection are clearly less favorable than in patients with medial temporal lobe epilepsy.[55–57] Most of the extratemporal cortical resections involve the frontal lobe. In nonlesional frontal lobe epilepsy, only a small proportion of patients are rendered seizure-free.[55,56] About 20% of patients with partial epilepsy have extratemporal (predominantly frontal lobe) seizures. One long-term study of operative outcome that relied heavily on preoperative, chronic intracranial EEG monitoring with depth electrodes revealed that approximately 20% of patients were seizure-free; however, most of the patients had some decrease in seizures.[56] The lesions in these patients have various degrees of gliosis. The problems associated with extratemporal surgery include accurate identification of the epileptogenic zone and the potential morbidity related to resection. Possible reasons

for the relatively dismal outcome in these patients are the absence of abnormality seen on neuroimaging studies, the limitations of intracranial and extracranial EEG studies, the variable ictal behavior, and the potentially large region of epileptogenicity. Ictal extracranial EEG recordings may not reveal an electrographic alteration during an extratemporal seizure, even when consciousness is impaired. The epileptogenic zone in these patients may not be well-localized or circumscribed. The surgical strategy in these patients relies heavily on intracranial EEG recordings to delineate the limits of the epileptic brain tissue. However, even aggressive attempts to resect the epileptogenic zone may be associated with unfavorable operative outcome. The anatomical location of eloquent or functional cortex may further limit the ability of the neurosurgeon to completely resect the epileptogenic zone.

THE RATIONALE FOR THE PREOPERATIVE EVALUATION

The rationale for the preoperative evaluation is to determine the localization of the epileptogenic zone, the underlying abnormality likely associated with the partial seizure disorder, and the functional importance of the epileptic cortex.[28] A comprehensive neurologic history and examination are performed before proceeding with diagnostic studies. Also, observers of seizure activity should be interviewed. Specific details of ictal behavior may provide information that may indicate the lateralization and localization of the epileptogenic zone in patients with partial epilepsy. The patient should be questioned about medication history and the presence of antiepileptic drug toxicity. The neurologic history may also reveal the likely cause of the seizure disorder.

The preliminary evaluation is conducted in an outpatient setting. A sleep/awake EEG recording, MRI of the head, neuropsychologic studies, visual perimetry, and language examination are performed. The MRI study should be performed to allow adequate assessment of hippocampal lesion in mesial temporal sclerosis. The results of the initial evaluation may indicate whether the patient has a surgically remediable partial epileptic syndrome. Subsequently, the patient is admitted to the epilepsy monitoring unit for long-term extracranial ictal EEG recordings. Treatment with antiepileptic drugs is often discontinued or reduced, depending on the frequency and type of seizure activity and drug level determinations. Usually, several seizures are recorded before a decision is made about the likely localization of the epileptogenic zone. Selected candidates should undergo a PET or ictal SPECT study.[22,23]

After evaluating the patient with noninvasive methods, the data are reviewed at an epilepsy surgical conference or directly with the neurosurgeon. Several treatment options are discussed with the patient, including investigational drug studies, "newer" antiepileptic drug medication, and epilepsy surgery. Surgical candidates may proceed to epilepsy surgery or chronic intracranial EEG monitoring, depending on the results of the noninvasive evaluation. The indications for intracranial EEG studies are discussed in Chapter 15.

DECISION ABOUT WHO SHOULD UNDERGO HEMISPHERECTOMY

Partial hemispherectomy and multilobar cortical resections are performed for intractable epilepsy in patients with diffuse hemispheric epileptic syndromes.[13,17] Multilobar cortical resection may be required in selected patients to excise the epileptogenic zone and to significantly reduce seizure tendency. Patients with hemiparesis may have a widespread region of epileptogenesis associated with a "damaged" hemisphere. The pathologic processes that may be amenable to this surgical treatment include prenatal and postnatal vascular occlusions, tuberous sclerosis, hemimegalencephaly, chronic encephalitis of Rasmussen, extensive cortical dysplasia, and Sturge-Weber syndrome.[13] All these patients have evidence of diffuse hemispheric neurologic deficits. The

neurologic deficit, including hemiplegia and homonymous hemianopia, is usually maximal in these patients preoperatively. The rationale for the preoperative evaluation is to establish the unilateral nature of the seizure activity. In these patients, MRI is essential for demonstrating the structural abnormality associated with the intractable seizure disorder. PET imaging is useful in identifying a region of nonepileptic cortical dysfunction in children with infantile spasms.[58,59] Interictal EEG not uncommonly may reveal bilateral epileptiform abnormalities. Candidates for hemispherectomy have prominent hemiparesis, with little or no useful fine finger movement. Focal resection of the cortex in these patients is unlikely to be associated with a favorable seizure outcome. The epileptic brain tissue in these patients is lateralized but not well localized. A large cortical resection may not produce additional neurologic morbidity, but it may render a patient seizure-free. The operative strategy in these patients often includes "functional" hemispherectomy, that is, a partial but functionally complete resection in which the frontal and occipital poles are disconnected from the rest of the brain but their blood supply remains intact.[17,31,60] The results of a multicenter study indicated that about two-thirds of patients undergoing hemispherectomy are rendered seizure-free and that only 11.6% do not have improvement.[37] It is important to note that not all patients with hemiparesis and intractable partial epilepsy require hemispherectomy. Temporal lobe cortical resection may be efficacious in patients with partial seizures of temporal lobe origin.

WHEN TO CONSIDER MULTIPLE SUBPIAL TRANSECTIONS

One of the most recent developments in the surgical management of partial epilepsy is the technique of "multiple subpial transections (MST)," introduced by Morrell et al.[18] These investigators have explained the rationale for MST and reviewed the experience at their institution.[18] This surgical procedure has been shown to be efficacious and safe in patients with epileptogenic zones that involve functional cortex. The procedure has been performed with surprisingly low morbidity in patients with partial seizures arising from primary motor cortex and eloquent language regions of the brain. Focal corticectomy in these patients would likely result in an unacceptable neurologic deficit. Multiple subpial transections may be particularly useful in patients with epilepsia partialis continua or Landau-Kleffner syndrome.

SURGICAL TREATMENT FOR SYMPTOMATIC GENERALIZED EPILEPSY

Patients with symptomatic generalized epilepsy may have medically refractory seizures associated with developmental delay. The unfavorable outcome of medical therapy in these patients has been established. Tonic or atonic seizures may be associated with drop attacks that are physically disabling. Drop attack seizures occur without warning, and patients cannot anticipate the fall, which results in injury. Drop attack is a type of seizure that causes considerable concern because of the possible head trauma and bodily injury due to an unanticipated fall. Persons with secondary generalized epilepsy may require protective head gear (for example, a bicycle helmet), because of the frequent drop attacks that may occur when the patient is ambulatory and in an upright position. It is unfortunate that wearing the helmet reminds patients and their families of the severity of the seizure disorder. Often, it is considered socially disabling.

Section of the corpus callosum, or corpus callosotomy, is mainly a palliative procedure that can decrease the frequency of tonic and atonic seizures.[19,20] Preoperative scalp-recorded EEGs usually reveal a widespread, synchronous, epileptiform abnormality consisting predominantly of generalized slow spike-and-wave or multifocal spike discharges. The ictal pattern during a drop attack may reveal an electrodecremental response. MRI may not reveal any intracranial focal lesion in patients being considered for corpus callosotomy. The rationale for this procedure is that it interrupts the commissural connections between the two cerebral hemispheres which may participate in the development of a secondary generalized seizure. Callosotomy is used as an alternative to focal cortical resection when the preoperative evaluation does not indicate that an anatomically localized region of epileptic brain tissue is amenable to excision. Paradoxically, simple or complex partial seizures (or both) may increase in frequency after this procedure.

The extent of the corpus callosum section is the most important surgical variable affecting seizure outcome. Postoperative MRI studies may be useful in objectively assessing the extent of resection. Intraoperative EEG recordings have not proved to be of prognostic importance. Postoperatively, most patients have less seizure activity; however, few patients are rendered seizure-free.[37] In one multicenter study, about 70% of the patients had improvement after callosotomy but about only 8% were seizure-free.[37] A marked decrease in atonic seizures may be of great benefit because of the potential decrease in physical injury associated with the seizures and because of the ability of the patient to participate in activities outside of the home (for example, sheltered workshop).

Most physicians consider callosotomy to be palliative in nature, with the operative goals different from those for patients having focal cortical resection for partial epilepsy. After callosotomy, most patients continue to require antiepileptic drug medication and to have persistent problems in intellectual performance. As is true for other surgical techniques for intractable epilepsy, morbidity may be related to the surgical treatment. The extent of callosotomy directly affects the likelihood of morbidity. Complete callosal transection produces a disconnection syndrome. The main concerns with callosotomy (even with an anterior transection) are decrease in verbal output, hemiparesis, and urinary incontinence. Advances in surgical methods have decreased operative morbidity. Fortunately, the complications mentioned above are usually short-term. Despite clear evidence that callosotomy is beneficial in the treatment of secondary generalized epilepsy, the performance of this procedure is limited to only a few epilepsy centers.

REFERENCES

1. Crandall PH. Neurosurgical management of the epilepsies. Postoperative management and criteria for evaluation. Adv Neurol 1975;8:265–79.

2. Drake J, Hoffman HJ, Kobayashi J, et al. Surgical management of children with temporal lobe epilepsy and mass lesions. Neurosurgery 1987;21:792–7.

3. Dreifuss FE. Goals of surgery for epilepsy. In: Engel J Jr, ed. Surgical treatment of the epilepsies. New York: Raven Press, 1987:31–49.

4. Engel J Jr. Seizures and epilepsy. Philadelphia: FA Davis Company, 1989: (a) 137–78; (b) 443–74.

5. McNaughton FL, Rasmussen T. Criteria for selection of patients for neurosurgical treatment. Adv Neurol 1975;8:37–48.

6. Penfield W, Jasper H. Epilepsy and the functional anatomy of the human brain. Boston: Little, Brown and Company, 1954.

7. Hauser A, Hesdorffer D. Prognosis. In: Hauser WA, Hesdorffer DC, eds. Epilepsy: frequency, causes, and consequences. New York: Demos, 1990:197–243.

8. Bengzon AR, Rasmussen T, Gloor P, et al. Prognostic factors in the surgical treatment of temporal lobe epileptics. Neurology 1968;18:717–31.

9. Cascino GD, Sharbrough FW, Hirschorn KA, et al. Surgery for focal epilepsy in the older patient. Neurology 1991;41:1415–7.

10. Falconer MA, Serafetinides EA. A follow-up study of surgery in temporal lobe epilepsy. J Neurol Neurosurg Psychiatry 1963;26:154–65.

11. Ojemann GA. Intraoperative tailoring of temporal lobe resections. In: Engel J Jr, ed. Surgical treatment of the epilepsies. 2nd ed. New York: Raven Press, 1993:481–8.

12. Wyllie E, Luders H, Morris HH III, et al. Clinical outcome after complete or partial cortical resection for intractable epilepsy. Neurology 1987;37:1634–41.

13. Andermann F, Freeman JM, Vigevano F, et al. Surgically remediable diffuse hemispheric syndromes. In: Engel J Jr, ed. Surgical treatment of the epilepsies. 2nd ed. New York: Raven Press, 1993:87–101.

14. Awad IA, Rosenfeld J, Ahl J, et al. Intractable epilepsy and structural lesions of the brain: mapping,

resection strategies, and seizure outcome. Epilepsia 1991;32:179–86.

15. Boon PA, Williamson PD, Fried I, et al. Intracranial, intraaxial, space-occupying lesions in patients with intractable partial seizures: an anatomoclinical, neuropsychological, and surgical correlation. Epilepsia 1991;32:467–76.

16. Cascino GD, Kelly PJ, Sharbrough FW, et al. Long-term follow-up of stereotactic lesionectomy in partial epilepsy: predictive factors and electroencephalographic results. Epilepsia 1992;33:639–44.

17. Rasmussen T, Villemure JG. Cerebral hemispherectomy for seizures with hemiplegia. Cleve Clin J Med 1989;56 Suppl 1:S62–8.

18. Morrell F, Whisler WW, Bleck TP. Multiple subpial transection: a new approach to the surgical treatment of focal epilepsy. J Neurosurg 1989;70:231–9.

19. Spencer SS. Corpus callosum section and other disconnection procedures for medically intractable epilepsy. Epilepsia 1988;29 Suppl 2:S85–99.

20. Wilson DH, Culver C, Waddington M, et al. Disconnection of the cerebral hemispheres. An alternative to hemispherectomy for the control of intractable seizures. Neurology 1975;25:1149–53.

21. Lüders HO, Awad I. Conceptual considerations. In: Lüders HO, ed. Epilepsy surgery. New York: Raven Press, 1992:51–62.

22. Berkovic SF, Newton MR, Rowe CC. Localization of epileptic foci using SPECT. In: Lüders HO, ed. Epilepsy surgery. New York: Raven Press, 1992: 251–6.

23. Engel J Jr, Brown WJ, Kuhl DE, et al. Pathological findings underlying focal temporal lobe hypometabolism in partial epilepsy. Ann Neurol 1982; 12:518–28.

24. Engel J Jr. The role of neuroimaging in the surgical treatment of epilepsy. Acta Neurol Scand Suppl 1988;117:84–9.

25. Commission on Classification and Terminology of the International League Against Epilepsy. Proposal for revised clinical and electroencephalographic classification of epileptic seizures. Epilepsia 1981;22:489–501.

26. Kotagal P. Psychomotor seizures: clinical and EEG findings. In: Wyllie E, ed. The treatment of epilepsy: principles and practice. Philadelphia: Lea & Febiger, 1993:378–92.

27. Wieser HG. Electroclinical features of the psychomotor seizure: a stereoelectroencephalographic study of ictal symptoms and chronotopographical seizure patterns including clinical effects of intracerebral stimulation. Stuttgart, Germany: Gustav Fischer, 1983.

28. Cascino GD. Surgical treatment of epilepsy. Neurology Chronicle 1993;3:1–8.

29. Dodrill CB, Wilkus RJ, Ojemann GA, et al. Multidisciplinary prediction of seizure relief from cortical resection surgery. Ann Neurol 1986;20:2–12.

30. Rasmussen TB. Surgical treatment of complex partial seizures: results, lessons, and problems. Epilepsia 1983;24 Suppl 1:S65–76.

31. Rasmussen T. Hemispherectomy for seizures revisited. Can J Neurol Sci 1983;10:71–8.

32. Shewmon DA, Sheilds D, Chugani HT, et al. Contrasts between pediatric and adult epilepsy surgery: rationale and strategy for focal cortical resection. J Epilepsy 1990;3 Suppl:141–55.

33. Ward AA. Perspectives for surgical therapy of epilepsy. In: Ward AA, Penry JK, Purpura DP, eds. Epilepsy. New York: Raven Press, 1983:371–90.

34. Duchowny M, Levin B, Jayakar P, et al. Temporal lobectomy in early childhood. Epilepsia 1992;33:298–303.

35. Holmes GL. The long-term effects of seizures on the developing brain: clinical and laboratory issues. Brain Dev 1991;13:393–409.

36. Mattson RH. Drug treatment of uncontrolled seizures. Epilepsy Res Suppl 1992;5:29–35.

37. Engel J Jr, Van Ness PC, Rasmussen TB, et al. Outcome with respect to epileptic seizures. In: Engel J Jr, ed. Surgical treatment of the epilepsies. 2nd ed. New York: Raven Press, 1993:609–21.

38. Jack CR Jr, Sharbrough FW, Cascino GD, et al. Magnetic resonance image-based hippocampal volumetry: correlation with outcome after temporal lobectomy. Ann Neurol 1992;31:138–46.

39. Spencer SS. Depth electroencephalography in selection of refractory epilepsy for surgery. Ann Neurol 1981;9:207–14.

40. Cascino GD, Jack CR Jr, Parisi JE, et al. Magnetic resonance imaging-based volume studies in temporal lobe epilepsy: pathological correlations. Ann Neurol 1991;30:31–6.

41. Gloor P. Mesial temporal sclerosis: historical background and an overview from a modern perspective. In: Lüders HO, ed. Epilepsy surgery. New York: Raven Press, 1992:689–703.

42. Mathieson G. Pathology of temporal lobe foci. Adv Neurol 1975;11:163–81.

43. Sloviter RS. The functional organization of the hippocampal dentate gyrus and its relevance to the pathogenesis of temporal lobe epilepsy. Ann Neurol 1994;35:640–54.

44. Kotagal P, Lüders H, Williams G, et al. Temporal lobe complex partial seizures: analysis of symptom clusters and sequences (abstract). Epilepsia 1988;29:661.

45. Jackson GD, Berkovic SF, Tress BM, et al. Hippocampal sclerosis can be reliably detected by magnetic resonance imaging. Neurology 1990;40:1869–75.

46. Bergen D, Bleck T, Ramsey R, et al. Magnetic resonance imaging as a sensitive and specific predictor of neoplasms removed for intractable epilepsy. Epilepsia 1989;30:318–21.

47. Blume WT, Girvin JP, Kaufmann JC. Childhood brain tumors presenting as chronic uncontrolled focal seizure disorders. Ann Neurol 1982;12:538–41.

48. Fish D, Andermann F, Olivier A. Complex partial seizures and small posterior temporal or extratemporal structural lesions: surgical management. Neurology 1991;41:1781–4.

49. Palmini A, Andermann F, Olivier A, et al. Focal neuronal migration disorders and intractable partial epilepsy: a study of 30 patients. Ann Neurol 1991;30:741–9.

50. Spencer DD, Spencer SS, Mattson RH, et al. Intracerebral masses in patients with intractable partial epilepsy. Neurology 1984;34:432–6.

51. Cascino GD. Epilepsy and brain tumors: implications for treatment. Epilepsia 1990;31 Suppl 3:S37–44.

52. Britton JW, Cascino GD, Sharbrough FW, et al. Low-grade glial neoplasms and intractable partial epilepsy: efficacy of surgical treatment. Epilepsia 1994;35:1130–5.

53. Dodick DW, Cascino GD, Meyer FB. Vascular malformations and intractable epilepsy: outcome after surgical treatment. Mayo Clin Proc 1994;69:741–5.

54. Yeh HS, Tew JM Jr, Gartner M. Seizure control after surgery on cerebral arteriovenous malformations. J Neurosurg 1993;78:12–8.

55. Cascino GD, Jack CR Jr, Parisi JE, et al. MRI in the presurgical evaluation of patients with frontal lobe epilepsy and children with temporal lobe epilepsy: pathologic correlation and prognostic importance. Epilepsy Res 1992;11:51–9.

56. Hajek M, Wieser HG. Extratemporal, mainly frontal, epilepsies: surgical results. J Epilepsy 1988;1:103–19.

57. Olivier A, Awad IA. Extratemporal resections. In: Engel J Jr, ed. Surgical treatment of the epilepsies. 2nd ed. New York: Raven Press, 1993:489–500.

58. Chugani HT, Shields WD, Shewmon DA, et al. Infantile spasms: I. PET identifies focal cortical dysgenesis in cryptogenic cases for surgical treatment. Ann Neurol 1990;27:406–13.

59. Shields D, Shewmon DA, Chugani HT, et al. The role of surgery in the treatment of infantile spasms. J Epilepsy 1990;3 Suppl:321–4.

60. Rasmussen T. Postoperative superficial hemosiderosis of the brain, its diagnosis, treatment and prevention. Trans Am Neurol Assoc 1973;98:133–7.

Selection of Candidates for Invasive Monitoring

Susan S. Spencer

Accurate localization of a resectable epileptogenic area enables potentially curative surgical treatment for patients with medically refractory partial epilepsy, who comprise at least 20% of patients with partial seizures.[1] The current pool of appropriate candidates for epilepsy surgery consists of about 100,000 persons and increases yearly. The theoretical possibility that some nonrefractory epilepsies might also be appropriately treated surgically could provide extended application of these concepts to many more patients.

Even in the context of the profound importance of neuroimaging in the diagnosis and treatment of epilepsy, the impact of this technique on the evaluation of patients for epilepsy surgery has been dramatic, making the evaluation more precise, less costly, less risky, and more rapid. Modifications of the evaluation of patients for epilepsy surgery have been insidious but parallel to and dependent on the rapid advances in neuroimaging. Most of this progress is a result of our ability to evaluate successfully an increasing number of patients without intracranial recording based primarily on the contributions of advanced neuroimaging.

REVIEW OF PATIENT EVALUATION PROTOCOLS FOR EPILEPSY SURGERY

The selection of patients for epilepsy surgery follows well-established guidelines outlined in this volume by Cascino. After a person is considered a surgical candidate, the means by which that person is evaluated must provide an accurate localization of the area of brain responsible for initiating the habitual and medically uncontrolled seizures. The fulfillment of this condition, based on many studies over several decades, is the most important factor contributing to successful amelioration of seizures after resection of an area identified as responsible for those seizures.[2–5] Early pioneers in epilepsy surgery operated almost entirely on the basis of the clinical symptoms, and most of their patients harbored gross structural lesions associated with previous trauma.[6] The advent of electroencephalography (EEG) brought a major change in the conceptual approach to epilepsy surgery,[7] because epilepsy could be better defined as a disease uniformly characterized by abnormal, excessive, electrical discharge of cerebral gray matter. Thus, treatment, whether medical or surgical, could be directed to this fundamental process. After medical treatment failed, and if resection of a portion of brain was contemplated, one had to prove as rigorously as possible the ability of that specific area to generate the abnormal electrical discharge and, further, to substantiate that this paroxysmal electrical activity was identical to that which caused the patient's spontaneous seizures. Electrical recording by EEG is the only way to do this,[8] so demonstration of localized EEG abnormality became the sine qua non of patient evaluation for epilepsy surgery. It remains so today.

Because EEG recording from surface electrodes may not demonstrate or accurately localize abnormalities in the interictal or ictal state[9,10] and because the ictal event is tied more directly to the seizures themselves, EEG techniques were modified to reflect more accurately the initial neuronal events that signal the seizure. More than 35 years ago, the technique of implanting electrodes within deep structures, including the temporal lobe and other regions, was developed and gained acceptance as an important modality for evaluating patients for epilepsy surgery. It provided a closer approximation to the early changes underlying the spontaneous seizure.[11–15] Considerably more localizing information was obtained from intracranial recording. Many paroxysmal electrical events were seen to occur in "deep structures" without evidence on the surface EEG. The surface EEG alteration sometimes was found to be falsely localized. Intracranial recording was able to increase availability of surgical treatment by providing the essential electrical localization otherwise lacking in many medically refractory epileptic patients.[16–18]

By 1975, the increasing use of and interest in epilepsy surgery prompted numerous publications of patient evaluation protocols, and the need for depth EEG or other intracranial recording was repeatedly addressed and modified over the years. The literature provides extensive material for reviewing the changes in patient evaluation for epilepsy surgery through the last two decades, which have been the years of most rapid advances in neuroimaging. The following review fosters an appreciation of the changes that neuroimaging has brought to the patient evaluation protocol for epilepsy surgery.

The range of abnormalities that could be demonstrated by neuroimaging techniques two decades ago, at the time when epilepsy surgery began to be used more frequently, was limited. The available techniques included only skull radiography, angiography, and pneumoencephalography. Furthermore, the few abnormalities that could be documented (usually an enlarged temporal horn) were not well correlated with EEG evidence of epileptogenesis. Walter[19] stated, "In the context of the evaluation of a seizure disorder, it should be kept in mind that there may well be a discrepancy between the demonstrable structural lesion and the epileptogenic focus." He concluded that depth electrode studies were invaluable in the evaluation of some patients for surgical treatment. This comment reflected the philosophy—in strict adherence to the proven need for electrographic localization before resective epilepsy surgery—to *require* intracranial EEG on essentially all candidates for epilepsy surgery. Other epilepsy surgery centers, following the Montreal tradition, used depth EEG only for selected patients with confusing scalp EEG localization but continued to select other patients by using scalp EEG supplemented by intraoperative EEG (electrocorticography).[20] It is fair to say that two decades ago, epilepsy surgery was seldom performed without *some* more invasive EEG investigation, either acute or chronic, beyond that supplied by surface recording.[8,20]

In 1981, Engel and colleagues[21] published a report on seven patients who were evaluated with 14 criteria for epilepsy surgery. The study was the preliminary step in a change in protocol at UCLA based on the use of positron emission tomography (PET). While reaffirming the guiding principle of patient selection for epilepsy surgery ("Epileptic excitability must still be demonstrated in order to identify a lesion as epileptogenic"), Engel proposed that if the findings of scalp EEG and tests of functional status, including neuropsychologic evaluation, intracarotid amobarbital test, and PET scan are concordant, then "it may not be necessary to risk depth electrode investigations." Ten years later, Engel and colleagues[22] verified in a larger group of patients that the demonstration of focal hypometabolism in one temporal lobe was highly predictive of seizure onset in medial temporal lobe structures recorded by depth electrodes. This solidified the first proposed change in patient selection for intracranial EEG prompted by neuroimaging. The combination of localized scalp EEG changes and fluorodeoxyglucose PET to the same temporal lobe was thought to be an excellent alternative to invasive study in many patients.

Simultaneously with these observations and modifications of the epilepsy surgery evaluation protocol, the development of computed tomography (CT) prompted further revision of the protocol. CT was shown to detect previously unsuspected, circumscribed, space-occupying lesions in 15% to 20% of the patients with refractory partial epilepsy who were being evaluated for surgical treatment. Spencer et al.[23] and Rich et al.[24] reported on groups of patients with such lesions and observed that most of the lesions were gliomas (some surprisingly high grade). Furthermore, they found that resection of the lesions was likely to cure the seizures and suggested that only minimal (but concordant) electrographic localization without intracranial EEG was a reasonable approach to this group of patients. By 1986, it became widely accepted protocol to define epileptogenicity of CT-detected space-occupying lesions with scalp EEG (albeit, defined less precisely than with depth EEG), and, without further invasive study, to remove such lesions with surrounding margins to normal tissue.[3,25] "Because resection of mass lesions with the surrounding gliotic tissue is associated with excellent seizure control, detection of such lesions limits the necessity for further invasive localizing study."[3]

Because of the greater sensitivity and specificity of magnetic resonance imaging (MRI), its advent as a widely used technique in epilepsy patients further modified the criteria for performing intracranial EEG, surprisingly toward *more* intracranial study in some lesional patients but also toward *less* intracranial study in others without space-occupying lesions.

Much depends on the localization of both the lesion and the epileptogenic area. The latter is usually close to the lesion but cannot be predicted without demonstrating EEG abnormalities and their field of distribution. Patients with frontal or occipital structural lesions may show predominant temporal epileptic discharges and a seizure pattern that does not permit more precise localization. There, too...the use of depth or subdural strip electrodes may be unavoidable.[26]

This apparent reversal in the concept of *less* localization being required with structural lesions came about because MRI was capable of revealing more than CT: not only the gliomas but also cavernous hemangiomas, hamartomas, cortical dysplasia, developmental abnormalities, and other atrophic lesions that held less strict correlation with scalp EEG localization. This permitted an approach to these lesions that was similar to the one that had evolved for the gliomatous lesions seen by CT.

Despite the earlier belief that "MR does not appear capable of identifying mesial temporal sclerosis,"[2] further study proved that it could identify such a lesion and could do so with a high degree of accuracy. MRI evidence of hippocampal atrophy was found to be highly predictive of medial temporal lobe epileptogenicity in selected and nonselected groups of patients verified to have this lesion by pathologic findings and intracranial EEG recording.[27–30] In 1993, Engel and Ojemann[31] reversed themselves, "At this point, definitive diagnosis and identification of the epileptogenic mesial temporal area can usually be made non-invasively, based largely on the pattern of ictal EEG onset, results of functional imaging, and visualization of an atrophic hippocampus on MR." This capability is now widely accepted and adopted. Hippocampal volumetric analysis provides standardization and quantification of what has become a landmark for the diagnosis of the medial temporal lobe atrophy that predicts cell loss and seizure onset in these temporal lobe structures.

Although more publications and protocols for epilepsy surgery evaluation have continued to appear and will certainly be modified by future developments in neuroimaging and other diagnostic studies, by 1993 considerable agreement had emerged on a basic philosophy of evaluation. This philosophy was molded by neuroimaging but respected the basic characteristics of the disease process being treated. MRI and PET are the neuroimaging cornerstones of these revised protocols, but they do not provide (independently or together) proven sufficient predictive value to stand alone, and intracranial EEG is still an option when other EEG data are not optimal. However, the approach to epilepsy surgery patients changed in a fundamental way. Evaluation now begins with neuroimaging, to which other criteria are applied, instead of commencing with EEG, to which other criteria are applied. MRI is now among the first studies performed on candidates for epilepsy surgery and virtually dictates the rest of the evaluation. "The early use of MRI has made previous evaluation protocols obsolete."[32]

Clear agreement exists (1) on the need for invasive EEG when confirmation of the epileptogenic nature of any MRI-identified lesion is lacking, (2) on the central role of neuroimaging in evaluation of patients for epilepsy surgery, and (3) on the reduced need for EEG precision because of neuroimaging findings. The various protocols now revolved around how many and which functional studies must demonstrate concordance with MRI and scalp EEG finding and whether discordance is acceptable for any method. The way in which epilepsy surgery protocols evolved can bias one to accept one neuroimaging technique as more predictive or essential than another not on the basis of careful clinical investigation but rather on the basis of availability, publicity, chronology, or tradition. Every effort should be made to substantiate and to standardize the presurgical evaluation on the basis of objective evidence as it emerges.

REVIEW OF THE CURRENT NEUROIMAGING TECHNIQUES IN RELATION TO THE EVALUATION OF PATIENTS FOR EPILEPSY SURGERY

Data are available to assess the sensitivity and specificity of the four major neuroimaging techniques currently used to evaluate patients for epilepsy surgery (namely, MRI, ictal single-photon emission computed tomography [SPECT], interictal SPECT, and PET) with respect to EEG, pathologic findings, or surgical outcome. Despite wide variability in the patient characteristics described in published reports, including chronicity of disease, age, localization, lesional presence, surgical procedures, instrumentation, pathologic analysis, and EEG techniques, the results support the current emphasis on MRI and PET in evaluating patients for epilepsy surgery. They also suggest an important, although still rudimentary, role for ictal SPECT. From these observations emerges a rational sequence and prioritization of procedures that could limit cost and confusion.

MRI is the only structural neuroimaging technique of the four techniques and, thus, has a unique place in epilepsy and epilepsy surgery evaluation. Its sensitivity in the detection, diagnosis, and definition of various developmental and foreign tissue lesions surpasses that of CT to the extent that CT is no longer used routinely in evaluating epilepsy patients (unless the patient cannot undergo MRI). As the possibility of resolving significant atrophic changes in hippocampal structures became evident, most epilepsy surgery centers changed their protocols for MRI evaluation of patients being considered for epilepsy surgery to include finer cuts and coronal T_1- and T_2-weighted images.[33] On the basis of the reports on 809 patients published through 1993, the sensitivity of MRI in temporal lobe epilepsy was 87%, and sensitivity was 55% in patients with extratemporal seizures.[34] Recognizing that EEG recordings in these patients may not always reflect accurately the location of the abnormal substrate of the epileptic process, we also examined pathologic verification and found MRI to have a sensitivity (86%) similar to that of pathologic findings in resected temporal lobes.[34] The ability of MRI to demonstrate medial temporal lobe atrophy may be improved with methods to quantitatively measure hippocampal size.[35] This modification of MRI for temporal lobe investigation is relatively new but holds great promise. Quantitative MRI assessment of hippocampal volume sensitivity was 86% sensitive to scalp EEG temporal lobe abnormalities in 153 reported patients and 94% sensitive to hippocampal lesions in 31 reported patients. At our institution, we investigated the results of hippocampal volumetric analysis with respect to intracranial EEG findings.[10] In a group of 56 patients with refractory epilepsy studied with intracranial EEG, we found 72% sensitivity and 66% specificity of quantitative evidence of hippocampal atrophy to medial temporal seizure onset. This finding is especially impressive in a group of patients in whom the lesion is difficult to localize because they did not have space-occupying lesions or surface EEG localization. In this study, quantitative MRI evidence of hippocampal atrophy was more sensitive than ictal or interictal scalp EEG, neuropsychologic assessment profile, and intracarotid amobarbital procedure in predicting onset of medial temporal lobe seizures documented by intracranial EEG. The detection rate for medial temporal lobe epilepsy might be improved further by using abnormal T_2 signal in medial temporal lobe structures as a marker for this epileptic process, but this application is still being standardized.[36]

Jack et al.[37] and Kuzniecky et al.[33] independently reported that MR evidence of hippocampal atrophy is also predictive of seizure outcome after epilepsy surgery. This is supported by quantitative MRI and intracranial EEG data for a previously reported group of 56 patients operated on at Yale. Of these patients, 41 had more than 1 year of postoperative follow-up. Hippocampal atrophy was highly and significantly predictive of a seizure-free state ($P < 0.001$). MRI documentation of space-occupying foreign tissue lesions in temporal or extratemporal areas is also highly correlated with surgical outcome, as judged by the cessation of seizures after removal of these lesions.[38,39] However, developmental and atrophic lesions, including dysplasia, focal atrophy, hamartomas, and gliosis, are *not* well correlated with seizure cessation after resection.[33,40–42]

PET and SPECT, which are distinct from MR because they measure functional rather than structural abnormalities, have also been used to evaluate patients with refractory epilepsy. As noted above, PET was the first of the new generation of neuroimaging techniques to be used when protocols for epilepsy surgery were modified, and with technical advances, the resolution of this method has increased.[21,22] PET studies with newer

compounds that allow assessment of neurotransmitters, amino acids, and various receptors may be the next wave of specific neuroimaging developments that hold promise for localizing epileptic tissue. The investigations that have been reported have used the ability of PET to map cerebral metabolism with fluorodeoxyglucose.

Fluorodeoxyglucose PET has been valuable in helping to avoid performing intracranial EEG recording in some patients with temporal lobe epilepsy, because the demonstration of decreased temporal lobe metabolism interictally is 95% sensitive to temporal lobe EEG abnormalities (312 reported patients through 1993).[34] However, the sensitivity is somewhat less to pathologic abnormalities in resected temporal lobe and to extratemporal EEG abnormalities. This remarkable level of sensitivity of PET to temporal lobe epileptic abnormalities is tarnished by its lack of definition of the nature of the underlying abnormality and by its diffuse distribution (the hypometabolism always extends beyond the medial temporal localization of epileptogenesis and the pathologic alterations, and often beyond the temporal lobe itself). The diffuse distribution of hypometabolism is not a result of technical factors, because current PET instruments have a resolution of 3 mm. Instead, it likely reflects a widespread functional effect of the medial temporal lobe/limbic epileptic process. The use of PET technique with other compounds to label receptors that may be more restricted in their alterations is a promise for the future. Nevertheless, fluorodeoxyglucose PET demonstration of temporal lobe hypometabolism has been reported by some authors to correlate with surgical success in terms of seizure control after temporal lobectomy.[43,44] PET findings have not been correlated with outcome in extratemporal epilepsy, and the yield of the technique in these patients makes it considerably less useful.

SPECT, the most recent addition to the neuroimaging studies in evaluating patients for epilepsy surgery, usually is used to image cerebral blood flow, although newer applications for demonstrating benzodiazepine and dopamine receptors are emerging. Even with more highly developed PET instruments, comparative studies show that altered cerebral blood flow is less sensitive for identifying an epileptogenic zone than altered metabolism.[45,46] Interictal SPECT measurement of blood flow fulfills this prediction. Reports vary considerably, but interictal SPECT measurement of decreased cerebral blood flow was 79% sensitive to temporal lobe EEG abnormalities and 49% sensitive to extratemporal EEG abnormalities (in 539 patients reported through 1993).[34] Sensitivity to temporal lobe pathologic abnormalities was 73%, with 30% specificity. SPECT results are difficult to interpret because they vary between studies, are often multifocal, and may show increased or decreased perfusion interictally. There are not sufficient data to comment on the predictive value of SPECT for surgical outcome.

Ictal SPECT is the ultimate functional neuroimaging technique for epilepsy, because a tracer injected at the time of the seizure is trapped for many hours and provides a depiction of a functional variable, cerebral blood flow, that is known to be correlated with seizure discharge.[47,48] However, this technique has practical limitations. Even injection at the moment of seizure onset may show increased flow in all areas involved by the seizure over its first 1 to 2 minutes (this is the amount of time required for brain extraction of the radioligand). Albeit SPECT is an improvement over PET in this regard (PET averages metabolic activity over 40 minutes), it still is difficult to interpret ictal SPECT results. Some authors claim that even injection postictally provides accurate localization in temporal lobe epilepsy.[49] In a report on 108 patients, the sensitivity of ictal or postictal SPECT to temporal lobe EEG abnormalities was 93% and the specificity was 71%; its sensitivity to extratemporal EEG abnormalities was 56%. Techniques are being developed to digitally subtract interictal from ictal images, because baseline hypoperfusion might obscure increases at the time of the seizure.[50] Ictal SPECT results have not yet been correlated with seizure outcome.

Few critical comparative assessments of the three neuroimaging techniques (MRI, PET, and SPECT) exist. The results of performing these studies on 20 epilepsy surgery patients indicate that the three techniques are not entirely redundant.[51,52] However, the meaning of a single abnormality seen with one of these three neuroimaging techniques is not known; this occurs rarely enough (except for MRI) that isolated abnormalities on PET or SPECT still require further independent study for confirmation of localization in an individual patient.

IMPACT OF NEUROIMAGING ON PATIENT SELECTION FOR INTRACRANIAL RECORDING

The available literature supports a preeminent role for MRI in defining the macrostructural concomitants of epileptogenesis, certain of which have a high correlation with temporal or extratemporal epileptogenic zones and with predicting seizure cessation after their removal. It is reasonable to conclude that if EEG confirms the localization of these specific lesions found with MRI, the presence, absence, or even location of PET or SPECT demonstration of functional abnormality probably should not affect decisions about epilepsy surgery. In fact, this situation has evolved for patients with space-occupying lesions demonstrated by MRI. However, hippocampal atrophy does not have the same status. Perhaps because the recognition of quantitative or qualitative hippocampal atrophy is newer and despite the high correlation of hippocampal atrophy seen on MRI with outcome and medial temporal seizure onset, concordant PET and/or SPECT (or at least absence of dis-

cordance) as well as EEG findings are still often considered essential in selecting these patients for temporal lobe epilepsy surgery. For patients without MRI abnormalities, intracranial EEG can occasionally be avoided by the intelligent use of neuroimaging (for example, in patients with concordant functional imaging, surface EEG, and cognitive assessments). In these situations, however, the absence of localized and concordant functional impairment is almost as significant as its discordance, because multiple independent confirmation of localization by scalp EEG is absolutely required.

At our institution,[53–55] intracranial EEG is no longer required if (1) MRI demonstrates a space-occupying foreign tissue lesion (consistent with glioma or cavernous hemangioma) *and* scalp EEG is concordant with localization, regardless of PET, SPECT, and neuropsychologic localization; (2) MRI demonstrates hippocampal atrophy *and* scalp EEG is localized to the anterior or medial temporal lobe *and* no significant discordance is found on any tests of functional imaging or functional ability (the results of tests of focal functional deficit may or may not be localized); and (3) MRI findings are normal, but scalp ictal and interictal EEG abnormalities are localized to the anterior or midtemporal region *and* this localization is confirmed by functional assessment, including at least the demonstration of temporal lobe hypometabolism by PET, *and* no significant discordance from any functional study is present. We continue to require intracranial EEG if (1) scalp EEG findings are discordant with an MRI-documented lesion (space-occupying lesion or hippocampal atrophy); (2) scalp EEG temporal lobe localization is unconfirmed; (3) more than one MRI lesion is present (for example, space-occupying lesion and hippocampal atrophy); (4) MRI shows a large atrophic lesion or cortical dysplasia; and (5) mapping of functional areas in proximity to the suspected zone of epileptogenesis is necessary. These specific guidelines reflect only the changes in evaluation protocol for patients at our institution, where 10 years ago almost all patients considered for epilepsy surgery were studied with intracranial EEG. Our current guidelines illustrate the profound effect that neuroimaging has had in selecting patients for epilepsy surgery, and these guidelines are not markedly different from those of other medical centers.[31,56–58]

INTRACRANIAL TECHNIQUES MODIFIED BY NEUROIMAGING

Independent of the decision-making process about who needs intracranial EEG, neuroimaging has had a critical effect in modifying the intracranial EEG technique itself. Patients who require intracranial EEG despite the presence of a structural or functional abnormality (because of discordant data or lack of confirmation) benefit from a more logical selection of sites for intracranial electrode implantation based on the results of functional and structural neuroimaging. For example, a patient with unilateral hippocampal atrophy and a space-occupying lesion in the ipsilateral occipital lobe who has posterior temporal scalp EEG abnormalities will benefit from invasive recording with electrodes that sample the occipital lobe, medial temporal lobe, and temporal lobe neocortex, and some contralateral sites. Ignorance of the lesion in the occipital lobe may have prevented adequate representation of a potentially epileptogenic zone in this lobe in the recording array. Similarly, an area of cortical dysplasia in the temporal neocortex in a patient with temporal lobe scalp EEG localization and diffuse frontotemporal parietal hypometabolism seen with PET dictates intracranial study, with sampling of both the medial and lateral aspects of the temporal lobe.

MRI has also revolutionized the process of intracranial recording. Stereotaxic MRI-guided placement of MRI-compatible electrodes with subsequent verification of the exact anatomical distribution of contacts provides a level of precision not previously contemplated, with significant implications for interpretation and implementation of results.[59] Because at most epilepsy surgical centers intracranial electrode techniques are selected to suit an individual case, combinations of strip, grid, and depth electrodes are common. The meaning of relative localization and propagation of electrical discharges accompanying seizures is profound. Medial versus lateral temporal lobe seizure onset can be distinguished and defined, occipital lobe seizure onset with variable suprasylvian and infrasylvian propagation can be appreciated, and adjacent structural components of medial temporal lobe circuitry can be documented to contribute to seizure onset independently and interactively. These observations have brought more understanding of the epileptic process that can be applied to treatment. For example, from data obtained with depth electrodes in the hippocampus and with simultaneous subdural strips recording from the medial temporal regions, including the entorhinal cortex, we have shown specific types of entorhinal and hippocampal synergy that differentiate medial temporal lobe epilepsy from other epilepsies of neocortical temporal or extratemporal locations.[60]

CONCLUSION

Neuroimaging techniques are the most important influence on epilepsy surgery. They contribute understanding, localization, design of safe and effective resective procedures, and reduction of risk. The basic tenets of epilepsy surgery, including the requirement for electrical localization of the area of onset of spontaneous seizures, have by necessity survived this explosion of technology. A thorough understanding of the data and their meaning, with logical application to each situation, will help ensure that neuroimaging continues to help each patient considered for epilepsy surgery, while successively advancing our surgical and theoretical approaches.

CASE REPORTS

The following case reports illustrate the complex interrelationships between the various localizing studies in evaluating patients for epilepsy surgery. They were selected to provide a spectrum of situations, including patients with MRI-demonstrated lesions concordant with (case 1) scalp EEG findings and patients with hippocampal atrophy with concordant (case 2) and discordant (case 3) functional and electrophysiologic data. Although each case is unique, the reasoning process and the importance of neuroimaging are best understood in cases like these.

Case 1

A 47-year-old right-handed woman began having seizures at age 33. Her birth was by breech delivery. Although she had neonatal jaundice, her development was normal. Her seizures were characterized by a wave rising through her body, nausea, and an inability to interact normally with the environment. Initial treatment was with phenytoin and phenobarbital, but a rash and tongue swelling developed that required emergency treatment with epinephrine. The rash resolved after phenobarbital therapy was discontinued. The patient then received phenytoin monotherapy. The seizures did not respond to treatment despite increases in the dose. A single secondarily generalized seizure occurred 4 years after seizure onset.

In 1991, the patient had the first of several MRI scans, all of which showed a cystic lesion in the right medial temporal lobe. It was minimally enhancing with gadolinium and was unchanged over the years (Figure 15-1). After phenytoin therapy failed, the patient was given valproate, which alleviated the seizures but caused alopecia. Treatment with primidone had unacceptable side effects, and carbamazepine did not control the seizures. Trials with ethosuximide and clonazepam were not successful. The results of her neurologic examination were normal.

The patient was evaluated with intensive audiovisual EEG monitoring. The interictal EEG was consistently normal, and four seizures were recorded. Two of them occurred during sleep. The patient reported having a strange feeling before seizure onset that occurred during wakefulness; she did not completely lose contact but put her hand on her head. The EEG was similar in all these spells and was characterized by right temporal rhythmic delta discharge. The seizures lasted 1 to 2 minutes (Figure 15-2).

Neuropsychologic evaluation demonstrated a verbal IQ of 113 and a performance IQ of 99. There was evidence of left upper extremity motor impairment, poor

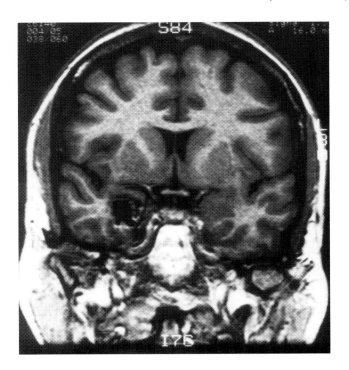

FIGURE 15-1. (Case 1). Cystic lesion consistent with cavernous hemangioma in the right medial temporal lobe.

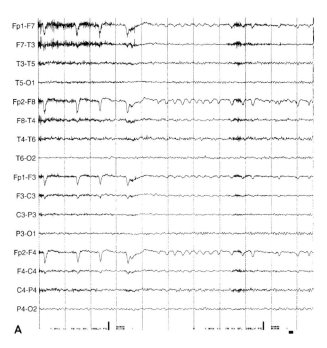

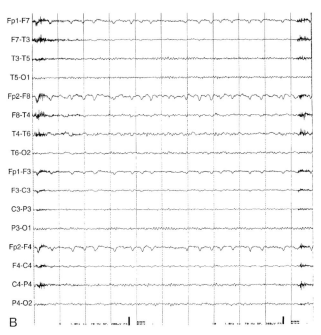

visual construction, and relative impairment of nonverbal reasoning. These findings were consistent with right temporal lobe dysfunction. MRI confirmed the right medial temporal cystic lesion. The intracarotid amobarbital procedure showed left hemisphere dominance for speech and intact memory function in the left hemisphere but inadequate memory function in the right hemisphere. On the basis of the concordance of electrographic, functional, and imaging characteristics, the lesion was resected. Pathologic examination showed a cavernous hemangioma. The patient has had no seizures during the more than 8 months of follow-up.

This case illustrates the concordance of electrographic and functional data with an MRI-identified lesion. This concordance allowed resection of the lesion without the need for intracranial monitoring. This type of lesion, that is, cavernous hemangioma, may not have been identified at an earlier time with CT. It is predominantly on the basis of the MRI-identified lesion that the resection was performed without further intracranial study, because the electrographic seizure discharge was atypical of temporal lobe epilepsy and no interictal EEG abnormality was present.

Case 2

A 28-year-old left-handed woman was referred for possible surgical treatment of medically intractable complex-partial seizures. The seizures began when the patient had

FIGURE 15-2. (Case 1). A–F. Continuous EEG segments (displayed with a longitudinal bipolar montage) recorded from patient in case 1 during a spontaneous seizure demonstrating right temporal slow discharge during the ictus. This localization is consistent with the location of the lesion shown in Figure 15-1. Fullscale, 200 µV; each division, 1 sec.

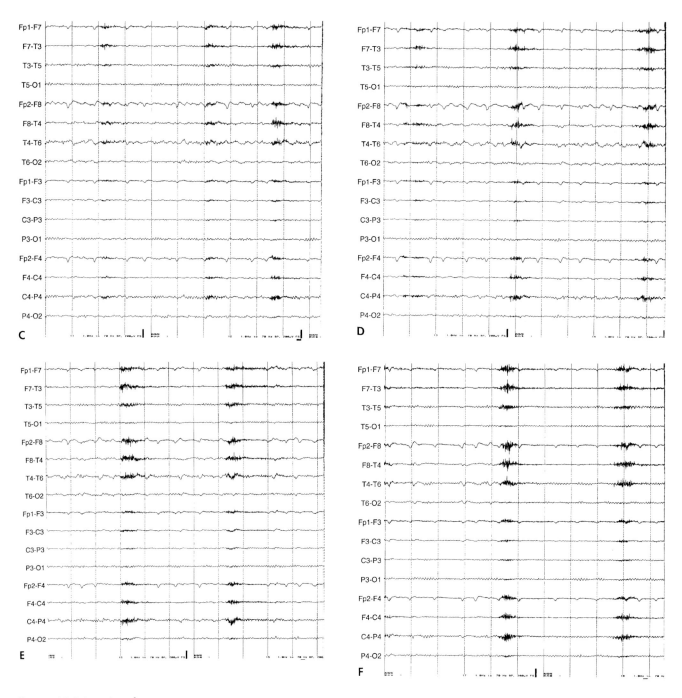

FIGURE 15-2 *(continued).*

a fever at age 2 years. She was seizure-free for 2 years after this initial febrile seizure and then had a second prolonged febrile seizure, at which time medical treatment was initiated. Six of her siblings also had febrile seizures and are currently seizure-free.

Her seizures continued unabated. They were characterized by a gastric aura that occasionally was followed by loss of contact and semipurposeful activity.

Phenytoin, phenobarbital, primidone, clonazepam, valproate, and carbamazepine alone and in various combinations were ineffective.

MRI showed atrophy of the body and tail of the left hippocampus, with increased T_2 signal consistent with hippocampal sclerosis (Figure 15-3). During intensive EEG audiovisual monitoring, four spontaneous seizures were recorded after reduction of medication.

Selection of Candidates for Invasive Monitoring

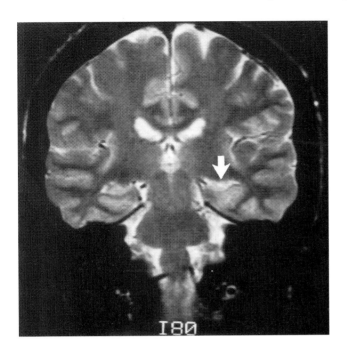

FIGURE 15-3. (Case 2). Coronal MRI showing left hippocampal atrophy (*arrow*).

The seizures were stereotyped, but their clinical characteristics were not lateralizing. During all her seizures, surface EEG demonstrated left temporal interictal abnormalities and left temporal ictal rhythmic discharge (Figure 15-4). Neuropsychologic evaluation showed an atypical pattern, with isolated language impairment and a decrease in verbal IQ compared with performance IQ

but intact verbal information acquisition and impaired visual information acquisition. It was thought that this pattern might be due to anomalous language representation. Interictal SPECT showed hypoperfusion of the left temporal lobe (Figure 15-5). PET scan demonstrated a marked decrease in metabolism of the left temporal lobe (Figure 15-6). Hippocampal volumetric analysis revealed a ratio at exactly 2 standard deviations below the norm, confirming significant hippocampal atrophy on the left.

Intracarotid amobarbital testing showed left speech dominance, with good memory function in the right hemisphere but absence of this function in the left hemisphere. No data were discordant. In view of the intracarotid amobarbital test results, the left temporal interictal and ictal scalp EEG abnormalities, the evidence of left hippocampal atrophy, the hypometabolism demonstrated with PET in the left temporal lobe, the history of febrile seizures, and stereotyped seizures consistent with a temporal lobe lesion, an anterior left medial temporal lobectomy was performed. The patient has been seizure-free for 6 months.

This case illustrates an ideal combination of localizing results in a patient without a space-occupying lesion. The concordance of these results allowed surgical resection to be performed without intracranial EEG study.

Case 3

A 48-year-old right-handed woman began having seizures at age 32. Her birth was normal, and she had no history of febrile seizures, meningitis, encephalitis, or

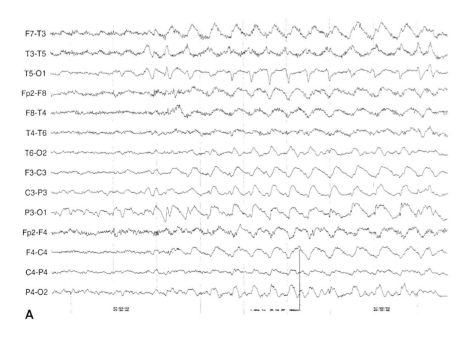

FIGURE 15-4 (Case 2). A–D. Continuous EEG segments (shown in longitudinal bipolar montage) during a spontaneous seizure in patient in case 2 showing early, predominantly left temporal, high-amplitude rhythmic slowing, followed by rhythmic 6- to 7-Hz left posterior temporal activity. The morphology and location of this discharge are consistent with, but somewhat atypical of, a mesial temporal seizure disorder on the left. Fullscale, 300 μV; each division, 1 sec.

A

FIGURE 15-4 *(continued).*

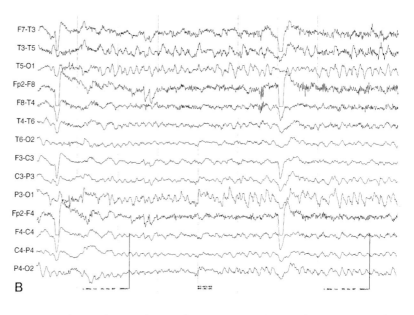

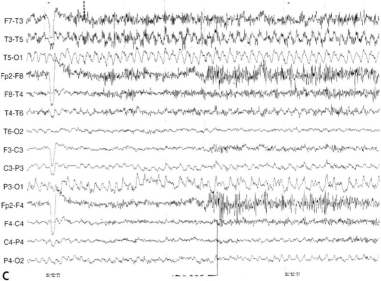

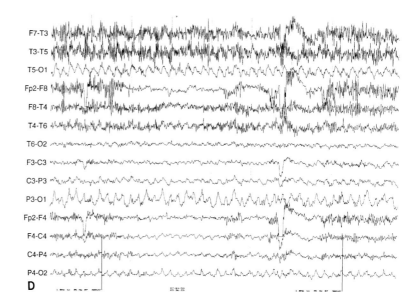

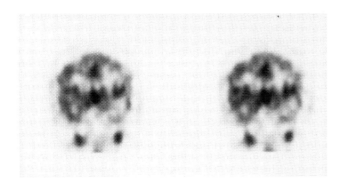

FIGURE 15-5. (Case 2). Interictal SPECT with HMPAO showing left temporal hypoperfusion.

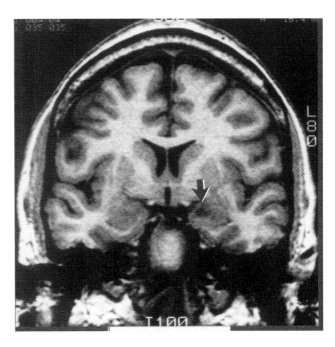

FIGURE 15-7. (Case 3). MRI depicting low-density lesion (*arrow*) in left anterior-medial temporal lobe.

head trauma. The seizures were characterized by a rising sensation in her epigastrium, followed by loss of contact, with lip-smacking, guttural sounds, and upper extremity automatisms. Despite treatment with primidone for 12 years, the seizures were not controlled and occurred every week. Subsequently, she received treatment with carbamazepine and, then, phenobarbital. Over the years, the aura receded and the seizures were sometimes secondarily generalized. On examination and initial evaluation, including EEG and MRI, no abnormality was apparent.

MRI demonstrated a hypodense lesion in the anterior left medial temporal lobe, involving the hippocampus, without gadolinium-DTPA enhancement (Figure 15-7). She was evaluated with intensive EEG audiovisual monitoring, at which time interictal EEG demonstrated rare right midtemporal spikes. Six seizures occurred during sleep; she had upper extremity automatisms. EEG showed rhythmic right hemisphere discharge at the time of the seizure, but this could not be localized further (Figure 15-8). Neuropsychologic evaluation

demonstrated a verbal IQ of 100, a performance IQ of 92, and a mild visual perceptual difficulty suggestive of dysfunction in the right hemisphere. Memory function was normal. An interictal SPECT scan demonstrated decreased perfusion in the right temporal region. Intracarotid amobarbital testing showed left hemisphere language dominance and intact memory bilaterally. Hippocampal volumetric analysis demonstrated a ratio not significantly different from normal. Because of the discordance of functional and electrographic information with the MRI-demonstrated lesion, an intracranial EEG study was planned to localize the

FIGURE 15-6. (Case 2). Interictal fluorodeoxyglucose PET demonstrating hypometabolism in left temporal lobe.

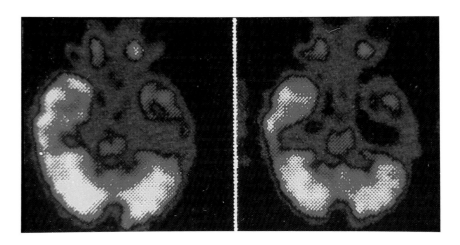

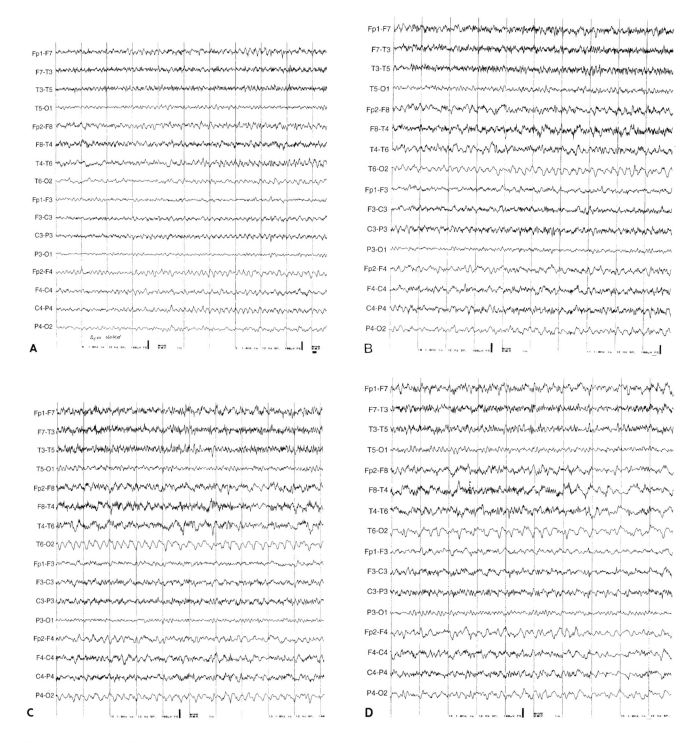

FIGURE 15-8. (Case 3). During a spontaneous seizure in patient in case 3, right temporal rhythmic slowing developed. A–E. Continuous EEG segments with longitudinal bipolar surface recording. Fullscale, 100 μV; each division, 1 sec.

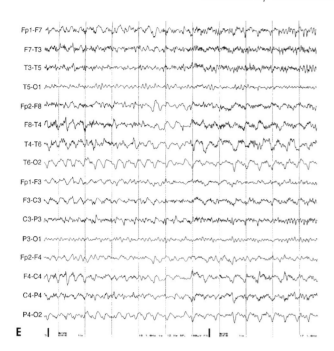

FIGURE 15-8 *(continued)*.

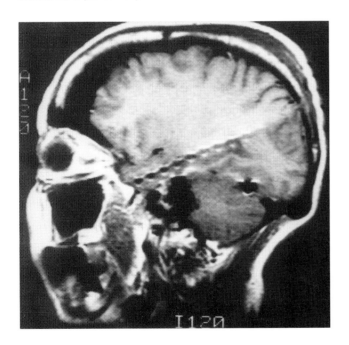

FIGURE 15-9. (Case 3). Intracranial EEG investigation included bilateral, 12 contact, medial temporal lobe depth electrodes inserted from posteriorly. Individual contacts are seen in this postimplantation MRI.

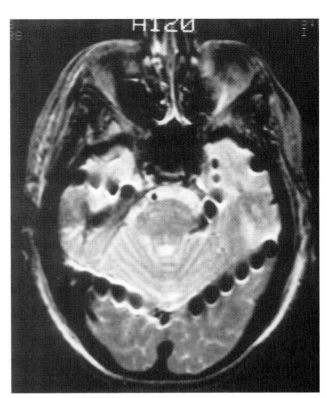

FIGURE 15-10. (Case 3). Subdural strips that sampled medial, inferior, and lateral temporal regions bilaterally were also implanted during the intracranial study in the patient in case 3. Locations of contacts are shown on this postimplantation MRI.

onset of the uncontrolled seizures. Biopsy of the left temporal lesion was performed at the time of electrode implantation.

The biopsy specimen revealed gliosis. Bilateral depth electrodes (Figure 15-9) and subdural electrodes (Figure 15-10) were inserted to record from the hip-pocampus, the anterior and posterior temporal lobe, and the frontopolar regions. Interictal intracranial recording demonstrated spikes that occurred focally in the right hippocampal region (recorded by the depth electrodes). Seven seizures beginning in the medial right anterior temporal region were similar clinically and electrographically (Figure 15-11). The clinical symptoms were similar to those of the seizures recorded with scalp electrodes. An anterior right medial temporal lobectomy was performed. At 9-month follow-up evaluation, the patient was seizure-free.

This case illustrates discordance between an MRI-demonstrated lesion and electrographic and functional studies. Biopsy was necessary to exclude a lesion that would require treatment independent of the patient's seizures. The area that was shown by intracranial recording to be responsible for the onset of the patient's habitual and uncontrolled seizures was resected. This case is typical of our experience that when the discordance between a focal MRI-demonstrated lesion and electrographic and functional evaluation is clear, the lesion is not a glioma.

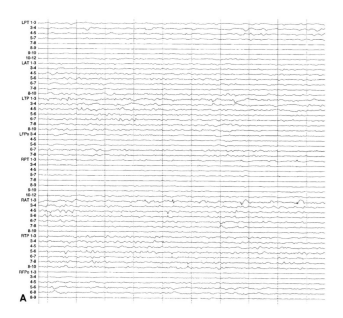

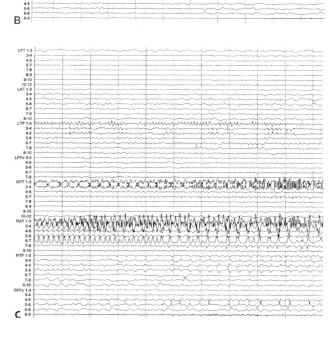

Figure 15-11. (Case 3). A–C. With hippocampal depth electrodes (*LPT, RPT*) and subdural strips in left and right anterior temporal (*LAT, RAT*), posterior temporal (*LTP, RTP*), and frontopolar regions (*LFP$_O$, RFP$_O$*), multiple seizures in patient in case 3 showed consistent right medial temporal onset, reflected in 1-3, 3-4 (*most anterior*) contacts of right hippocampal electrode (*RPT*) and simultaneously in most distal (*medial*) contacts of right anterior temporal subdural strip (*RAT, 1-3, 3-4*). The morphology is different in these locations, showing the typical low-voltage fast neocortical discharge in RAT and the slower periodic discharge in RPT.

REFERENCES

1. Spencer SS, Katz A. Arriving at the surgical options for intractable seizures. Semin Neurol 1990;10:422–30.

2. Engel J. Approaches to localization of the epileptogenic lesion. In: Engel J, ed. Surgical treatment of the epilepsies. New York: Raven Press, 1987:75–96.

3. Spencer SS. Surgical options for uncontrolled epilepsy. Neurol Clin 1986;4:669–95.

4. Luders HO, Awad I. Conceptual considerations. In: Luders HO, ed. Epilepsy surgery. New York: Raven Press, 1992:51–62.

5. Rossi GF. Considerations on the principles of surgical treatment of partial epilepsy. Brain Res 1975; 95:395–402.

6. Foerster O, Penfield W. Structural basis of traumatic epilepsy and results of radical operation. Brain 1930;53:99–119.

7. Bailey P, Gibbs FA. Surgical treatment of psychomotor epilepsy. JAMA 1951;145:365–70.

8. Gloor P. Contributions of electroencephalography and electrocorticography to the neurosurgical treatment of the epilepsies. Adv Neurol 1975;8:59–105.

9. Spencer SS, Williamson PD, Bridgers SL, et al. Reliability and accuracy of localization by scalp ictal EEG. Neurology 1985;35:1567–75.

10. Spencer SS, So NK, Engel J Jr, et al. Depth electrodes. In: Engel J Jr, ed. Surgical treatment of the epilepsies. 2nd ed. New York: Raven Press, 1993: 359–76.

11. Talairach J, Bancaud J, Bonis A, et al. Functional stereotaxic exploration of epilepsy. Confin Neurol 1962;22:328–30.

12. Bancaud J, Talairach J, Bonis A, et al. La stéréo-électroencéphalographie dan l'épilepsie: informations neurophysiopathologiques apportées par l'investigation

fonctionnelle stéreotaxique. Paris: Masson & Cie, Éditeurs, 1965.

13. Ajmone Marsan C, Van Buren JM. Epileptiform activity in cortical and subcortical structures in the temporal lobe of man. In: Baldwin M, Bailey P, eds. Temporal lobe epilepsy. Springfield, Illinois: Charles C Thomas, 1958:78–108.

14. Ajmone Marsan C, Abraham K. Considerations on the use of chronically implanted electrodes in seizure disorders. Confin Neurol 1966;27:95–110.

15. Abraham K, Ajmone Marsan C. Patterns of cortical discharges and their relation to routine scalp electroencephalography. Electroencephalogr Clin Neurophysiol 1958;10:447–61.

16. Spencer SS, Spencer DD, Williamson PD, et al. The localizing value of depth electroencephalography in 32 patients with refractory epilepsy. Ann Neurol 1982;12:248–53.

17. Spencer SS. Depth electrodes. Epilepsy Res 1992;Suppl 5:135–45.

18. Spencer SS. Depth electroencephalography in selection of refractory epilepsy for surgery. Ann Neurol 1981;9:207–14.

19. Walter RD. Principles of clinical investigation of surgical candidates. Adv Neurol 1975;8:49–58.

20. Olivier A, Gloor P, Andermann F, et al. The place of stereotactic depth electrode recording in epilepsy. Appl Neurophysiol 1985;48:395–9.

21. Engel J Jr, Rausch R, Lieb JP, et al. Correlation of criteria used for localizing epileptic foci in patients considered for surgical therapy of epilepsy. Ann Neurol 1981;9:215–24.

22. Engel J Jr, Henry TR, Risinger MW, et al. Presurgical evaluation for partial epilepsy: relative contributions of chronic depth-electrode recordings versus FDG-PET and scalp-sphenoidal ictal EEG. Neurology 1990;40:1670–7.

23. Spencer DD, Spencer SS, Mattson RH, et al. Intracerebral masses in patients with intractable partial epilepsy. Neurology 1984;34:432–6.

24. Rich KM, Goldring S, Gado M. Computed tomography in chronic seizure disorder caused by glioma. Arch Neurol 1985;42:26–7.

25. Engel J Jr, Crandall PH. Intensive neurodiagnostic monitoring with intracranial electrodes. Adv Neurol 1986;46:85–106.

26. Andermann F. Approaches to patient selection for resective procedures. In: Spencer SS, Spencer DD, eds. Surgery for epilepsy. Boston: Blackwell Scientific Publications, 1991:18–35.

27. Cascino GD, Jack CR Jr, Parisi JE, et al. Magnetic resonance imaging-based volume studies in temporal lobe epilepsy: pathological correlations. Ann Neurol 1991;30:31–6.

28. Berkovic SF, Andermann F, Olivier A, et al. Hippocampal sclerosis in temporal lobe epilepsy demonstrated by magnetic resonance imaging. Ann Neurol 1991;29:175–82.

29. Spencer SS, McCarthy G, Spencer DD. Diagnosis of medial temporal lobe seizure onset: relative specificity and sensitivity of quantitative MRI. Neurology 1993;43:2117–24.

30. Lencz T, McCarthy G, Bronen RA, et al. Quantitative magnetic resonance imaging in temporal lobe epilepsy: relationship to neuropathology and neuropsychological function. Ann Neurol 1992;31:629–37.

31. Engel J Jr, Ojemann GA. The next step. In: Engel J Jr, ed. Surgical treatment of the epilepsies. 2nd ed. New York: Raven Press, 1993:319–29.

32. Spencer SS. Temporal lobectomy: selection of candidates. In: Wyllie E, ed. The treatment of epilepsy: principles and practice. Philadelphia: Lea & Febiger, 1993:1062–74.

33. Kuzniecky R, Burgard S, Faught E, et al. Predictive value of magnetic resonance imaging in temporal lobe epilepsy surgery. Arch Neurol 1993;50:65–9.

34. Spencer SS. The relative contributions of MRI, SPECT, and PET imaging in epilepsy. Epilepsia 1994;35 Suppl 6:S72–89.

35. Jack CR Jr, Sharbrough FW, Twomey CK, et al. Temporal lobe seizures: lateralization with MR volume measurements of hippocampal formation. Radiology 1990;175:423–9.

36. Jackson GD, Connelly A, Duncan JS, et al. Detection of hippocampal pathology in intractable partial epilepsy: increased sensitivity with quantitative magnetic resonance T_2 relaxometry. Neurology 1993;43:1793–9.

37. Jack CR Jr, Sharbrough FW, Cascino GD, et al. Magnetic resonance image-based hippocampal volumetry: correlation with outcome after temporal lobectomy. Ann Neurol 1992;31:138–46.

38. Kuzniecky RI, Cascino GD, Palmini A, et al. Structural neuroimaging. In: Engel J Jr, ed. Surgical treatment of the epilepsies. 2nd ed. New York: Raven Press, 1993:197–209.

39. Cascino GD, Jack CR Jr, Parisi JE, et al. MRI in the presurgical evaluation of patients with frontal lobe epilepsy and children with temporal lobe epilepsy: pathologic correlation and prognostic importance. Epilepsy Res 1992;11:51–9.

40. Kuzniecky R, Garcia JH, Faught E, et al. Cortical dysplasia in temporal lobe epilepsy: magnetic resonance imaging correlations. Ann Neurol 1991; 29:293–8.

41. Palmini A, Andermann F, Aicardi J, et al. Diffuse cortical dysplasia, or the 'double cortex' syndrome: the clinical and epileptic spectrum in 10 patients. Neurology 1991;41:1656–62.

42. Otsubo H, Hwang PA, Jay V, et al. Focal cortical dysplasia in children with localization-related epilepsy: EEG, MRI, and SPECT findings. Pediatr Neurol 1993;9:101–7.

43. Radtke RA, Hanson MW, Hoffman JM, et al. Temporal lobe hypometabolism on PET: predictor of seizure control after temporal lobectomy. Neurology 1993;43:1088–92.

44. Theodore WH, Sato S, Kufta C, et al. Temporal lobectomy for uncontrolled seizures: the role of positron emission tomography. Ann Neurol 1992;32:789–94.

45. Leiderman DB, Balish M, Sato S, et al. Comparison of PET measurements of cerebral blood flow and glucose metabolism for the localization of human epileptic foci. Epilepsy Res 1992;13:153–7.

46. Yamamoto YL, Ochs R, Gloor P, et al. Patterns of rCBF and focal energy metabolic changes in relation to electroencephalographic abnormality in the inter-ictal phase of partial epilepsy. In: Baldy-Moulinier M, Ingvar DH, Meldrum BS, eds. Cerebral blood flow, metabolism and epilepsy. London: John Libbey, 1983:51–62.

47. Raichle ME, Grubb RL Jr, Gado MH, et al. Correlation between regional cerebral blood flow and oxidative metabolism: in vivo studies in man. Arch Neurol 1976;33:523–6.

48. Lebrun-Gradié P, Baron J-C, Soussaline F, et al. Coupling between regional blood flow and oxygen utilization in the normal human brain: a study with positron tomography and oxygen 15. Arch Neurol 1983;40:230–6.

49. Rowe CC, Berkovic SF, Sia STB, et al. Localization of epileptic foci with postictal single photon emission computed tomography. Ann Neurol 1989;26:660–8.

50. Spencer S, Zubal G, Hoffer P, et al. Subtraction technique for epilepsy localization using SPECT (abstract). Epilepsia 1993;34 Suppl 6:121.

51. Coubes P, Awad IA, Antar M, et al. Comparison and spacial correlation of interictal HMPAO-SPECT and FDG-PET in intractable temporal lobe epilepsy. Neurol Res 1993;15:160–7.

52. Stefan H, Bauer J, Feistel H, et al. Regional cerebral blood flow during focal seizures of temporal and frontocentral onset. Ann Neurol 1990;27:162–6.

53. Spencer DD, Pappas CTE. Surgical decisions regarding medically intractable epilepsy. Clin Neurosurg 1992;38:548–66.

54. Spencer DD, Inserni J. Temporal lobectomy. In: Luders HO, ed. Epilepsy surgery. New York: Raven Press, 1991:553–54.

55. Williamson PD. Evaluation of patients for epilepsy surgery at the West Haven VA/Yale-New Haven Epilepsy Unit. In: Spencer SS, Spencer DD, eds. Surgery for epilepsy. Boston: Blackwell Scientific Publications, 1991:36–52.

56. Sperling MR, O'Connor MJ, Saykin AJ, et al. A noninvasive protocol for anterior temporal lobectomy. Neurology 1992;42:416–22.

57. Risinger MW. Electroencephalographic strategies for determining the epileptogenic zone. In: Luders HO, ed. Epilepsy surgery. New York: Raven Press, 1991:337–47.

58. Wyllie E, Awad I. Intracranial EEG and localization studies. In: Wyllie E, ed. The treatment of epilepsy: principles and practice. Philadelphia: Lea & Febiger, 1993:1023–38.

59. Spencer DD, McCarthy G, Luby M, et al. MRI stereotactic placement of intracranial electrodes. In: Shorvon S, ed. Advanced magnetic resonance imaging and epilepsy. New York: Plenum Press, 1994:149–53.

60. Spencer SS, Spencer DD. Entorhinal-hippocampal interactions in medial temporal lobe epilepsy. Epilepsia 1994;35:721–7.

Use of Magnetic Resonance Imaging in Surgical Strategies for Epilepsy

Kenneth P. Vives, Nayef Al-Rodhan,
and Dennis D. Spencer

Magnetic resonance imaging (MRI) has generally revolutionized our neurologic diagnostic capabilities, but the field of surgery for medically intractable seizures has been singularly affected. To offer surgical resection or disconnection for chronic epilepsy, one must address the need for precise localization of an epileptogenic region. Also the neurologic and cognitive function contained in that volume of tissue and the potential morbid consequence of resection or disconnection have to be predicted with a high degree of accuracy.

MRI is used to address each of these issues. The superb anatomical resolution and the quantitative power of the computer to manipulate the brain images has led to accurate placement of depth electrodes and to more precise correlation of electrophysiologic events. As a corollary to this, coregistration with other dynamic imaging, such as positron emission tomographic (PET) scans and single-photon emission computed tomographic (SPECT) scans, has begun to colocalize structural and functional alterations in epileptogenic regions. Functional MRI (*f*MRI) holds promise for noninvasively defining neurologic and cognitive processing within and around the presumptive epileptogenic area.

As yet, how structural abnormalities (atrophy, congenital cortical variations, etcetera) are associated with epileptogenesis is not clearly understood. Clinical, pathologic, and outcome data indicate that about 80% of patients with epilepsy who receive surgical treatment have a structural abnormality seen on MRI. Although electroclinical correlation is critical to confirm the epileptogenic potential of a lesion, resection strategies begin with the imaged abnormality.

SUBSTRATE CONCEPT

The convergence of anatomy and pathology as illustrated in the partial epilepsies by MRI has led us to use the substrate concept to reclassify the partial epilepsies. "Substrate" denotes the epileptogenic pathologic process plus the anatomical cerebral location, which dictates the behavioral expression of the seizure. It is increasingly evident that most partial epilepsies have a potentially well-defined substrate.[1] The substrates are divided into the following categories: sclerosis (neuronal loss and gliosis), neoplasia, vascular malformations, developmental abnormalities, and indeterminate (usually with gliosis from trauma or other acquired insults) (Table 16-1). Each of these substrates may have its own epileptic pathogenesis. Importantly, MRI is critical in categorizing the substrates, because the surgical approach may be altered by what is known about the epileptogenesis of the abnormality and its anatomical constraints.

In this chapter, the substrate concept is used to illustrate (1) how MRI has been used to guide surgeons and (2) how a logic tree of rational approaches to chronic partial epilepsy can be created.

SCLEROSIS (MESIAL TEMPORAL SCLEROSIS)

Generically, sclerosis is neuronal cell loss and gliosis. Most frequently, it is identified with disease in the medial temporal lobe. This is not to say that gliosis associated with epilepsy in regions outside of the temporal lobe is not also consequent to or associated with specific forms of neuronal loss. This is a reasonable assumption, but neuronal loss in such areas has not been frequently described qualitatively or quantitatively. The pathologic entity of mesial temporal lobe sclerosis has long been associated with temporal lobe epilepsy, and in the last decade, it has been refined as an entity that may be due to events occurring in very early childhood or infancy, such as infection, febrile seizures, ischemia, or trauma, that is expressed primarily in the medial temporal lobe electrophysiologically, with ictal onset in the hippocampus, amygdala, entorhinal cortex triangle during depth electrode studies.[2,3] The examination of the resected hippocampal tissue has revealed specific patterns of neuronal cell loss, particularly reorganization in the dentate gyrus, that has further refined the concept of sclerosis.[4,5] This pattern is expected in patients with the syndrome of medial temporal lobe epilepsy, and seizure control is excellent in many of these patients after a limited anteromedial temporal resection.

TABLE 16-1. Substrate Classification Scheme: Partial Epilepsies Classified by Substrate and Revealed by MRI

Pathologic substrate	Anatomical location
Sclerosis (neuronal loss and gliosis)	Primarily medial temporal
Neoplasia	Cortically based, any lobe
Vascular	Any lobe
Developmental	Any lobe
Indeterminate (primarily gliosis)	Any lobe

By the mid to late 1980s, MRI was capable of identifying mesial temporal sclerosis preoperatively as hippocampal atrophy and T_2 signal change. In the last few years, careful correlative studies have confirmed the MRI predictions of medial temporal lobe sclerosis and the good response of seizure control with limited resection of the atrophic medial structures (that is, the hippocampus, amygdala, and parahippocampus, including entorhinal cortex).[6]

In patients with medial temporal lobe epilepsy, MRI can clearly direct surgeons to resect a specific volume, but only after the anatomical abnormality has been confirmed, either directly or indirectly, as the epileptogenic substrate. If unilateral hippocampal atrophy is the only abnormality, the directed resection can be performed if the preoperative localizing data are concordant. These data consist of the medical history and physical examination findings and the results of scalp audiovisual electroencephalographic (EEG) monitoring, neuropsychologic testing, and the intracarotid amobarbital (Amytal) procedure.

MRI-defined medial temporal lobe atrophy has become a major criterion at our medical center for noninvasively selecting patients for anteromedial temporal resection. It must be accompanied by one of the other two major criteria: scalp interictal localized spikes and unilateral ictal onset. These major criteria must then be corroborated by at least two of our minor criteria: PET and SPECT scans, intracarotid amobarbital procedure, neuropsychologic evaluation, and the clinical symptoms of the seizures. If any of the criteria are contradictory, invasive electrode studies are performed. Figures 16-1 and 16-2 illustrate this evaluation procedure in the form of a logic tree, and the following cases are examples of the procedure.

Case: Unilateral Atrophy

The patient is a 38-year-old (at the time of initial evaluation) left-handed woman. At the age of 2 years, she had onset of seizures that consisted of an epigastric aura followed by the loss of contact, spitting, and bilateral hand

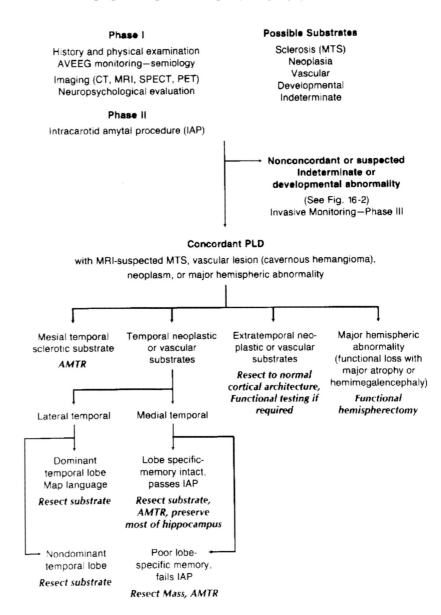

FIGURE 16-1. Logic tree for concordant preoperative localizing data. (*AMTR*) anteromedial temporal resection, (*AVEEG*) audiovisual electroencephalography, (*CT*) computed tomography, (*MRI*) magnetic resonance imaging, (*MTS*) mesial temporal sclerosis, (*PET*) positron emission tomography, (*SPECT*) single-photon emission computed tomography.

automatisms. The symptoms changed over the years so that she no longer experienced the aura and often had a generalized tonic extension of her body, followed by falling. Seizures averaged three per month despite adequate trials of numerous medications. The results of her neurologic examination were normal, and an interictal EEG revealed left temporal spikes. During ictal monitoring, she had four seizures with different clinical manifestations, but all of them arose from the left hemisphere, two clearly from the temporal area. This was thought to represent unifocal disease with variable spread patterns. MRI revealed marked left hippocampal atrophy, but no T_2 signal change, accompanied by left temporal neocortical atrophy (Figure 16-3). The results of neuropsychologic examination were suggestive of bilateral temporal dysfunction, predominantly on the left. The intracarotid

amobarbital procedure showed left speech dominance and intact memory bilaterally. A left anteromedial temporal resection was performed, and the pathologic examination of the resected specimen showed a gliotic hippocampus with near total cell loss in the CA1 area. The patient has been seizure-free for more than 3 years.

Case: Bilateral Atrophy

A 24-year-old right-handed man had a history of neonatal seizures of unclear cause and an episode of hemophilus influenza meningitis at the age of 6 months. At age 14, he had two tonic-clonic seizures and went on to develop complex partial seizures that began with a strange feeling in his forehead, followed by loss of contact, lip smacking, eye fluttering, and automatisms of the right hand. Despite tri-

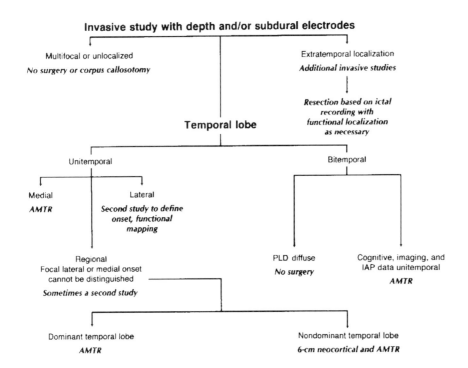

Invasive study with depth and/or subdural electrodes

Multifocal or unlocalized
No surgery or corpus callosotomy

Extratemporal localization
Additional invasive studies

*Resection based on ictal
recording with
functional localization
as necessary*

Temporal lobe

Unitemporal

Bitemporal

Medial
AMTR

Lateral
*Second study to define
onset, functional
mapping*

Regional
Focal lateral or medial onset
cannot be distinguished
Sometimes a second study

PLD diffuse
No surgery

Cognitive, imaging, and
IAP data unitemporal
AMTR

Dominant temporal lobe
AMTR

Nondominant temporal lobe
6-cm neocortical and AMTR

FIGURE 16-2. Logic tree for nonconcordant preoperative localizing data.
Abbreviations as in Figure 16-1.

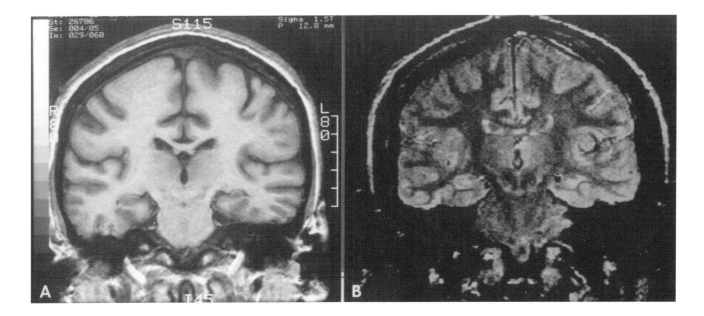

FIGURE 16-3. A. Coronal T$_1$-weighted MRI scan of patient with unilateral left hippocampal atrophy. The neocortex of the left
temporal lobe was also atrophied; note elevation of the floor of the left middle cranial fossa. B. Coronal proton density-weighted
MRI scan of another patient showing T$_2$ signal change in the left hippocampus. These changes are not present in A.

als with multiple medications, his seizures persisted at a rate
of 5 to 10 per month. Continuous audiovisual EEG monitoring showed interictal spike-wave phenomena diffusely
but greater on the right. He had five seizures, all of which
generalized rapidly but had predominant build-up on the
right. MRI revealed bilateral symmetrical hippocampal
atrophy (Figure 16-4). Neuropsychologic evaluation indi-

cated right hemispheric dysfunction. He was admitted for
intracranial monitoring with bilateral depth probes through
the hippocampi and multiple subdural strips with wide coverage. Interictally, he had independent right frontal and
bilateral hippocampal spikes. He had eight seizures, which
clearly began in the right hippocampus, whose symptoms
were typical of his usual seizures. He also had four seizures

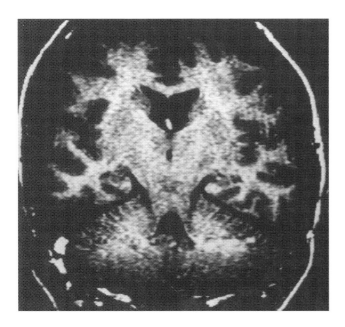

FIGURE 16-4. Coronal T_1-weighted MRI scan of patient with bilateral hippocampal atrophy.

originating in the left hippocampus, all of which were subclinical. Because of the concordance of the neuropsychologic data and the clinical seizures arising from the right, a right anteromedial temporal resection was performed. Pathologically, the hippocampus revealed severe sclerosis. At 2.5 years postoperatively, the patient is seizure-free and takes reduced amounts of anticonvulsants.

VASCULAR, NEOPLASTIC, AND DEVELOPMENTAL SUBSTRATES

Diagnosis

Clearly, MRI is superior to CT in sensitivity and specificity for diagnosing lesions in epilepsy.[7-14] MRI usually defines the substrate by identifying the lesion, illustrating its location and relationship to other brain structures, and providing clues to the pathologic diagnosis. Still, distinguishing among the different lesions associated with epilepsy is often difficult. Because specific diagnosis frequently is critical to surgical planning, this problem is discussed below for each substrate.

Invasive Study Design

The preoperative evaluation of vascular, neoplastic, and developmental substrates demands the same concordance of preoperative localizing data as in mesial temporal lobe epilepsy if the patient is to undergo resection without invasive electrode studies. However, neoplasm or vascular anomaly alone is frequently a sufficiently compelling reason for resection. In developmental abnormalities, the affected cortex may be diffuse and not clearly delineated by MRI or other modalities, and invasive study is almost always warranted. In neoplasms or vascular anomalies with nonconcordant data (that is, all seizures have onset in the opposite hemisphere), an invasive study with subdural and depth strip electrodes is also planned, usually with coverage of both hemispheres but with concentration on the area of the lesion. Prolonged electrophysiologic monitoring and mapping in nonconcordant cases may not reveal that the structural lesion is the source of epileptic activity.[2,15-18] Resection of the epileptogenic area alone may or may not achieve seizure control,[15] but in these rare cases, the lesion itself may require resection, as an issue separate from epilepsy.

Mapping of Cortical Function

MRI may identify a lesion in or adjacent to the cerebral cortex, which, if resected, may cause an unacceptable neurologic deficit. Thus, the resection may have to be altered with regard to margins, although the success of lesion extirpation or epilepsy control may be diminished. In cases in which the MRI-identified lesion involves primary language cortices, a subdural grid may be considered at the time of invasive study to allow functional mapping at the bedside or, in cases with concordant preoperative localizing data, language mapping may be performed at the time of the cortical resection.[19-25] When MRI reveals a lesion in or adjacent to primary sensory or motor cortex, the Rolandic fissure may be identified by MRI[26] or fMRI[27-30] and its relationship verified by direct mapping with brain surface somatosensory evoked potentials[31-33] or direct stimulation of motor cortex[34-38] with a bipolar electrode (or both). Functional mapping of a lesion located by MRI in the occipital cortex may be performed if the surgeon intends to restrict the resection to spare visual pathways or primary cortex to prevent visual deficit.

Assessment of Surgical Resection and Follow-Up Study

MRI may also be used to assess the completeness of resection and for follow-up evaluation. The frequency and number of follow-up MRI studies are dictated by the histopathologic features of the substrate. Our protocol for patients with low-grade tumors is to perform MRI studies annually for about 10 years postoperatively and then every other year thereafter. Higher grade tumors need more frequent follow-up study, but vascular or developmental substrates may not require MRI evaluations postoperatively.

Resective Techniques

Considerable controversy exists about the amount of tissue that needs to be removed in addition to the MRI-delineated lesion to achieve the best seizure outcome.

Much of the literature in which these techniques are discussed is heavily weighted toward neoplastic substrates, but many of the principles and issues for this may be applied to the other substrates. Generally, three different approaches are used: MRI-guided limited lesionectomy, MRI-guided lesionectomy to normal margins, and electrocorticographically tailored resection.

Magnetic Resonance Imaging–Guided Limited Lesionectomy

Complete resection of the lesion is desirable to optimize seizure outcome.[8,15,39] This may not be possible if it involves areas of cortex that if removed would produce unacceptable neurologic deficit. Stereotactically guided lesion resection has been discussed in several articles from the Mayo Clinic.[9,40–42] Overall, 57% to 60% of the patients who had stereotactically guided lesion resection were seizure-free postoperatively.[41,42] The results for patients with low-grade gliomas were slightly better, with a seizure-free rate of 82%, but the difference was not significant.[40] The results indicate that, at the same institution, the outcome is similar to that of electrocorticographically tailored resection.[9,40] In a combined series of stereotactic and open surgery, no significant difference was found between partial and total resection on seizure outcome.[9] The presence of distant interictal foci on extracranial EEG was not a predictor of poor outcome.[9,42] Seizure outcome was better in patients with extratemporal lesions, as compared with those with temporal lesions.[42] Potentially, stereotactic resection may be associated with decreased morbidity in comparison with conventional surgical techniques in selected patients undergoing resection for epilepsy.[43,44]

One study examining lesionectomy alone found that complete lesion resection resulted in a 90% seizure-free outcome, regardless of the extent of the interictal spikes.[15] The electrocorticographic results were not predictive of seizure outcome,[45] and excision of the lesion without resection of the epileptogenic zone can produce favorable results.[46,47]

Magnetic Resonance Imaging–Guided Lesionectomy with Margins

Lesionectomy with pathologic examination of the margins in frozen tissue sections is used at the Yale Medical School to guide resection for neoplasms associated with epilepsy. Specimens are taken from the margins of the resection bed and frozen sections are examined to confirm that the tumor was totally extirpated. MRI may be useful in these cases by delineating a T_2 signal change surrounding the neoplasm that may represent gliosis or tumor cells. This together with one of the new frameless stereotactic devices may simplify the method. With MRI-guided lesionectomy, 83% of patients were rendered seizure-free with resection to tumor-free margins.[8] In a recent report by Fried et al.[48] of gliomas, 82% of the patients became seizure-free; subtotal resection was associated with a poorer outcome. This concept may be extended to the low-flow vascular malformations to include in the margins all hemosiderin-stained tissue. However, in developmental, gliotic, or high-flow arteriovenous malformation substrates, a clear delineation between abnormal and normal tissue is often not possible, even with examination of frozen sections.

Lesionectomy with Tailored Cortical Resection

Secondary epileptogenesis refers to the genesis of independent seizure activity in regions of brain remote from a primary lesion as a result of repetitive seizure damage.[49–51] This is partly the basis for electrocorticographically based tailored resections. Some authors think that the interictal events recorded intraoperatively are a reflection of cortex with the ability to generate seizures; these areas are then considered for resection in addition to the lesion itself.[25,52–56] Considerable controversy remains over this issue; its use varies from medical center to medical center.

Surgeons following this dictum will nearly always resect at least as much surrounding cortex as in the Yale resection of margins and may resect considerably more, depending on the extent of interictal spiking and functional brain. The results are comparable to prior technique (79% of patients became seizure-free or had a marked reduction in seizures versus 91% who became seizure-free).[52,55] In a nonrandomized analysis at the Mayo Clinic comparing lesionectomy alone with electrocorticographically directed resection, the outcome was not significantly different for the two methods.[9] Confounding variables in studies that attempt to compare these two methods include surgical candidacy criteria and differences in how electrocorticography is used to guide the resection. With electrocorticographic guidance, larger areas of brain tissue are resected and, in some circumstances, may result in an inferior functional outcome.[57]

Dual Pathology

Dual pathology is concerned with the identification of two substrates in a patient with seizures. Previous reports have noted cases in which pathologic changes in the hippocampus were associated with extrahippocampal lesions.[9,49,58–64] The UCLA series[63,64] demonstrated severe hippocampal cell loss associated with extrahippocampal heterotopias, but only mild hippocampal cell loss was associated with gliomas. Patients with severe hippocampal cell loss were less likely to become seizure-free.[64] In a similar study at Yale, patients with temporal lobe neoplasms had a significant mild cell loss compared with control subjects, and the age of seizure onset was correlated with the degree of cell loss.[63,65] The location of the lesion appears to be an important determinant of the degree of associated hippocampal damage.[5,58,63,65,66]

Hippocampal atrophy, as documented by volumetric MRI studies, has been observed more frequently in patients with unsatisfactory outcome after lesionectomy alone.[67] Also, several reports have described patients in whom seizure control was achieved after mesial temporal resection but who previously had had a poor outcome after temporal lobe lesionectomy without hippocampectomy.[9,67–69] On the basis of these data, a strategy can be developed as follows: if the patient has a medial temporal lobe tumor, hippocampectomy in addition to lesionectomy may be considered based on the presence of hippocampal atrophy seen on MRI and, in particular, on evidence of the absence of significant function of that hippocampus, as shown by the intracarotid amobarbital procedure and neuropsychologic evaluation. In patients with extramedial temporal lobe lesions who do not fulfill the above criteria, lesionectomy with margins may be performed initially. Further resection of the hippocampus may be undertaken at a later time if seizures recur and are demonstrated to originate in the medial temporal lobe.

VASCULAR MALFORMATIONS

The spectrum of cerebral vascular malformations include arteriovenous malformations, cavernous hemangiomas, venous angiomas, and capillary telangiectasias.[70–72] The ones most often associated with epilepsy are arteriovenous malformations and cavernous hemangiomas, at a rate of 4 to 5:1.[73,74] Seizures are the most common presenting symptom in patients with cavernous malformations[75–77] and second to hemorrhage as a presenting symptom in patients with arteriovenous malformations.[78–80] About 3% of patients considered for surgical resection for intractable epilepsy have a vascular malformation that causes their seizures.[73] Venous angiomas are common in the normal population and may be found incidentally in patients with epilepsy.[70] Although capillary telangiectasias may occur with other vascular lesions associated with epilepsy, they are rarely the sole cause of seizures.

Magnetic Resonance Imaging Characteristics

The high rate of flow through arteriovenous malformations often creates a flow void on MRI imaging, but this is not true for cavernous hemangiomas. These flow voids should be differentiated from signal loss due to calcium. Feeding arteries and draining veins may also be visualized by comparing precontrast and postcontrast scans. Magnetic resonance angiography (MRA) may provide additional information about arteriovenous malforma-

tions.[81–83] Arteriovenous malformations that are not revealed with angiography (angiographically occult arteriovenous malformations) are thought to behave similarly to cavernous hemangiomas.[84]

Cavernous hemangiomas appear as discrete mass lesions on MRI. Descriptions of the appearance of the core of these lesions vary but, as a rule, they have a peripheral rim of marked hypointensity[85–87] due to hemosiderosis and gliosis of the surrounding brain tissue.[87,88]

Resective Strategies

In considering resection in patients with vascular malformations, physicians must take into account not only the potential for curing the seizures but the annual rate of hemorrhage (1 to 3%)[89] of untreated vascular lesions. The morbidity and mortality of resection for arteriovenous malformations are greater than those for other lesions in the same location. Some early reports indicated a poor seizure outcome,[90–94] but recent reports have shown that 70% to 83% of patients were rendered seizure-free after resection of arteriovenous malformation.[69,95] Complete excision of the lesion appears to produce the best outcome.[95] MRI may be helpful in delineating the surrounding gliotic brain that should be resected to more normal margins.

Significant hemorrhage is less likely with cavernous hemangiomas than with arteriovenous malformations. Unique characteristics of these lesions seen on MRI are their frequent multiplicity and the features of hemosiderin-staining of the surrounding brain. No study has considered the need for resecting the surrounding hemosiderin-stained brain to effect "total lesionectomy." Because hemosiderin-stained tissue may be implicated in epileptogenesis, it is included in our resection to achieve "normal" tissue margins. The outcome after resection is often "cure" or adequate seizure control.[73,96] Multiple cavernous hemangiomas seen on MRI may prompt an invasive study to determine whether one or more malformations are epileptogenic. MRI is a useful guide in such a study. When the electrophysiologic source is identified, the outcome for seizures in these patients may be favorable. In two series, complete resection of the lesion rendered about 75% of the patients seizure-free and another 15% to 27% had a significant decrease in seizure tendency.[73,74]

Case

A 49-year-old right-handed woman had onset of seizures at age 32. Before this onset, she recalled having episodes of "wave-like" sensations. During her seizures, she was pale and stared. Despite maximal medical treatment, she had several seizures per month, and she complained of significant deterioration in her ability to work. She was admitted for continuous audiovisual EEG monitoring,

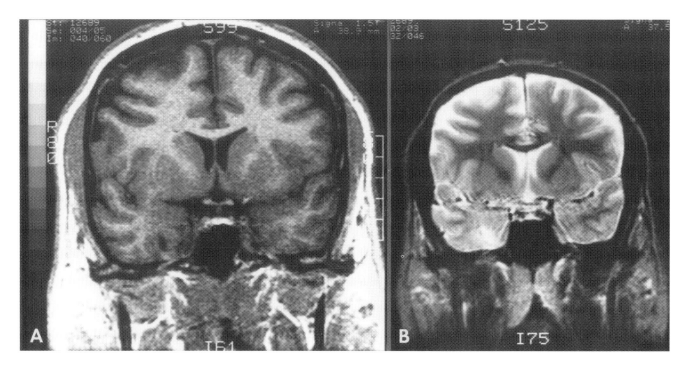

FIGURE 16-5. Coronal MRI scans of a patient with a right medial temporal lobe cavernous hemangioma. A. T$_1$-weighted scan. B. T$_2$-weighted scan.

during which time four seizures were recorded; all showed a right temporal onset and build-up. Neuropsychologic examination was notable for impairments resulting in poor visual construction and nonverbal reasoning. MRI revealed a cystic lesion in the right anteromedial temporal lobe consistent with a vascular lesion (Figure 16-5). The intracarotid amobarbital procedure revealed no abnormal flow, left speech dominance, and absence of memory in the right hemisphere. The patient underwent a right anteromedial temporal resection that spared the posterior hippocampus. All associated areas of gliotic, hemosiderin-stained brain were excised with the lesion. Pathologic examination of frozen and permanent sections showed a leptomeningeal-based cavernous hemangioma and a normal-appearing pes hippocampus. Except for one episode of a questionable aura, she has been seizure-free for 1 year postoperatively. The neuropsychologic examination was repeated and did not show a decline in any area.

NEOPLASMS

Primary brain tumors are the cause of intractable epilepsy in 10% to 30% of patients undergoing surgical resection for intractable epilepsy.[39,58,66,97] Seizures of long duration are the presenting symptom in most patients with low-grade cerebral neoplasms.[9,39,46,97,98] With the advent of MRI, an increasing number of these lesions have been identified.[13,66] The clinical manifestations of

TABLE 16-2. Neoplasms Often Associated with Epilepsy

Pure glial origin
Astrocytomas
Oligodendrogliomas
Oligoastrocytomas
Neuronoglial origin
Gangliogliomas
Dysembryoplastic neuroepithelial tumors

these lesions are indistinguishable from those of other substrates for epilepsy; the location of the tumor dictates the symptoms.[99] Surgical management of these lesions is directed to curing the epilepsy and tumor.

Pathologic and Magnetic Resonance Imaging Characteristics of Neoplasms

Two major subdivisions of neoplasms are associated with epilepsy: pure gliomas and neuronoglial neoplasms (Table 16-2). Within the gliomas, there is a continuous spectrum of histologic features from pure astrocytic tumors to pure oligodendrocytic tumors. All these tumors may harbor characteristics indicative of a more aggressive nature. In comparison with vascular malformations, neoplasms are less frequent in patients with epilepsy, occurring in about 9% to 17% of patients in surgical series for truly intractable epilepsy.[15,48,100] These astrocytomas may have a lineage different from that of their white matter counterparts and, accordingly, have a different, more benign clinical course.[48,101]

Gangliogliomas are lesions that contain abnormal appearing neurons as well as astrocytic and oligodendrocytic components.[102] They are uncommon tumors that are often classified as congenital and that are believed to have a benign course,[12,103,104] although rarely more aggressive features have been observed.[105–107] Gangliogliomas account for up to 38% of neoplasms resected for epilepsy.[39] Daumas-Duport et al.[108] have described a new class of neoplasm, dysembryoplastic neuroepithelial tumor, on the basis of the pathologic examination of surgical resection specimens from patients with epilepsy. The frequency of occurrence of this tumor in surgical series is debated.[9,39,45,109]

Typically, the neoplasms associated with epilepsy are well circumscribed and small. Infrequently, they produce a mass effect on the surrounding tissue. On T_1-weighted images, they are often well-defined hypointense lesions, although an isodense appearance may also be observed, but on T_2-weighted images, they appear hyperintense. The tumors rarely show enhancement with gadolinium. If enhancement occurs, it should be regarded as a possible indicator of a more aggressive tumor, although up to 50% of malignant gliomas in patients 30 to 50 years old may fail to enhance on CT after the administration of contrast agent.[110] The most frequent location of these lesions is the cerebral cortex, especially in the temporal lobe.[9,39,46,48,66,108]

In many cases it is difficult, if not impossible, to distinguish among low-grade tumors with MRI.[111–113] Of major importance, these lesions may be confused with developmental disorders (discussed below), which frequently require invasive study to delineate the ictal region. When any question arises with regard to the cause of the lesion, the concordance criteria of other clinical variables must be stringent to ensure that a given lesion is responsible for the patient's epilepsy.

Resective Strategies

The goals of resection are not restricted only to controlling the seizures but also to controlling the neoplasm. Consensus has not been reached about the efficacy of surgical resection for the control of low-grade gliomas or about the outcome for different techniques used for resection when the goal is to eliminate the seizures.

Low-grade tumors can undergo malignant transformation.[39,114,115] Thus, if total resection is possible, it would be desirable for controlling the tumor; studies have shown that more extensive resection correlates with longer survival.[99,116–122] Not all investigators have embraced such an aggressive stance and some, instead,

recommend a more conservative approach.[98,123–126] In several studies, age was identified as an important independent risk factor, with younger patients having increased survival time.[99,120,127] Considerable debate remains about adjuvant treatment for low-grade gliomas.[119,128] Radiotherapy may be considered in patients with subtotal resections[99,121,129,130] and in older patients.[99,124,129,131]

Case: Ganglioglioma

A 23-year-old left-handed man had onset of seizures at the age of 15. The initial seizures were of a generalized nature, but subsequent ones began with a warning of "chest heaviness," followed by a loss of contact, lip smacking, and head shaking. He had several seizures daily despite trials of multiple medications. Interictal EEG revealed isolated right temporal spikes. During ictal monitoring, six seizures occurred, and although none were lateralizing, they all consistently began with right arm automatisms and left facial twitching. The results of neuropsychologic testing were suggestive of right hemispheric dysfunction. MRI revealed a right inferomedial temporal mass consistent with a low-grade glioma (Figure 16-6). The intracarotid amobarbital procedure showed left speech dominance and the absence of memory on the right. The patient underwent right anteromedial temporal resection. The intraoperative findings were notable for an abnormally large vein of Labbé that, in comparison with its normal location, was far anterior and a tough lesion with multiple cysts located in the anterior fusiform gyrus. Pathologic examination of permanent sections revealed a ganglioglioma. At 1 year postoperatively, the patient is seizure-free.

Case: Oligodendroglioma

A 45-year-old right-handed woman was first evaluated after a motor vehicle accident, at which time CT showed a right posterior frontal abnormality. Six weeks after the accident, she had onset of seizures, which consisted of stereotypical turning of the head to the left and upward extension of the left arm, followed by falling and left-sided clonic activity, but there was no aura or loss of contact. Left upper extremity Todd's paralysis occurred postictally. The patient received treatment with multiple medications, none of which controlled the seizures; however, seizure frequency was reduced to about one per month. The results of neurologic examination were normal, but MRI showed a large right frontal mass, hypointense on T_1-weighted scans and hyperintense on T_2-weighted scans, that included the supplementary motor cortex (Figure 16-7 A). Functional MRI showed that both motor and sensory leg areas were posterior to the mass and not involved by it (Figure 16-7 B and C). The results of neuropsychologic evaluation were normal.

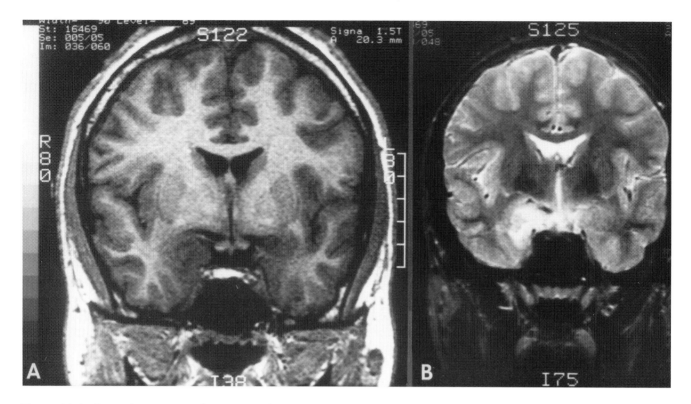

FIGURE 16-6. Coronal MRI scans of a patient with a right medial temporal lobe mass. Pathologic examination after resection revealed a ganglioglioma. A. T_1-weighted scan. B. T_2-weighted scan.

The patient underwent a right frontal craniotomy for excision of the mass. Somatosensory evoked potentials and direct cortical stimulation verified the *f*MRI findings. The mass extended to but did not involve the primary motor cortex. A gross total resection was obtained with normal frozen section margins. Pathologic examination of the tissue revealed an oligodendroglioma. Postoperatively, the patient had significant left-sided weakness, and, despite continued improvement, she tends to neglect her left arm. She had three seizures in the first 3 postoperative months, but adjustments in medication appear to have improved seizure control. MRI was repeated and did not reveal evidence of recurrence.

DEVELOPMENTAL DISORDERS

Increasingly, developmental abnormalities are becoming associated with medically refractory epilepsy. Studies suggest that they comprise between 4.3% and 25% of cases of chronic epilepsy (the wide range is influenced somewhat by the age ranges included in the different studies).[132–135] Developmental abnormalities are a diverse group of disorders that may be caused by derangement of neuronal migration from the ventricular zone to the marginal zone. Although many of the severe forms of these malformations are diagnosed in child-

hood, more subtle variations are being discovered in adults with epilepsy, largely because of advances in high-resolution imaging techniques. A brief review of the normal development of the human cerebral cortex and an overview of the classification, morphology, and histopathology of these disorders are discussed below.

Resective Strategies Based on Magnetic Resonance Imaging Findings

The developmental abnormalities can be grouped together on the basis of their predominant histologic feature. One group has defects predominantly in lamination, another group has relatively normal-appearing neurons in abnormal locations, and still another group has predominantly abnormal-appearing neurons (Table 16-3). None of these features occurs in isolation, and more than one of them may be present in a patient.

About 12.5% of patients with focal imaging signs suggestive of a developmental abnormality have seizures that are not controlled with optimal drug therapy and should be considered for resection.[136] Although many of the severe disorders are readily apparent on MRI, the more subtle focal cortical dysplasias and microdysgeneses may not be detected visually. In a blinded retrospective review of MRI studies of epilepsy patients at the Yale Medical

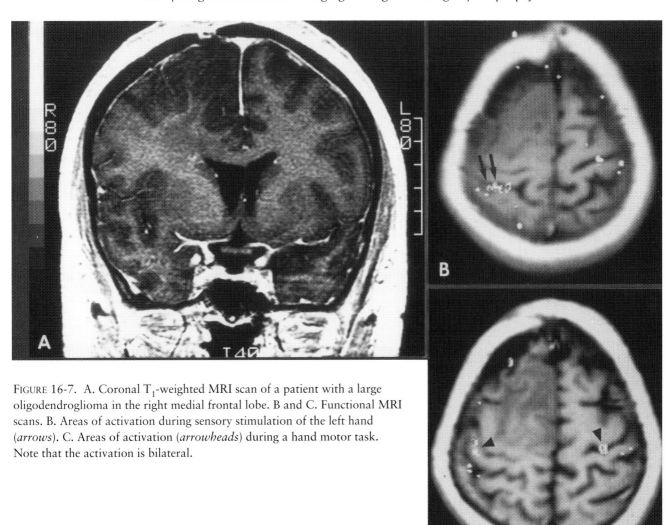

FIGURE 16-7. A. Coronal T_1-weighted MRI scan of a patient with a large oligodendroglioma in the right medial frontal lobe. B and C. Functional MRI scans. B. Areas of activation during sensory stimulation of the left hand (*arrows*). C. Areas of activation (*arrowheads*) during a hand motor task. Note that the activation is bilateral.

TABLE 16-3.   Classification of Developmental Abnormalities

Primarily defective gyration
    Polymicrogyria
    Pachygyria/lissencephaly
    Schizencephaly
Primarily misplaced neurons
    Microdysgenesis
    Gray matter heterotopia
Primarily abnormal neurons/glia
    Focal cortical dysplasia
    Hemimegalencephaly
Hamartomas

School, only 10 of 24 patients with a pathologically diagnosed developmental abnormality had such a condition listed as the primary lesion suspected on the basis of MRI (unpublished data). Many of the developmental abnormalities may look similar on MRI (Table 16-4). Currently, with MRI, six different developmental entities can be distinguished: (1) focal cortical developmental abnormalities, including focal pachygyria, macrogyria, cortical dysplasia of Taylor, and polymicrogyria; (2) nodular heterotopias; (3) laminar heterotopias, including band heterotopia; (4) hemimegalencephaly; (5) lissencephaly; and (6) schizencephaly. In some instances, polymicrogyria may be separated from the first group. However, the extent and type of the lesions as defined by MRI may not correlate with the severity or type of seizures.[137]

    These disorders are often multifocal or diffuse.[137] Generally, the precision of localizing data is dependent on how well circumscribed the lesion is, the rate of recruit-

TABLE 16-4.   Relationship of MRI to Histopathologic Substrate

MRI diagnosis	Histopathologic substrate
Lissencephaly	Pachygyria (four-layered cortex)
Schizencephaly	Polymicrogyria
Laminar or nodular heterotopia	Gray matter heterotopia
Hamartoma	Focal cortical dysplasia of Taylor
	Glial hamartoma
Macrogyria	Pachygyria
	Polymicrogyria
	Focal cortical dysplasia of Taylor
	Microdysgenesis?
Polymicrogyria	Polymicrogyria
Nonspecific cortical dysplasia	Polymicrogyria
	Focal cortical dysplasia of Taylor
	Microdysgenesis
Hemimegalencephaly, diffuse bilateral cortical dysplasia	Similar to focal cortical dysplasia of Taylor

ment of surrounding normal tissue, and the path of spread. Many of these disorders are often seen in the perisylvian or perirolandic[138–141] areas, thus making assessment of the boundaries of epileptogenic, lesional, and functional tissue critical. Unique to the developmental abnormalities is that the area of electrographic abnormality (ictal or interictal or both) and the MRI abnormality may not be the same; sometimes, it is located at the edge of the lesion or altogether separate from the lesion. Intracranial study is required most frequently for precise ictal localization; however, evidence indicates that the lesion should also be resected completely whenever possible.[142]

Primarily Defective Gyration

Polymicrogyria

Polymicrogyria is characterized by multiple small fused gyri that form a region of thickened cortex. It is distinguished from ulegyria, which is gyral atrophy with sulcal widening. Polymicrogyria may be focal or widespread, and the patient's functional status may be related to the amount of cortex involved. Although grossly the cortex appears thickened, the microscopic cortical thickness of each fused gyrus is less than normal. The gyri typically contain abnormally folded cortex, but the folds may affect only the superficial layers of the cortex.[143]

The terms "lissencephaly" and "pachygyria" refer to brains with flattened gyri. They differ from each other only in degree; lissencephaly refers to brains with a complete lack of gyri, whereas pachygyria refers to a decreased number of broad flattened gyri with shallow sulci.[143] Both abnormalities have decreased white matter and a thickened cortex consisting of only four layers.[144–146] These malformations most often are accompanied by severe neurologic deficits that present in early childhood. Similar histopathologic features may be found in less severely malformed brains that have only focal gyral flattening and broadening[143] (which must be distinguished from other causes of macrogyria) or in other named syndromes.[145,147,148]

Patients with lissencephaly are often severely affected and have a short life-span; they are not considered surgical candidates.[149] Patients with pachygyria or polymicrogyria commonly have seizure onset in mid-childhood (age 10 years), although this is somewhat variable with the extent of disease.[132,149] Many patients have complex partial seizures, but myoclonic seizures or focal sensory seizures may occur.[132,149] The EEG may show focal interictal changes or generalized abnormalities.[132] Several distinct clinical seizure types have been associated with the suspected involvement of the central sulcus or operculum in polymicrogyria, but not all the reported cases have had pathologic confirmation.[138,140,141,150] The patients with bilateral involvement of the somatosensory cortices are considered candidates for possible corpus callosotomy.

Often, patients with pachygyria are mentally retarded; present with delayed development, seizures, and failure-to-thrive; and live only into early adulthood.[149] MRI frequently reveals only macrogyria, although newer generation machines may reveal other abnormalities. The patients often have generalized tonic-clonic seizures, atonic seizures, or focal motor seizures and may have focal interictal EEG abnormalities.[132] On MRI, they show thickened broad gyri with a broad base, reverse gray matter-to-white matter ratio, and a decreased number of white matter digitations.[149,151,152] No study has examined the outcome of resection for the above-mentioned focal entities in isolation.

Case

At the time of operation, the patient was a 32-year-old right-handed male potato farmer. He was born 6 weeks prematurely (birth weight, 4.5 lb). Despite this, he had a normal development and no history of febrile seizures. At age 11, he experienced trauma to his left eye with a baseball bat. At age 13, he had his first seizure, which was reportedly generalized. Thereafter, frequent daily seizures developed that were of different types. Two of the types were complex partial in nature, had no warning, and frequently involved falling. Another type was generalized, but it occurred only one to three times yearly. Postictally, he had Todd's paralysis on the left side. He underwent continuous audiovisual EEG monitoring that

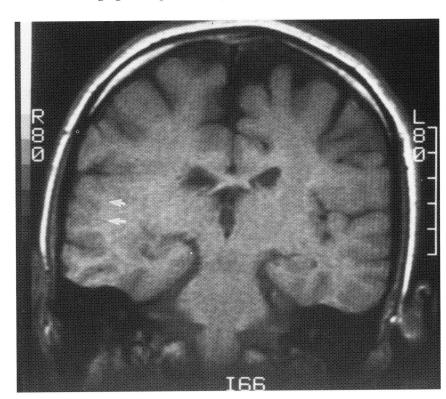

FIGURE 16-8. Coronal T_1-weighted MRI scan showing an area of thickened cortex and polymicrogyria in the midposterior right temporal lobe (*arrows*). Also note atrophy in the superomedial parietal lobe on the left.

revealed right midtemporal spike activity. He had four seizures while being monitored, and they revealed a bilateral onset, followed by a predominant right-sided build-up. MRI revealed diffuse atrophy and a right temporo-occipital area of polymicrogyria (Figure 16-8). The intracarotid amobarbital procedure revealed left-sided speech, intact memory in the left hemisphere, and the absence of memory in the right hemisphere. Neuropsychologic evaluation was significant for a verbal IQ of 86, performance IQ of 89, problems with visual-spatial memory, and slowness and disorganization, which gave evidence of frontal lobe dysfunction.

Because of the nonconcordance of these data, the patient underwent an intracranial study that revealed simultaneous right hippocampal and right temporal neocortical seizure onset. No ictal events arose from the area of the abnormality seen on MRI. A standard anteromedial temporal resection, without resection of the MRI-identified lesion, was performed. Pathologic examination revealed an area of cortical neuronal loss and subcortical gliosis. Postoperatively, the patient continued to have seizures. Repeat neuropsychologic examination showed substantial improvement in his performance IQ and no new deficits.

Schizencephaly

In 1946, Yakovlev and Wadsworth[153,154] reported on five patients with cerebral malformations that had in common an abnormal congenital cleft extending through the full thickness of the cerebrum, resulting in a pial-ependymal seam. This was referred to as "schizencephaly."[153,154] They divided their patients into two groups: (1) those with clefts with closed lips, and (2) those with clefts with open lips and hydrocephalus. The cerebral cortex lining these clefts showed a lack of lamination, similar to that seen in unlayered polymicrogyria. In addition, schizencephalies are often associated with gray matter heterotopias.[143,153,154] More severe cases may also be associated with pontine and pyramidal tract deformities. Cases of unilateral schizencephaly may be associated with a more subtle developmental abnormality in a homologous position in the contralateral hemisphere.[155]

Patients with schizencephaly make up a small proportion of patients evaluated for lesional epilepsy. The diagnosis of this disorder has been made with MRI in patients from 1 month[152] to 37 years old.[156] Between 60% and 100% of the patients reported had seizure disorders, although a selected population was reported.[132,152,155,157,158] In one series, the seizures of 9 of 15 patients were well controlled with medication.[155] The demonstration of gray matter lining the cleft, the pathognomonic finding of the pial-ependymal seam, and the absence of a clear gray matter–white matter junction was of particular interest. A full set of coronal and sagittal images in addition to the standard axial ones were useful, because without a full study some of these lesions may have been missed.[151,157] Surgical resection for this disorder has been reported for four patients. Two of them had temporal lobectomy and two had frontotemporal resections. Two of the four resections involved, at least partly, the area of schizencephaly. Pathologic examination revealed gliosis in three of the patients and polymicrogyria in the other one. In two of the patients seizure frequency was decreased 80%, and the other two have had only one postoperative seizure each. Follow-up was from 1 to 3 years.[156,159]

Schizencephaly clearly demonstrates the value of delineating the ictal epileptogenic area before resection. Because none of the patients reported on have been rendered seizure-free, it cannot be assumed that the resections completely removed all the substrate. The localization of the ictal epileptogenic region to an area away from the MRI-defined abnormality in some patients and seizure improvement after resection of the ictal region only are evidence of the variable expression of this disease.

Case

A 23-month-old girl without strong hand preference at the time of operation was delivered by cesarean section without complication after full-term gestation. Her development was normal until the age of 2 months, when she experienced her first spell, which consisted of increased tone and deviation of the head to the left side. The seizures occurred with increasing frequency until she was admitted to the hospital at age 4 months in status epilepticus. At that time, EEG revealed right posterior seizure onset and interictal spikes and slow waves from the same area. The seizures were poorly controlled with phenobarbital and carbamazepine. They developed a more complex partial semiology, with the patient seeking out her mother with a preoccupied anxious look that was followed by blank staring, tonic head deviation to the left side, lip smacking, and left tonic arm posturing. Postictally, she had Todd's paralysis on the left side. Her family history revealed a paternal first cousin who had died during infancy because of seizures. The patient underwent continuous audiovisual EEG monitoring, during which her interictal EEG showed right temporal slow waves, right anterior temporal spikes, and rare right central spikes. She had six seizures that had a stereotyped clinical onset 5 minutes after the electrographic onset. All these seizures showed a right temporal rhythmic theta discharge. MRI showed an abnormal sulcus in the right temporal lobe that extended to a persistent hippocampal fissure and was consistent with temporal schizencephaly (Figure 16-9). An abnormally configured right hippocampus, thickened cortex in the right temporal lobe and pole, and abnormal signal in the subjacent white matter were also present. Resection was guided by the three-dimensional MRI reconstruction: 7.2 cm of the middle and inferior temporal gyri were resected, followed by a medial resection of the malformed hippocampus. Pathologic examination revealed gliosis and giant neu-

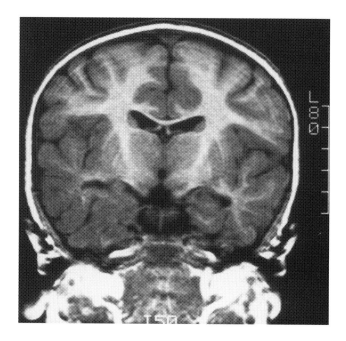

FIGURE 16-9. Coronal T_1-weighted MRI scan showing a grossly malformed right temporal lobe with a schizencephalic sulcus extending to the hippocampal fissure. The gray matter of the temporal lobe is also thickened. Note the deep collateral sulcus and enlarged temporal horn on the left.

rons, but the findings were not consistent with polymicrogyria or focal cortical dysplasia. At 10 months' follow-up the patient had been seizure-free since resection and was taking phenobarbital; no neurologic deficit had occurred.

Misplaced Neurons

Microdysgenesis

Microdysgenesis refers to slight disturbances in cortical architecture in patients with primary generalized epilepsy, Lennox-Gastaut syndrome, or West's syndrome.[160–166] The lesions have been described in some resection specimens.[167,168] They consist of one or more of the following: (1) increased number of dystopic neurons in the molecular layer, (2) increased number of dystopic neurons in the subcortical white matter, (3) indistinct border between layers I and II, (4) indistinct gray matter–white matter border, and (5) columnar arrangement of neurons.[164,169] Many neuropathologists believe that the findings described above are variations of normal cortical architecture.[164,170] Several recent studies have included age- and sex-matched autopsy controls and are more convincing with respect to the dystopic layer I or subcortical white neurons.[160,161,167] Of note is that these disorders were defined originally in the context of epilepsy rather than at autopsy. These findings in patients with primary generalized epilepsies and in some patients with presumed focal epilepsies raise the question of whether these aberrantly located neurons are epileptogenic or are simply indicators of an undefined process.

Gray Matter Heterotopias

Gray matter heterotopias are masses of gray matter abnormally located in the white matter. The more common nodular form consists of nodular masses of gray matter separated by myelinated fibers. They commonly are located at the angles of the lateral ventricles or at the inferolateral surface of the temporal horn. They may occur in isolation or in combination with other disorders such as lissencephaly,[149] hemimegalencephaly (see below), or polymicrogyria.[143] Laminar heterotopias are linear masses of gray matter separated from the overlying cortex by a thin layer of white matter that has normal digitations. The overlying cortex may be normal or macrogyric. This type of heterotopia may be localized, but more often it is diffuse.[171–173] The microscopic organization of the overlying cortex (1) may be normal (the phenomenon of band heterotopia with normal overlying cortex is termed "double cortex"[172]), (2) the upper layers may be preserved and lower layers disorganized,[172] or (3) the four layers usually associated with pachygyria may be present.[143,172] The heterotopia usually has a relatively normal, albeit disorganized, mixture of neurons and glia; many pyramidal cells may be seen, but well-differentiated ganglion cells may also be found.[172,173]

Seizures are the most common presenting symptom in patients with heterotopic gray matter.[174] In those with the nodular form, the seizures typically have onset in late childhood and are of multiple types; up to two-thirds of patients have tonic-clonic seizures.[136,174–176] The results of neurologic examination in the patients are usually normal, and developmental delay is rare. Many patients have a normal interictal EEG, although the ictal EEG may show a rapid bilateral onset.[174,176] MRI reveals nodular periventricular masses isointense with gray matter on T_1, T_2, and proton density scans.[149,151,177] Multiple bilateral lesions are present in most patients.[174] Although data about outcome are scarce, patients with the bilateral form of heterotopia should be considered for callosotomy if the EEG shows rapid generalization or synchronous bilateral ictal onset and the patient falls during a seizure.[176] Patients with unilateral heterotopia in accessible areas may be considered for resection of the lesion delineated by MRI after invasive study reveals that the lesion is in or near the area of ictal onset.

Patients with laminar heterotopias, or "band heterotopias," usually present with seizures at an earlier age.[136,171–173,178] Up to 90% have evidence of developmental delay.[172,173] Again, there are various seizure types, with a preponderance of generalized tonic-clonic, atonic, and drop seizures[171–173,178]; less than 20% are well controlled with optimal medical treatment.[172] The interictal EEG may show diffuse or multifocal abnormalities[171–173,178] and many of these patients have been classified as having Lennox-Gastaut syndrome. Some with focal heterotopia such as double cortex may be amenable to localization with conventional monitoring.[136,172,173] Corpus callosotomy is advocated for those patients with drop attacks; substantial improvement occurs in about two-thirds of the patients.[134,172]

Primarily Abnormal Neurons and Glia

Focal Cortical Dysplasia

Focal cortical dysplasia was first described by Taylor et al.[179] in a 1971 review of the pathologic findings in the brains of 10 patients with epilepsy. The gross morphological features of the brain are not disturbed in this disorder. Microscopically, there is a loss of the normal lamination of the cortex, and the gray matter–white matter junction may be indistinct. In the gray matter are large bizarre neurons with abnormally clumped Nissl substance (ganglion cells). In 7 of the 10 patients described by Taylor et al.,[179] large cells with small and often multiple nuclei and abundant opalescent cytoplasm ("balloon cells") occurred in the deeper cortical layers or in the subcortical white matter. This pattern is similar to that seen in tuberous sclerosis or in its forme fruste,[180] but without calcification. These microscopic features may be found in association with hemimegalencephaly[181,182] or they may exist in isolation.

In the earlier literature, focal cortical dysplasia was used loosely in describing abnormal structure of the cerebral cortex. In this section, the term is used exclusively to refer to the complex of findings described by Taylor et al.[179] and does not include the findings listed above for microdysgenesis. Much of the literature pertaining to the clinical course of focal cortical dysplasia consists of series of patients without histologic confirmation of the disorder as described by Taylor et al.[179]; thus, some of the patients in these series may have had polymicrogyria or pachygyria instead of focal cortical dysplasia.

The age of seizure onset in patients with focal cortical dysplasia is usually early childhood, although in up to one-half, onset may be after age 10. Also, as many as half of the patients have developmental delay.[132,134,136,183] Focal cortical dysplasia is the most common pathologic diagnosis in resection specimens from children younger than 12 years.[134]

The EEG findings associated with focal cortical dysplasia vary.[135,137,183–185] PET and SPECT have shown promise in further delineating the abnormal cortex in patients in whom EEG or MRI has not been helpful.[186,187] MRI abnormalities have been reported in 70% to 90% of the patients, but different generations of machines were used among and even within these studies.[135,137,183,184,188] The most frequent findings are macrogyria, thickened cortex, loss of differentiation of gray matter and white matter, and, in some cases, increased signal on T_2-weighted imaging in the thickened cortex or the subjacent white matter.[135,136,183,189] In many patients, there is multilobar or bilateral involvement,[135,189] and there is an increased incidence in the involvement of the rolandic and sylvian fissures.[137,189] Most patients have interictal scalp EEG abnormalities that extend outside the region of abnormality seen on MRI.[183]

The outcome after surgical resection of these lesions has varied. Bruton[59] reported a poor outcome for all eight of his patients, but Taylor et al.[179] reported improvement in 80% of their patients. In the more recent studies, 35% to 50% of the patients became seizure-free or almost seizure-free and another 35% to 50% had no worthwhile improvement. Total resection of the MRI-defined abnormality appears to be the most important goal in the surgical treatment of these patients.[142]

Case

At the time of operation, the patient was a 34-year-old right-handed man. His gestation, birth, and development were normal. At the age of 5 years, he experienced his first seizure while he had chickenpox, but the seizure was not associated with increased temperature. He went on to have several seizures per day characterized by an aura of a feeling of nervousness and flushing, followed by loss of contact, walking in circles, and postictal sleepiness. These eventually evolved into two separate seizure types. One type was typified by brief tonic posturing without any loss of contact and postictal "palpitations," of which he would have several per day. The other type occurred only once or twice a month and was characterized by arising from bed at night with garbled speech and loss of contact. All seizures were resistant to multiple medications. Chronic scalp recordings revealed no interictal abnormalities and only diffuse desynchronization at the onset of all seven recorded seizures. MRI showed thickened cortex (Figure 16-10 A) and increased T_2 signal in the left medial frontal lobe. The hippocampal volumetric measurements were normal. Intracranial study demonstrated multifocal interictal abnormalities and a left inferomesial frontal onset of seizures consistent with the MRI abnormality. With three-dimensional MRI reconstruction (Figure 16-10 B and C) as a guide, an area 3.4 × 1.8 cm was resected. Pathologic examination of the resected tissue revealed focal cortical dysplasia, as described by Taylor et al.[179] At 6 months' follow-up, the patient was seizure-free.

Hemimegalencephaly

Hemimegalencephaly is characterized by diffuse hypertrophy of one side of the brain. The hypertrophy may be confined to one lobe or involve the whole hemisphere.

The microscopic findings may range from those of true lissencephaly to those of pachygyria and polymicrogyria and often are associated with multiple heterotopias of the gray matter.[151,190,191] The microscopic changes described for each of the disorders above may be seen in hemimegalencephaly. In addition, neuronal cytomegaly and balloon cells similar to those seen in focal cortical dysplasia of Taylor et al.[179] or tuberous sclerosis[180] are often seen.[181,182] Areas of less obvious polymicrogyria or neuronal heterotopias may be seen in the contralateral "normal" side.[190] A bilateral form of hemimegalencephaly may occur[192] separate from the megalencephaly described by DeMeyer.[193] However, some of the cases of suspected bilateral hemimegalencephaly[194] have been shown with high-resolution MRI to have band heterotopia.[172] The cause of these malformations is not clear. The similarities between the microscopic morphologic features of hemimegalencephaly and tuberous sclerosis raise the question of whether an inherited genetic propensity or somatic mutation may be responsible.[181] The bizarre cells and enlarged hemispheres seen in some of the patients indicate that these malformations may be part of a spectrum between hamartomatous lesions and neoplasia.[195]

The clinical manifestations of hemimegalencephaly often include the onset of seizures during infancy and developmental delay. Often, there is a mild-to-moderate hemiparesis on the contralateral side.[195,196] In one series, almost half of the patients had an associated phakomatosis, most commonly linear sebaceous nevus syndrome.[197] The seizure types seen include focal motor seizures with secondary generalization, frequent brief tonic seizures, drop attacks, and focal myoclonus.[195,196] Interictal EEG often shows hemihypsarrhythmia or diffuse epileptiform activity, either unilateral or bilateral, with triphasic features; burst suppression is common.[196–198] MRI usually shows a grossly enlarged hemisphere with distorted thickened cortex, loss of white matter digitations, and ipsilateral ventricular dilatation. In T_2-weighted images, there is often an increased signal in deep cortex similar to that seen in focal cortical dysplasia.[151] The opposite hemisphere frequently shows subtle abnormalities.[190] The bilateral form of hemimegalencephaly has many of the same features, but has bilateral EEG alterations, and neurologic deterioration is more progressive.[192] Patients with unilateral deformities should be considered for hemispherectomy if there is unilateral ictal onset and psychomotor retardation. Postoperatively, many of the patients have immediate cessation of seizures and developmental improvement.[197,199]

Case

At 1 month before birth, ultrasonography demonstrated hemimegalencephaly in a child. (At 16 weeks of gestation, ultrasonographic results were considered normal.) Birth was at full term, and 2 hours after delivery, seizures

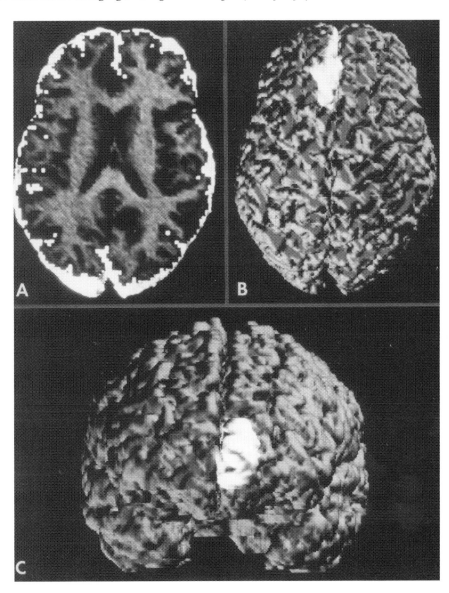

FIGURE 16-10. A. Three-dimensional reconstruction MRI scan with an axial T$_1$-weighted slice showing area of thickened cortex in the medial left frontal lobe. B and C. Full three-dimensional reconstructions viewed superiorly (B) and anteriorly (C) assisted in guiding resection of the lesion (*indicated in white*).

developed; thereafter, the child was in status epilepticus until the age of 2 weeks. His early course was complicated further by an episode of bowel obstruction that required resection and ileostomy. During this time, scalp EEG showed a left occipital onset of seizures, with spread to frontal regions and subsequent spread to the right hemisphere. MRI showed diffuse left hemispheric enlargement, cortical thickening, and high signal intensity in the subjacent white matter (Figure 16-11). During continuous audiovisual EEG monitoring, the ictal onset was seen as a rhythmic high-amplitude build-up of 5 or 6 Hz in the left posterior region, spreading to the left occipital and left temporal regions. After allowing about 3 months for the patient to increase in weight and to decrease the risks of the operation, a staged anatomical hemispherectomy was performed. Pathologic examination of the resected tissue revealed diffuse involvement of the cortex, with changes typically seen in focal cortical

dysplasia of Taylor et al.[179] At latest follow-up, about age 2½, the boy was seizure-free and hemiplegic but otherwise developmentally appropriate.

Hamartomas

Hamartoma is defined as a focal excessive accumulation of cells normally present in that location. Although the cells are mature, their organization is not normal, and they form a "tumorous" mass. This definition has caused considerable confusion. Recently, Vital et al.[200] described two classes of what previously had been termed "hamartomas." They distinguished lesions that contained neuronal elements from those that did not. Lesions containing neurons were classified as focal cortical dysplasia (as described by Taylor et al.[179]), microdysgenesis, or low-grade neoplasms. Previously, some of these lesions had been referred to as "neuronoglial hamartomas."

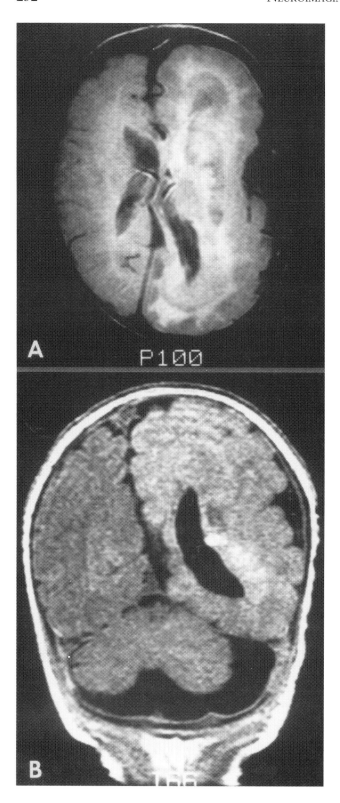

FIGURE 16-11. Axial (A) and coronal (B) T_1-weighted MRI scans showing diffuse left hemispheric changes consistent with hemimegalencephaly.

Lesions with only glial elements were classified as astrocytic hamartomas, oligodendroglial hamartomas, and mixed oligoastrocytic hamartomas. Often, it is difficult to distinguish among this disorder, severe focal cortical dysplasia of Taylor, and slow-growing tumors of the central nervous system, that is, the low-grade gliomas, gangliogliomas, and dysembryoplastic neuroepithelial tumors. In keeping with this classification, we consider glial hamartomas separate entities, and any lesion that may be considered hamartomatous and contains neuronal elements is classified into a more specific category. Classically, these lesions have been grouped together with the developmental disorders, but their histologic similarities to low-grade gliomas raise the question of whether they belong in that group or are a transitional form. Separate from the telencephalic lesions that cause epilepsy are hypothalamic hamartomas, which commonly are associated with gelastic epilepsy and precocious puberty (they are not discussed here).

The age of patients with this diagnosis is from 2 to 23 years. Most of them have complex partial seizures. On MRI, the lesions often are seen as focal increases in T_2 signal and up to 30% exhibit mass effect. They must be differentiated from low-grade neoplasms. The approach to resection of hamartomas is similar to that for low-grade tumors: resection to negative margins. Generally, the prognosis for glial hamartomas appears to be better than that for other developmental abnormalities.

INDETERMINATE SUBSTRATES

The group of indeterminate substrates comprises other diagnoses about which the least is known pathogenetically and surgical outcome may not be predicted. Included in this group are nonspecific cortical atrophy, infection, and trauma. Although MRI may demonstrate atrophy or areas of gliosis, they are often ill defined. Typically, noninvasive electrophysiologic findings are diffuse, and invasive studies are often required to delineate an evasive ictal volume.

The findings of major areas of cortical atrophy and tissue loss are believed to be due to an in-utero insult, such as infection or infarction. The treatment of these conditions is similar to that described for developmental abnormalities.[201] The long-term consequences of postnatal intracerebral infection often include epilepsy.[202–204] The areas affected are poorly defined except in cases of cysticercosis, tuberculosis, or other examples of rare fungal or parasitic infections in which an individual mass or cyst may be visualized with MRI and removed with good result.[205,206] The usual course of Rasmussen's encephalitis results in holohemispheric involvement; thus, hemispherectomy is often performed to alleviate the seizures.[182,207,208] Trauma-induced epilepsy accounts for about 20% of patients with epilepsy, although most of these patients have generalized seizures.[202,209] MRI may delineate an area of focal gliosis and hemosiderin staining that may have a role in epileptogenesis.[209,210] The presence of such an area can guide invasive studies and resection in patients with trauma-related partial seizures.

SUMMARY

The work-up of surgical candidates has been aided considerably by MRI. A simplified approach is shown in Figures 16-1 and 16-2. This is by no means complete and some patients may warrant a modified approach, but such constructs as illustrated can help clarify the necessary steps required to effect a substrate-directed resection for patients with intractable epilepsy.

REFERENCES

1. Spencer DD. Classifying the epilepsies by substrate. Clin Neurosci 1994;2:104–9.

2. Engel J Jr, Driver MV, Falconer MA. Electrophysiological correlates of pathology and surgical results in temporal lobe epilepsy. Brain 1975;98:129–56.

3. Spencer SS, Spencer DD, Williamson PD, et al. The localizing value of depth electroencephalography in 32 patients with refractory epilepsy. Ann Neurol 1982;12:248–53.

4. de Lanerolle NC, Brines M, Williamson A, et al. Neurotransmitters and their receptors in human temporal lobe epilepsy. Epilepsy Res Suppl 1992;7:235–50.

5. Kim JH, Guimaraes PO, Shen MY, et al. Hippocampal neuronal density in temporal lobe epilepsy with and without gliomas. Acta Neuropathol (Berl) 1990;80:41–5.

6. Spencer DD, Spencer SS, Mattson RH, et al. Access to the posterior medial temporal lobe structures in the surgical treatment of temporal lobe epilepsy. Neurosurgery 1984;15:667–71.

7. Avrahami E, Cohn DF, Neufeld M, et al. Magnetic resonance imaging (MRI) in patients with complex partial seizures and normal computerized tomography (CT) scan. Clin Neurol Neurosurg 1987;89:231–5.

8. Boon PA, Williamson PD, Fried I, et al. Intracranial, intraaxial, space-occupying lesions in patients with intractable partial seizures: an anatomoclinical, neuropsychological, and surgical correlation. Epilepsia 1991;32:467–76.

9. Britton JW, Cascino GD, Sharbrough FW, et al. Low-grade glial neoplasms and intractable partial epilepsy: efficacy of surgical treatment. Epilepsia 1994;35:1130–5.

10. Bronen RA. Epilepsy: the role of MR imaging. AJR Am J Roentgenol 1992;159:1165–74.

11. Cascino GD, Jack CR Jr, Hirschorn KA, et al. Identification of the epileptic focus: magnetic resonance imaging. Epilepsy Res Suppl 1992;5:95–100.

12. Celli P, Scarpinati M, Nardacci B, et al. Gangliogliomas of the cerebral hemispheres. Report of 14 cases with long-term follow-up and review of the literature. Acta Neurochir (Wien) 1993;125:52–7.

13. Ormson MJ, Kispert DB, Sharbrough FW, et al. Cryptic structural lesions in refractory partial epilepsy: MR imaging and CT studies. Radiology 1986;160:215–9.

14. Sperling MR, Wilson G, Engel J Jr, et al. Magnetic resonance imaging in intractable partial epilepsy: correlative studies. Ann Neurol 1986;20:57–62.

15. Awad IA, Rosenfeld J, Ahl J, et al. Intractable epilepsy and structural lesions of the brain: mapping, resection strategies, and seizure outcome. Epilepsia 1991;32:179–86.

16. Goldring S, Gregorie EM. Surgical management using epidural recordings to localize the seizure focus: review of 100 cases. J Neurosurg 1984;60:457–66.

17. Ives JR, Gloor P. A long term time-lapse video system to document the patients spontaneous clinical seizure synchronized with the EEG. Electroencephalogr Clin Neurophysiol 1978;45:412–6.

18. Morris HH III, Luders H, Hahn JF, et al. Neurophysiological techniques as an aid to surgical treatment of primary brain tumors. Ann Neurol 1986;19:559–67.

19. Devinsky O, Perrine K, Llinas R, et al. Anterior temporal language areas in patients with early onset of temporal lobe epilepsy. Ann Neurol 1993;34:727–32.

20. Haglund MM, Berger MS, Shamseldin M, et al. Cortical localization of temporal lobe language sites in patients with gliomas. Neurosurgery 1994;34:567–76.

21. Ojemann G, Ojemann J, Lettich E, et al. Cortical language localization in left, dominant hemisphere. An electrical stimulation mapping investigation in 117 patients. J Neurosurg 1989;71:316–26.

22. Ojemann GA. Functional mapping of cortical language areas in adults. Intraoperative approaches. Adv Neurol 1993;63:155–63.

23. Ojemann GA. Individual variability in cortical localization of language. J Neurosurg 1979;50:164–9.

24. Ojemann GA. Mapping of neuropsychological language parameters at surgery. Int Anesthesiol Clin 1986;24:115–31.

25. Pilcher WH, Silbergeld DL, Berger MS, et al. Intraoperative electrocorticography during tumor resection: impact on seizure outcome in patients with gangliogliomas. J Neurosurg 1993;78:891–902.

26. Berger MS, Cohen WA, Ojemann GA. Correlation of motor cortex brain mapping data with magnetic resonance imaging. J Neurosurg 1990;72:383–7.

27. Connelly A, Jackson GD, Frackowiak RS, et al. Functional mapping of activated human primary cortex with a clinical MR imaging system. Radiology 1993;188:125–30.

28. McCarthy G, Blamire AM, Rothman DL, et al. Echo-planar magnetic resonance imaging studies of frontal cortex activation during word generation in humans. Proc Natl Acad Sci USA 1993;90:4952–6.

29. Puce A, Constable RT, Luby ML, et al. Function magnetic resonance imaging of sensory and motor cortex: comparison with electrophysiological location. J Neurosurg (in press).

30. Stehling MK, Turner R, Mansfield P: Echo-planar imaging: magnetic resonance imaging in a fraction of a second. Science 1991;254:43–50.

31. Dinner DS, Luders H, Lesser RP, et al. Cortical generators of somatosensory evoked potentials to median nerve stimulation. Neurology 1987;37:1141–5.

32. Gregorie EM, Goldring S. Localization of function in the excision of lesions from the sensorimotor region. J Neurosurg 1984;61:1047–54.

33. Lueders H, Lesser RP, Hahn J, et al. Cortical somatosensory evoked potentials in response to hand stimulation. J Neurosurg 1983;58:885–94.

34. Berger MS, Kincaid J, Ojemann GA, et al. Brain mapping techniques to maximize resection, safety, and seizure control in children with brain tumors. Neurosurgery 1989;25:786–92.

35. Burchiel KJ, Clarke H, Ojemann GA, et al. Use of stimulation mapping and corticography in the excision of arteriovenous malformations in sensorimotor and language-related neocortex. Neurosurgery 1989;24:322–7.

36. LeRoux PD, Berger MS, Haglund MM, et al. Resection of intrinsic tumors from nondominant face motor cortex using stimulation mapping: report of two cases. Surg Neurol 1991;36:44–8.

37. Lesser RP, Luders H, Klem G, et al. Extraoperative cortical functional localization in patients with epilepsy. J Clin Neurophysiol 1987;4:27–53.

38. Uematsu S, Lesser R, Fisher RS, et al. Motor and sensory cortex in humans: topography studied with chronic subdural stimulation. Neurosurgery 1992;31:59–71.

39. Morris HH, Estes ML, Gilmore R, et al. Chronic intractable epilepsy as the only symptom of primary brain tumor. Epilepsia 1993;34:1038–43.

40. Cascino GD. Epilepsy and brain tumors: implications for treatment. Epilepsia 1990;31 Suppl 3:S37–44.

41. Cascino GD, Kelly PJ, Hirschorn KA, et al. Stereotactic resection of intra-axial cerebral lesions in partial epilepsy. Mayo Clin Proc 1990;65:1053–60.

42. Cascino GD, Kelly PJ, Sharbrough FW, et al. Long-term follow-up of stereotactic lesionectomy in partial epilepsy: predictive factors and electroencephalographic results. Epilepsia 1992;33:639–44.

43. Kelly PJ. Computer-assisted stereotaxis: new approaches for the management of intracranial intra-axial tumors. Neurology 1986;36:535–41.

44. Kelly PJ. Volumetric stereotactic surgical resection of intra-axial brain mass lesions. Mayo Clin Proc 1988;63:1186–98.

45. Kirkpatrick PJ, Honavar M, Janota I, et al. Control of temporal lobe epilepsy following en bloc resection of low-grade tumors. J Neurosurg 1993;78:19–25.

46. Goldring S, Rich KM, Picker S. Experience with gliomas in patients presenting with a chronic seizure disorder. Clin Neurosurg 1986;33:15–42.

47. Hirsch JF, Sainte Rose C, Pierre-Kahn A, et al. Benign astrocytic and oligodendrocytic tumors of the cerebral hemispheres in children. J Neurosurg 1989;70:568–72.

48. Fried I, Kim JH, Spencer DD. Limbic and neocortical gliomas associated with intractable seizures: a distinct clinicopathological group. Neurosurgery 1994;34:815–23.

49. Falconer MA, Driver MV, Serefetinides EA. Temporal lobe epilepsy due to distant lesions: two cases relieved by operation. Brain 1962;85:521–34.

50. Falconer MA, Kennedy WA. Epilepsy due to small focal temporal lesions with bilateral independent spike-discharging foci: a study of seven cases relieved by operation. J Neurol Neurosurg Psychiatry 1961;24:205–12.

51. Morrell F. Secondary epileptogenesis in man. Arch Neurol 1985;42:318–35.

52. Berger MS, Ghatan S, Haglund MM, et al. Low-grade gliomas associated with intractable epilepsy: seizure outcome utilizing electrocorticography during tumor resection. J Neurosurg 1993;79:62–9.

53. Gonzalez D, Elvidge AR. On the occurrence of epilepsy caused by astrocytoma of the cerebral hemispheres. J Neurosurg 1962;19:470–82.

54. Rasmussen T. Surgical treatment of complex partial seizures: results, lessons, and problems. Epilepsia 1983;24 Suppl 1:S65–76.

55. Rasmussen T. Surgery of epilepsy associated with brain tumors. Adv Neurol 1975;8:227–39.

56. Wyllie E, Luders H, Morris HH III, et al. Clinical outcome after complete or partial cortical resection for intractable epilepsy. Neurology 1987;37:1634–41.

57. Sass KJ, Spencer DD, Kim JH, et al. Verbal memory impairment correlates with hippocampal pyramidal cell density. Neurology 1990;40:1694–7.

58. Babb TL, Brown WJ. Pathological findings in epilepsy. In: Engel J, ed. Surgical treatment of the epilepsies. New York: Raven Press, 1987:511–40.

59. Bruton CJ. The neuropathology of temporal lobe epilepsy. Oxford: Oxford University Press, 1988.

60. Cavanagh JB. On certain small tumours encountered in the temporal lobe. Brain 1958;81:389–405.

61. Drake J, Hoffman HJ, Kobayashi J, et al. Surgical management of children with temporal lobe epilepsy and mass lesions. Neurosurgery 1987;21:792–7.

62. Fish D, Andermann F, Olivier A. Complex partial seizures and small posterior temporal or extratemporal structural lesions: surgical management. Neurology 1991;41:1781–4.

63. Levesque MF, Nakasato N, Vinters HV, et al. Surgical treatment of limbic epilepsy associated with extrahippocampal lesions: the problem of dual pathology. J Neurosurg 1991;75:364–70.

64. Naksato N, Levesque MF, Babb TL. Seizure outcome following standard temporal lobectomy: correlation with hippocampal neuron loss and extrahippocampal pathology. J Neurosurg 1992;77:194–200.

65. Fried I, Kim JH, Spencer DD. Hippocampal pathology in patients with intractable seizures and temporal lobe masses. J Neurosurg 1992;76:735–40.

66. Spencer DD, Spencer SS, Mattson RH, et al. Intracerebral masses in patients with intractable partial epilepsy. Neurology 1984;34:432–6.

67. Cascino GD, Jack CR Jr, Parisi JE, et al. Operative strategy in patients with MRI-identified dual pathology and temporal lobe epilepsy. Epilepsy Res 1993;14:175–82.

68. Costantino A, Vinters HV. A pathologic correlate of the 'steal' phenomenon in a patient with cerebral arteriovenous malformation. Stroke 1986;17:103–6.

69. Yeh HS, Tew JM Jr, Gartner M. Seizure control after surgery on cerebral arteriovenous malformations. J Neurosurg 1993;78:12–8.

70. McCormick WF. The pathology of vascular ("arteriovenous") malformations. J Neurosurg 1966;24:807–16.

71. Steiger HJ, Tew JM Jr. Hemorrhage and epilepsy in cryptic cerebrovascular malformations. Arch Neurol 1984;41:722–4.

72. Stein BM, Mohr JP. Vascular malformations of the brain (editorial). N Engl J Med 1988;319:368–70.

73. Awad IA, Robinson JR. Cavernous malformations and epilepsy. In: Awad IA, Barrow DL, eds. Cavernous malformations. Park Ridge, IL: American Association of Neurological Surgeons, 1993:49–64.

74. Dodick DW, Cascino GD, Meyer FB. Vascular malformations and intractable epilepsy: outcome after surgical treatment. Mayo Clin Proc 1994;69:741–5.

75. Churchyard A, Khangure M, Grainger K. Cerebral cavernous angioma: a potentially benign condition? Successful treatment in 16 cases. J Neurol Neurosurg Psychiatry 1992;55:1040–5.

76. MacKenzie I. The clinical presentation of the cerebral angioma: a review of 50 cases. Brain 1953;76:184–214.

77. Robinson JR, Awad IA, Little JR. Natural history of the cavernous angioma. J Neurosurg 1991;75:709–14.

78. Crawford PM, West CR, Chadwick DW, et al. Arteriovenous malformations of the brain: natural history in unoperated patients. J Neurol Neurosurg Psychiatry 1986;49:1–10.

79. Ondra SL, Troupp H, George ED, et al. The natural history of symptomatic arteriovenous malformations of the brain: a 24-year follow-up assessment. J Neurosurg 1990;73:387–91.

80. Pasqualin A, Scienza R, Cioffi F, et al. Treatment of cerebral arteriovenous malformations with a combination of preoperative embolization and surgery. Neurosurgery 1991;29:358–68.

81. Carriero A, Tartaro A, Dragani M, et al. Magnetic resonance angiography compared with basic magnetic resonance in intracranial vascular diseases. J Neuroradiol 1994;21:30–9.

82. Marchal G, Bosmans H, Van Fraeyenhoven L, et al. Intracranial vascular lesions: optimization and clinical evaluation of three-dimensional time-of-flight MR angiography. Radiology 1990;175:443–8.

83. Nussel F, Wegmuller H, Huber P. Comparison of magnetic resonance angiography, magnetic resonance imaging and conventional angiography in cerebral arteriovenous malformation. Neuroradiology 1991;33:56–61.

84. Awad IA, Robinson JR Jr, Mohanty S, et al. Mixed vascular malformations of the brain: clinical and pathogenetic considerations. Neurosurgery 1993;33:179–88.

85. Barker CS. Magnetic resonance imaging of intracranial cavernous angiomas: a report of 13 cases with pathological confirmation. Clin Radiol 1993;48:117–21.

86. Rigamonti D, Drayer BP, Johnson PC, et al. The MRI appearance of cavernous malformations (angiomas). J Neurosurg 1987;67:518–24.

87. Tomlinson FH, Houser OW, Scheithauer BW, et al. Angiographically occult vascular malformations: a correlative study of features on magnetic resonance imaging and histological examination. Neurosurgery 1994;34:792–9.

88. Perl J, Ross JS. Diagnostic imaging of cavernous malformations. In: Awad IA, Barrow DL, eds. Cavernous malformations. Park Ridge, IL: American Association of Neurological Surgeons, 1993:37–48.

89. Kraemer DL, Awad IA. Vascular malformations and epilepsy: clinical considerations and basic mechanisms. Epilepsia 1994;35 Suppl 6:S30–43.

90. Crawford PM, West CR, Shaw MD, et al. Cerebral arteriovenous malformations and epilepsy: factors in the development of epilepsy. Epilepsia 1986;27:270–5.

91. Drake CG. Cerebral arteriovenous malformations: considerations for and experience with surgical treatment in 166 cases. Clin Neurosurg 1979;26:145–208.

92. Forster DM, Steiner L, Hakanson S. Arteriovenous malformations of the brain. A long-term clinical study. J Neurosurg 1972;37:562–70.

93. Murphy MJ. Long-term follow-up of seizures associated with cerebral arteriovenous malformations. Results of therapy. Arch Neurol 1985;42:477–9.

94. Parkinson D, Bachers G. Arteriovenous malformations. Summary of 100 consecutive supratentorial cases. J Neurosurg 1980;53:285–99.

95. Piepgras DG, Sundt TM Jr, Ragoowansi AT, et al. Seizure outcome in patients with surgically treated cerebral arteriovenous malformations. J Neurosurg 1993;78:5–11.

96. Kraemer DL, Lee NS, Griebel ML, et al. Surgical outcome in epilepsy patients with occult vascular malformations treated by lesionectomy (abstract). Epilepsia 1993;34 Suppl 6:S27–8.

97. Penfield W, Erickson TC, Tarlov I. Relation of intracranial tumors and symptomatic epilepsy. Arch Neurol Psychiatry 1940;44:300–15.

98. Smith DF, Hutton JL, Sandemann D, et al. The prognosis of primary intracerebral tumours presenting with epilepsy: the outcome of medical and surgical management. J Neurol Neurosurg Psychiatry 1991;54:915–20.

99. Laws ER Jr, Taylor WF, Clifton MB, et al. Neurosurgical management of low-grade astrocytoma of the cerebral hemispheres. J Neurosurg 1984;61:665–73.

100. Plate KH, Wieser HG, Yasargil MG, et al. Neuropathological findings in 224 patients with temporal lobe epilepsy. Acta Neuropathol (Berl) 1993;86:433–8.

101. Piepmeier JM, Fried I, Makuch R. Low-grade astrocytomas may arise from different astrocyte lineages. Neurosurgery 1993;33:627–32.

102. Courville CB. Gangliogliomas. A further report with special reference to those occurring in the temporal lobe. Arch Neurol Psychiatry 1931;25:309–26.

103. Demierre B, Stichnoth FA, Hori A, et al. Intracerebral ganglioglioma. J Neurosurg 1986;65:177–82.

104. Johannsson JH, Rekate HL, Roessmann U. Gangliogliomas: pathological and clinical correlation. J Neurosurg 1981;54:58–63.

105. Isla A, Alvarez F, Gutierrez M, et al. Gangliogliomas: clinical study and evolution. J Neurosurg Sci 1991;35:193–7.

106. Smith NM, Carli MM, Hanieh A, et al. Gangliogliomas in childhood. Childs Nerv Syst 1992;8:258–62.

107. Ventureyra E, Herder S, Mallya BK, et al. Temporal lobe gangliogliomas in children. Childs Nerv Syst 1986;2:63–6.

108. Daumas-Duport C, Scheithauer BW, Chodkiewicz JP, et al. Dysembryoplastic neuroepithelial tumor: a surgically curable tumor of young patients with intractable partial seizures. Report of thirty-nine cases. Neurosurgery 1988;23:545–56.

109. Wolf HK, Campos MG, Zentner J, et al. Surgical pathology of temporal lobe epilepsy. Experience with 216 cases. J Neuropathol Exp Neurol 1993;52:499–506.

110. Chamberlain MC, Murovic JA, Levin VA. Absence of contrast enhancement on CT brain scans of patients with supratentorial malignant gliomas. Neurology 1988;38:1371–4.

111. Peretti-Viton P, Perez-Castillo AM, Raybaud C, et al. Magnetic resonance imaging in gangliogliomas and gangliocytomas of the nervous system. J Neuroradiol 1991;18:189–99.

112. Raymond AA, Halpin SF, Alsanjari N, et al. Dysembryoplastic neuroepithelial tumor. Features in 16 patients. Brain 1994;117:461–75.

113. Vali AM, Clarke MA, Kelsey A. Dysembryoplastic neuroepithelial tumour as a potentially treatable cause of intractable epilepsy in children. Clin Radiol 1993;47:255–8.

114. Muller W, Afra D, Schroder R. Supratentorial recurrences of gliomas. Morphological studies in relation to time intervals with astrocytomas. Acta Neurochir (Wien) 1977;37:75–91.

115. Vertosick FT Jr, Selker RG, Arena VC. Survival of patients with well-differentiated astrocytomas diagnosed in the era of computed tomography. Neurosurgery 1991;28:496–501.

116. Ammirati M, Vick N, Liao YL, et al. Effect of the extent of surgical resection on survival and quality of life in patients with supratentorial glioblastomas and anaplastic astrocytomas. Neurosurgery 1987;21:201–6.

117. Ciric I, Ammirati M, Vick N, et al. Supratentorial gliomas: surgical considerations and immediate postoperative results. Gross total resection versus partial resection. Neurosurgery 1987;21:21–6.

118. Fadul C, Wood J, Thaler H, et al. Morbidity and mortality of craniotomy for excision of supratentorial gliomas. Neurology 1988;38:1374–9.

119. Morantz RA. Radiation therapy in the treatment of cerebral astrocytoma. Neurosurgery 1987;20:975–82.

120. North CA, North RB, Epstein JA, et al. Low-grade cerebral astrocytomas. Survival and quality of life after radiation therapy. Cancer 1990;66:6–14.

121. Soffietti R, Chio A, Giordana MT, et al. Prognostic factors in well-differentiated cerebral astrocytomas in the adult. Neurosurgery 1989;24:686–92.

122. Weir B, Grace M. The relative significance of factors affecting postoperative survival in astrocytomas, grades one and two. Can J Neurol Sci 1976;3:47–50.

123. Cairncross JG, Laperriere NJ. Low-grade glioma. To treat or not to treat? Arch Neurol 1989;46:1238–9.

124. Recht LD, Lew R, Smith TW. Suspected low-grade glioma: is deferring treatment safe? Ann Neurol 1992;31:431–6.

125. Shapiro WR. Low-grade gliomas: when to treat? (editorial). Ann Neurol 1992;31:437–8.

126. Shaw EG. Low-grade gliomas: to treat or not to treat? A radiation oncologist's viewpoint. Arch Neurol 1990;47:1138–40.

127. Piepmeier JM. Observations on the current treatment of low-grade astrocytic tumors of the cerebral hemispheres. J Neurosurg 1987;67:177–81.

128. Imperato JP, Paleologos NA, Vick NA. Effects of treatment on long-term survivors with malignant astrocytomas. Ann Neurol 1990;28:818–22.

129. Garcia DM, Fulling KH, Marks JE. The value of radiation therapy in addition to surgery for astrocytomas of the adult cerebrum. Cancer 1985;55:919–27.

130. Leibel SA, Sheline GE, Wara WM, et al. The role of radiation therapy in the treatment of astrocytomas. Cancer 1975;35:1551–7.

131. Shaw ER, Daumas-Duport C, Scheithauer BW, et al. Radiation therapy in the management of low-grade supratentorial astrocytomas. J Neurosurg 1989;70:853–61.

132. Brodtkorb E, Nilsen G, Smevik O, et al. Epilepsy and anomalies of neuronal migration: MRI and clinical aspects. Acta Neurol Scand 1992;86:24–32.

133. Dietrich RB, el Saden S, Chugani HT, et al. Resective surgery for intractable epilepsy in children: radiologic evaluation. AJNR Am J Neuroradiol 1991;12:1149–58.

134. Kuzniecky R, Murro A, King D, et al. Magnetic resonance imaging in childhood intractable partial epilepsies: pathologic correlations. Neurology 1993;43:681–7.

135. Otsubo H, Hwang PA, Jay V, et al. Focal cortical dysplasia in children with localization-related epilepsy: EEG, MRI, and SPECT findings. Pediatr Neurol 1993;9:101–7.

136. Palmini A, Andermann F, Olivier A, et al. Neuronal migration disorders: a contribution of modern neuroimaging to the etiologic diagnosis of epilepsy. Can J Neurol Sci 1991;18 Suppl 4:580–7.

137. Guerrini R, Dravet C, Raybaud C, et al. Epilepsy and focal gyral anomalies detected by MRI: electroclinico-morphological correlations and follow-up. Dev Med Child Neurol 1992;34:706–18.

138. Ambrosetto G, Tassinari CA. Sleep-related focal motor seizures in bilateral central macrogyria (letter). Ann Neurol 1990;28:840–2.

139. Graff-Radford NR, Bosch EP, Stears JC, et al. Developmental Foix-Chavany-Marie syndrome in identical twins. Ann Neurol 1986;20:632–5.

140. Kuzniecky R, Andermann F, Tampieri D, et al. Bilateral central macrogyria: epilepsy, pseudobulbar palsy, and mental retardation—a recognizable neuronal migration disorder. Ann Neurol 1989;25:547–54.

141. Kuzniecky R, Berkovic S, Andermann F, et al. Focal cortical myoclonus and rolandic cortical dysplasia: clarification by magnetic resonance imaging. Ann Neurol 1988;23:317–25.

142. Palmini A, Andermann F, Olivier A, et al. Focal neuronal migration disorders and intractable partial epilepsy: results of surgical treatment. Ann Neurol 1991;30:750–7.

143. Friede RL. Developmental neuropathology. New York: Springer-Verlag, 1975:330–46.

144. Dobyns WB. Developmental aspects of lissencephaly and the lissencephaly syndromes. Birth Defects 1987;23:225–41.

145. Dobyns WB, Kirkpatrick JB, Hittner HM, et al. Syndromes with lissencephaly. II: Walker-Warburg and cerebro-oculo-muscular syndromes and a new syndrome with type II lissencephaly. Am J Med Genet 1985;22:157–95.

146. Dobyns WB, Stratton RF, Greenberg F. Syndromes with lissencephaly. I: Miller-Diecker and Norman-Roberts syndromes and isolated lissencephaly. Am J Med Genet 1984;18:509–26.

147. Dobyns WB, Gilbert EF, Opitz JM. Further comments on the lissencephaly syndromes. Am J Med Genet 1985;22:197–211.

148. Dobyns WB, Stratton RF, Parke JT, et al. Miller-Dieker syndrome: lissencephaly and monosomy 17p. J Pediatr 1983;102:552–8.

149. Byrd SE, Osborn RE, Bohan TP, et al. The CT and MR evaluation of migrational disorders of the brain. Part I. Lissencephaly and pachygyria. Pediatr Radiol 1989;19:151–6.

150. Ambrosetto G. Treatable partial epilepsy and unilateral opercular neuronal migration disorder. Epilepsia 1993;34:604–8.

151. Barkovich AJ, Chuang SH, Norman D. MR of neuronal migration anomalies. AJNR Am J Neuroradiol 1987;8:1009–17.

152. Osborn RE, Byrd SE, Naidich TP, et al. MR imaging of neuronal migrational disorders. AJNR Am J Neuroradiol 1988;9:1101–6.

153. Yakovlev PI, Wadsworth RC. Schizencephalies: a study of the congenital clefts in the cerebral mantle. I. Clefts with fused lips. J Neuropathol Exp Neurol 1946;5:116–30.

154. Yakovlev PI, Wadsworth RC. Schizencephalies: a study of the congenital clefts in the cerebral mantle. II. Clefts with hydrocephalus and lips separated. J Neuropathol Exp Neurol 1946;5:169–206.

155. Barkovich AJ, Kjos BO. Schizencephaly: correlation of clinical findings with MR characteristics. AJNR Am J Neuroradiol 1992;13:85–94.

156. Leblanc R, Tampieri D, Robitaille Y, et al. Surgical treatment of intractable epilepsy associated with schizencephaly. Neurosurgery 1991;29:421–9.

157. Byrd SE, Osborn RE, Bohan TP, et al. The CT and MR evaluation of migrational disorders of the brain. Part II. Schizencephaly, heterotopia and polymicrogyria. Pediatr Radiol 1989;19:219–22.

158. Page LK, Brown SB, Gargano FP, et al. Schizencephaly: a clinical study and review. Childs Brain 1975;1:348–58.

159. Landy HJ, Ramsay RE, Ajmone-Marsan C, et al. Temporal lobectomy for seizures associated with unilateral schizencephaly. Surg Neurol 1992;37:477–81.

160. Meencke HJ. The density of dystopic neurons in the white matter of the gyrus frontalis inferior in epilepsies. J Neurol 1983;230:171–81.

161. Meencke HJ. Neuron density in the molecular layer of the frontal cortex in primary generalized epilepsy. Epilepsia 1985;26:450–4.

162. Meencke HJ, Gerhard C. Morphological aspects of aetiology and the course of infantile spasms (West-syndrome). Neuropediatrics 1985;16:59–66.

163. Meencke HJ, Janz D. Neuropathological findings in primary generalized epilepsy: a study of eight cases. Epilepsia 1984;25:8–21.

164. Meencke HJ, Janz D. The significance of micro-dysgenesia in primary generalized epilepsy: an answer to the considerations of Lyon and Gastaut. Epilepsia 1985;26:368–71.

165. Meencke HJ, Janz D, Cervos-Navarro J. Neuropathology of primary generalized epilepsies with awak-

ening grand mal. Acta Neuropathol Suppl (Berl) 1981;7:378–80.

166. Meencke HJ, Veith G. Migration disturbances in epilepsy. Epilepsy Res Suppl 1992;9:31–9.

167. Hardiman O, Burke T, Phillips J, et al. Microdysgenesis in resected temporal neocortex: incidence and clinical significance in focal epilepsy. Neurology 1988; 38:1041–7.

168. Nordburg C, Sourander P, Silfvenius H, et al. Mild cortical dysplasia in patients with intractable seizures: a histological study. In: Wolf P, Dam M, Janz D, et al, eds. Advances in epileptology. New York: Raven Press, 1987;29–33.

169. Meencke HJ. Pathology of childhood epilepsies. Cleve Clin J Med 1989;56 Suppl pt 1:S111–20.

170. Lyon G, Gastaut H. Considerations on the significance attributed to unusual cerebral histological findings recently described in eight patients with primary generalized epilepsy. Epilepsia 1985;26:365–7.

171. Livingstone JH, Aicardi J. Unusual MRI appearance of diffuse subcortical heterotopia or "double cortex" in two children. J Neurol Neurosurg Psychiatry 1990;53:617–20.

172. Palmini A, Andermann F, Aicardi J, et al. Diffuse cortical dysplasia, or the 'double cortex' syndrome: the clinical and epileptic spectrum in 10 patients. Neurology 1991;41:1656–62.

173. Ricci S, Cusmai R, Fariello G, et al. Double cortex. A neuronal migration anomaly as a possible cause of Lennox-Gastaut syndrome. Arch Neurol 1992;49:61–4.

174. Smith AS, Weinstein MA, Quencer RM, et al. Association of heterotopic gray matter with seizures: MR imaging. Work in progress. Radiology 1988;168:195–8.

175. Reutens DC, Berkovic SF, Kalnins RM, et al. Localised neuronal migration disorder and intractable epilepsy: a prenatal vascular aetiology. J Neurol Neurosurg Psychiatry 1993;56:314–6.

176. Stearns M, Wolf AL, Barry E, et al. Corpus callosotomy for refractory seizures in a patient with cortical heterotopia: case report. Neurosurgery 1989;25:633–5.

177. Hayden SA, Davis KA, Stears JC, et al. MR imaging of heterotopic gray matter. J Comput Assist Tomogr 1987;11:878–9.

178. Landy HJ, Curless RG, Ramsay RE, et al. Corpus callosotomy for seizures associated with band heterotopia. Epilepsia 1993;34:79–83.

179. Taylor DC, Falconer MA, Bruton CJ, et al. Focal dysplasia of the cerebral cortex in epilepsy. J Neurol Neurosurg Psychiatry 1971;34:369–87.

180. Perot P, Weir B, Rasmussen T. Tuberous sclerosis. Surgical therapy for seizures. Arch Neurol 1966;15:498–506.

181. De Rosa MJ, Secor DL, Barsom M, et al. Neuropathologic findings in surgically treated hemimegalencephaly: immunohistochemical, morphometric, and ultrastructural study. Acta Neuropathol (Berl) 1992;84:250–60.

182. Farrell MA, DeRosa MJ, Curran JG, et al. Neuropathologic findings in cortical resections (including hemispherectomies) performed for the treatment of intractable childhood epilepsy. Acta Neuropathol (Berl) 1992;83:246–59.

183. Palmini A, Andermann F, Olivier A, et al. Focal neuronal migration disorders and intractable partial epilepsy: a study of 30 patients. Ann Neurol 1991; 30:741–9.

184. Hirabayashi S, Binnie CD, Janota I, et al. Surgical treatment of epilepsy due to cortical dysplasia: clinical and EEG findings. J Neurol Neurosurg Psychiatry 1993;56:765–70.

185. Quirk JA, Kendall B, Kingsley DP, et al. EEG features of cortical dysplasia in children. Neuropediatrics 1993;24:193–9.

186. Chugani HT, Shields WD, Shewmon DA, et al. Infantile spasms: I. PET identifies focal cortical dysgenesis in cryptogenic cases for surgical treatment. Ann Neurol 1990;27:406–13.

187. Kuzniecky R, Mountz JM, Wheatley G, et al. Ictal single-photon emission computed tomography demonstrates localized epileptogenesis in cortical dysplasia. Ann Neurol 1993;34:627–31.

188. Kuzniecky R, Garcia JH, Faught E, et al. Cortical dysplasia in temporal lobe epilepsy: magnetic resonance imaging correlations. Ann Neurol 1991; 29:293–8.

189. Barkovich AJ, Kjos BO. Nonlissencephalic cortical dysplasias: correlation of imaging findings with clinical deficits. AJNR Am J Neuroradiol 1992;13:95–103.

190. Cochrane DD, Poskitt KJ, Norman MG. Surgical implications of cerebral dysgenesis. Can J Neurol Sci 1991;18:181–95.

191. Robain O, Floquet C, Heldt N, et al. Hemimegalencephaly: a clinicopathological study of four cases. Neuropathol Appl Neurobiol 1988;14:125–35.

192. Kazee AM, Lapham LW, Torres CF, et al. Generalized cortical dysplasia. Clinical and pathologic aspects. Arch Neurol 1991;48:850–3.

193. DeMeyer W. Megalencephaly in children. Clinical syndromes, genetic patterns, and differential diagnosis from other causes of megalocephaly. Neurology 1972;22:634–43.

194. Marchal G, Andermann F, Tampieri D, et al. Generalized cortical dysplasia manifested by diffusely thick cerebral cortex. Arch Neurol 1989;46:430–4.

195. Townsend JJ, Nielsen SL, Malamud N. Unilateral megalencephaly: hamartoma or neoplasm? Neurology 1975;25:448–53.

196. Vigevano F, Bertini E, Boldrini R, et al. Hemimegalencephaly and intractable epilepsy: benefits of hemispherectomy. Epilepsia 1989;30:833–43.

197. Vigevano F, Di Rocco C. Effectiveness of hemispherectomy in hemimegalencephaly with intractable seizures. Neuropediatrics 1990;21:222–3.

198. Konkol RJ, Maister BH, Wells RG, et al. Hemimegalencephaly: clinical, EEG, neuroimaging, and IMP-SPECT correlation. Pediatr Neurol 1990;6:414–8.

199. Rasmussen T, Villemure JG. Cerebral hemispherectomy for seizures with hemiplegia. Cleve Clin J Med 1989;56 Suppl 1:S62–8.

200. Vital A, Marchal C, Loiseau H, et al. Glial and neuronoglial malformative lesions associated with medically intractable epilepsy. Acta Neuropathol (Berl) 1994;87:196–201.

201. Di Rocco C, Caldarelli M, Guzzetta F, et al. Surgical indication in children with congenital hemiparesis. Childs Nerv Syst 1993;9:72–80.

202. Bergamini L, Bergamasco B, Benna P, et al. Acquired etiological factors in 1,785 epileptic subjects: clinical-anamnestic research. Epilepsia 1977;18:437–44.

203. Marks DA, Kim J, Spencer DD, et al. Characteristics of intractable seizures following meningitis and encephalitis. Neurology 1992;42:1513–8.

204. Vinters HV, De Rosa MJ, Farrell MA. Neuropathologic study of resected cerebral tissue from patients with infantile spasms. Epilepsia 1993;34:772–9.

205. Stern WE. Neurosurgical considerations of cysticerocosis of the central nervous system. J Neurosurg 1981;55:382–9.

206. Vazquez V, Sotelo J. The course of seizures after treatment for cerebral cysticercosis. N Engl J Med 1992; 327:696–701.

207. Andermann F. Clinical indications for hemispherectomy and callosotomy. Epilepsy Res Suppl 1992;5:189–99.

208. Vining EP, Freeman JM, Brandt J, et al. Progressive unilateral encephalopathy of childhood (Rasmussen's syndrome): a reappraisal. Epilepsia 1993;34:639–50.

209. Yablon SA. Posttraumatic seizures. Arch Phys Med Rehabil 1993;74:983–1001.

210. Moriwaki A, Hattori Y, Hayashi Y, et al. Development of epileptic activity induced by iron injection into rat cerebral cortex: electrographic and behavioral characteristics. Electroencephalogr Clin Neurophysiol 1992;83:281–8.

Clinical Applications of Neuroimaging: Surgical Planning in Pediatrics

Elaine Wyllie

Recent developments in neuroimaging have had significant impact on the strategy for selecting pediatric candidates for epilepsy surgery. Increasingly, pediatric surgical candidates are identified on the basis of the presence of an important structural lesion detected with magnetic resonance imaging (MRI) or positron emission tomography (PET), sometimes without clearly localized findings on electroencephalography (EEG). This review focuses on four specific clinical settings in pediatric epilepsy in which neuroimaging has a key role in defining surgical strategy: focal neuronal migration disorders, Sturge-Weber syndrome, Rasmussen's chronic focal encephalitis, and temporal lobe epilepsy.

FOCAL ABNORMALITIES OF NEURONAL MIGRATION

Hemimegalencephaly, or unilateral megalencephaly, is enlargement of all or part of one cerebral hemisphere and its ventricular system, with thick flat gyri, shallow sulci, and abnormal white matter. Patients with hemimegalencephaly may have devastating epilepsy, with very frequent seizures arising from the affected hemisphere.[1–7] Infants may also have developmental delay and hemiparesis. EEG typically shows ictal and interictal epileptiform discharges, predominantly or exclusively from the affected hemisphere, and PET shows hypometabolism in the hemimegalencephalic cortex.

Epilepsy surgery may produce a marked decrease in seizure frequency. Functional hemispherectomy[8–12] may be appropriate in patients with involvement of a whole hemisphere, and lobar or multilobar resection in those with involvement of part of one hemisphere (Figure 17-1). The operation developed by Rasmussen[8] and Villemure[12] at the Montreal Neurologic Institute has been shown in follow-up studies to be safe and effective, without the late neurologic complications reported for complete anatomical resections. This operation involves resection of central and temporal regions, complete corpus callosotomy, and complete transection of the white matter from the remaining frontal and parieto-occipital cortex. A further modification to the procedure involves resecting only the central region, with transection of the white matter from the remaining temporal cortex. Both operations functionally isolate the hemisphere, although they do not involve complete anatomical resection of all cortical regions.

Focal cortical dysplasia was first described in epilepsy surgery specimens in 1971 by Taylor and colleagues.[13] Since then, several series have confirmed that cortical dysplasia is an important pathologic substrate in patients with focal epilepsy[14–23] and that resection of the dysplastic region may lead to dramatic improvement in seizure frequency.

Typical features of focal cortical dysplasia on MRI include focal areas of cortical thickening and indistinct differentiation between gray matter and white matter (Figure 17-2 and 17-3).[24–27] However, MRI findings may be normal in patients with pathologically demonstrated focal cortical dysplasia,[15,28] especially if the abnormality is only minimal and microscopic. PET may show hypometabolism in the affected cortical region (Figure 17-4) and may be more sensitive than MRI in identifying an area of focal cortical dysplasia.[18,28]

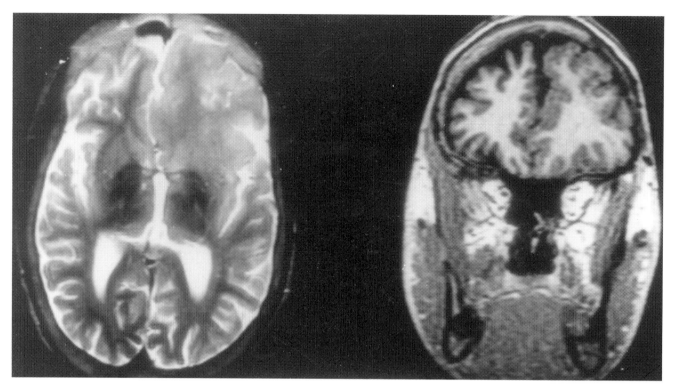

FIGURE 17-1. MRI showing partial hemimegalencephaly with dysplasia throughout the left frontal lobe. The cortex was thickened and had an abnormal gyral pattern. The volume of the entire left frontal lobe was increased compared with that of the right lobe. Right focal motor seizures began when the patient was 2 years old and occurred daily. The patient had moderately severe mental retardation but no hemiparesis. Preoperative scalp EEG showed ictal and interictal epileptiform discharges over the left frontal lobe, and PET showed hypometabolism in that area. The patient had left frontal lobectomy at age 15 years, with complete removal of the area seen to be abnormal on MRI and at intraoperative inspection. The patient had no new neurologic deficit postoperatively. Seizures persisted but were markedly decreased, with dramatic improvement in quality of life. (From Wyllie et al.[28] By permission of Butterworth-Heinemann.)

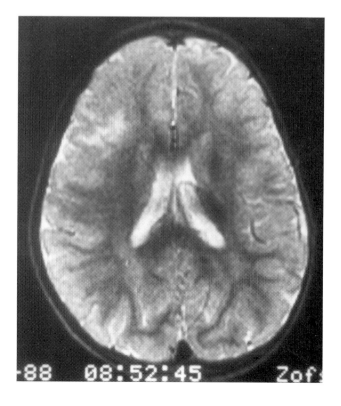

◀ FIGURE 17-2. MRI showing an area of focal cortical dysplasia in the right frontal lobe in a 21-month-old boy with mild developmental delay, normal motor function, and intractable left hemiconvulsions, 10 to 50 daily, since age 10 months. EEG showed ictal and interictal epileptiform discharges over the right frontal lobe. Extensive right frontal lobectomy performed when he was 22 months old produced no new neurologic deficit and marked improvement in seizure frequency (a brief seizure every 1 to 4 months), with reduced dose of antiepileptic medication.

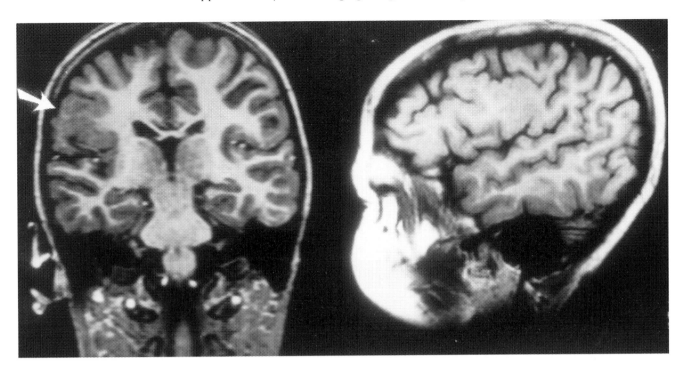

FIGURE 17-3. MRI showing cortical dysplasia (*arrow*) in the right frontocentral region in a 7-year-old girl with mental retardation and intractable seizures since age 13 months. The dysplastic cortex just above the right midposterior sylvian fissure is thickened and poorly sulcated. The patient had daily tonic and left frontal motor seizures since age 1 year, with moderately severe mental retardation and no hemiparesis. Interictal PET showed extensive hypometabolism throughout the anterior right hemisphere (Figure 17-4), and EEG showed ictal and interictal epileptiform discharges over the right frontocentral region. At age 7 years, the patient had partial right frontal lobectomy. Seizures persisted but were markedly improved in frequency and severity, and she made developmental progress. Resection of remaining right frontal cortex was offered, but the family felt that reoperation was not required. (From Wyllie et al. [28] By permission of Butterworth-Heinemann.)

The typical clinical setting of focal cortical dysplasia is severe extratemporal epilepsy that began in infancy or early childhood, usually in the setting of mental retardation or significant developmental delay, often with MRI evidence of the focal neuronal migration abnormality.[16,28] These patients, usually with daily seizures, often present for extratemporal resection or hemispherectomy in infancy, childhood, or adolescence. EEG may reveal ictal and interictal epileptiform discharges predominantly or exclusively over the dysplastic region. Histopathologic findings include clusters of atypical cortical neurons, disrupted cortical laminar architecture, increased number of neurons in the molecular layer, and neuronal heterotopia in the white matter.

In a series of patients with focal cortical dysplasia examined at The Cleveland Clinic Foundation, the rate of seizure-free outcome after extratemporal resection or hemispherectomy was modest (53% of patients).[28]

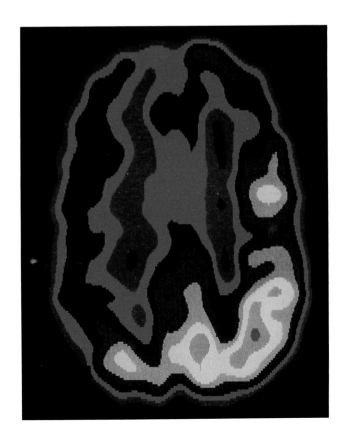

FIGURE 17-4. ▶ Preoperative interictal 2-fluorodeoxyglucose-PET scan from the patient in Figure 17-3 showing extensive right hemisphere hypometabolism.

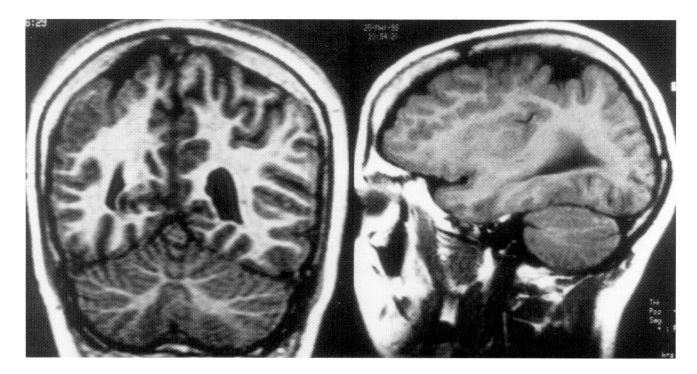

FIGURE 17-5. MRI showing cortical dysplasia in the right superior parietal area, with an area of thickened cortex inferior to an area of polymicrogyria dipping in a rounded cleft. The patient was 15 years old and had congenital left hemiparesis, mental retardation, and weekly left focal motor seizures since age 6 months. Interictal PET showed hypometabolism in the right superior parietal area, and EEG showed ictal and interictal epileptiform discharges over the same area. After right frontoparietal resection, the patient was seizure-free but without significant change in the severity of the left hemiparesis. (From Wyllie et al.[28] By permission of Butterworth-Heinemann.)

However, several of the patients with persistent seizures had a marked reduction in seizure frequency and major improvement in quality of life (cases shown in Figures 17-1 through 17-3). This was especially clear among the infants with catastrophic epilepsy, who had dozens of seizures every day preoperatively and only a few seizures weekly or monthly postoperatively. Palmini and colleagues[17] also reported encouraging results after operation. Successful outcome may be related to the completeness of the resection of the cortical region seen to be abnormal on MRI and intraoperative visual inspection.[17]

Focal cortical dysplasia may also be a cause of temporal lobe epilepsy.[15,28] In the series from The Cleveland Clinic Foundation,[28] these patients, compared with those with extratemporal cortical dysplasia, typically had epilepsy that began later in childhood or adolescence, had seizures less frequently, and were not mentally retarded. MRI gave evidence of the neuronal migration abnormality less often, but PET showed temporal hypometabolism. In many cases, EEG findings were similar to those in patients with mesial temporal epilepsy due to other causes, such as hippocampal sclerosis, with sphenoidal maximum sharp waves and temporal EEG seizure patterns. Whereas cortical dysplasia was usually suspected preoperatively in the patients with extratemporal epilepsy, it

was typically an unexpected histopathologic finding in the older, intellectually normal patients with temporal lobe epilepsy. The rate of seizure-free outcome postoperatively was good (77% of patients), and the histopathologic findings were usually less severe than among the patients with extratemporal epilepsy. In the series reported by Kuzniecky and colleagues,[15] MRI revealed the temporal cortical dysplasia in 7 of 10 patients.

Focal polymicrogyria refers to a cortical region with an excessive number of abnormal small gyri (Figure 17-5).[20,29] Histologic findings include ischemic laminar necrosis in cortical layer V and normal-appearing layers II, III, and IV, suggesting a postmigratory ischemic mechanism. Although no large operative series of patients with this specific abnormality is available, the case presented in Figure 17-5 illustrates the potential for good operative outcome.

A special group includes patients with focal cortical dysplasia and those with infantile spasms. Chugani and colleagues[18] reported a small series of patients with infantile spasms and hypsarrhythmia, often with a preceding history of focal seizures, who had resolution of spasms after resection of a focal area of cortical dysplasia identified with PET. Some patients also had MRI evidence of focal neuronal migration disorder and EEG evidence of focal dysfunction, such as abnormal back-

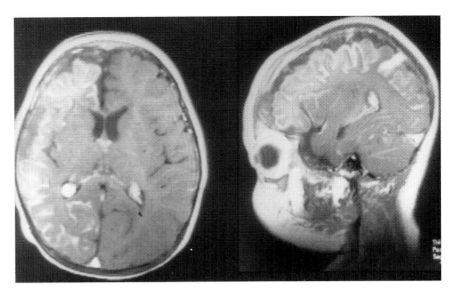

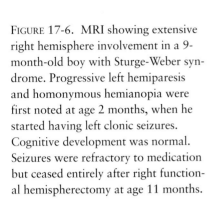

FIGURE 17-6. MRI showing extensive right hemisphere involvement in a 9-month-old boy with Sturge-Weber syndrome. Progressive left hemiparesis and homonymous hemianopia were first noted at age 2 months, when he started having left clonic seizures. Cognitive development was normal. Seizures were refractory to medication but ceased entirely after right functional hemispherectomy at age 11 months.

ground rhythms over the affected area. Increasingly, experience indicates that patients with intractable infantile spasms should be evaluated carefully for the possibility of a potentially resectable focal abnormality, such as dysplasia, low-grade tumor, or other structural lesion.

STURGE-WEBER SYNDROME

Sturge-Weber syndrome involves progressive cortical atrophy in part or all of one hemisphere, with facial nevus (port-wine stain) of the upper face, contralateral hemiparesis and hemianopia, seizures, and, often, mental retardation.[30] Meningeal angiomatosis and intracranial calcifications of the affected hemisphere are rarely present at birth but are almost always present by the end of the second decade[31] (Figure 17-6). The associated epilepsy is often intractable, with focal or secondarily generalized seizures arising from the affected hemisphere.

Patients with intractable epilepsy may benefit remarkably from epilepsy surgery. EEG typically shows pronounced asymmetry of background rhythms, decreased over the affected hemisphere, with ictal and interictal epileptiform discharges from the same side. PET scan typically reveals marked hypometabolism in the atrophic cortical regions. Lobar or multilobar resection may be appropriate for patients with intractable epilepsy due to localized involvement of part of one hemisphere, whereas functional hemispherectomy would be more appropriate in the setting of whole hemisphere involvement. Seizure-free outcome may be expected for the majority of cases.[32,33]

Some infants have a rapidly progressive course, with evolution to dense motor and visual deficit and intractable seizures within the first year of life. For these patients, early functional hemispherectomy may be beneficial. By relieving the seizures and reducing the burden of high doses of antiepileptic medications, early surgical

therapy in refractory cases may help to maximize the child's developmental potential.

RASMUSSEN'S CHRONIC FOCAL ENCEPHALITIS

The four key elements of Rasmussen's chronic focal encephalitis, as characterized by Rasmussen and colleagues at the Montreal Neurologic Institute,[34–36] are (1) onset of partial seizures in childhood (14 months to 14 years old); (2) slowly progressive neurologic deterioration with hemiparesis, mental retardation, homonymous hemianopia, and dysphasia (if the dominant hemisphere is involved); (3) slowly progressive brain atrophy, predominantly unilateral (Figure 17-7); and (4) histopathologic features suggesting viral encephalitis. EEG typically shows lateralized or localized seizures over the most atrophic hemisphere, although bilateral interictal slowing and sharp waves may also be present. PET scan shows hypometabolism in the affected hemisphere (Figure 17-8).

Treatment with standard medications usually does not provide seizure control, and many patients have recurrent epilepsia partialis continua. Some patients have had significant improvement with high doses of steroids,[36] but functional hemispherectomy is indicated for patients with intractable seizures, severe hemiplegia, and homonymous hemianopia. Rasmussen and Andermann[35] reported that 76% of patients were seizure-free or had rare attacks after functional hemispherectomy. These authors noted much less successful outcome after more limited cortical excisions.

In young children with intractable seizures and rapid progression, it may be appropriate to perform functional hemispherectomy even before a complete hemiparesis has evolved.[35] Because the course of this relentless syndrome is toward eventual hemiparesis in any event, early surgical therapy would not add to the

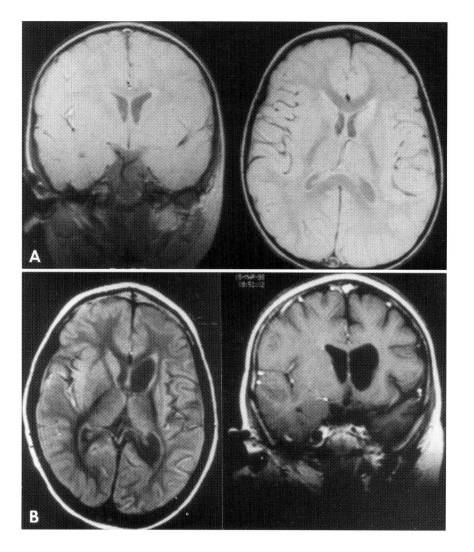

FIGURE 17-7. MRI of a boy with Rasmussen's chronic focal encephalitis showing progressive left hemisphere atrophy. A. At age 3 years. B. At 6 years. Progressive right hemiparesis and intractable right focal motor and secondarily generalized seizures began at age 2 years. EEG showed ictal and interictal epileptiform discharges over the left hemisphere, and interictal PET showed extensive left hemisphere hypometabolism (Figure 17-8). Right functional hemispherectomy performed at age 7 years produced a seizure-free outcome.

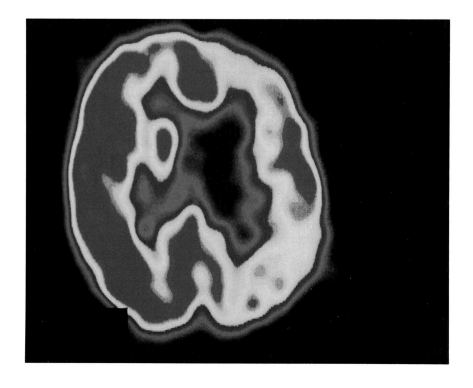

FIGURE 17-8. Interictal 2-fluoro-deoxyglucose PET scan showing extensive left hemisphere hypometabolism in the same patient as in Figure 17-7 at age 6 years.

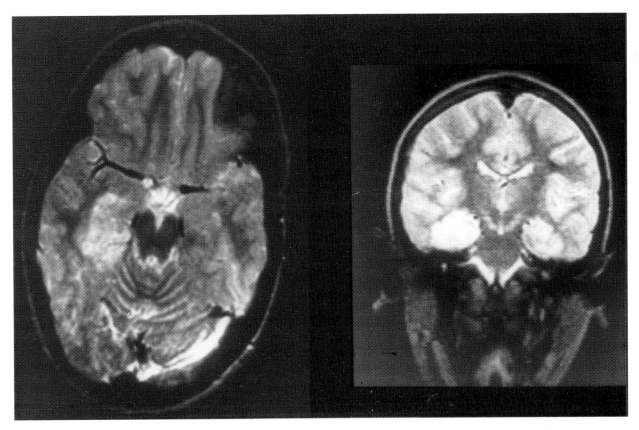

FIGURE 17-9. MRI showing right temporal ganglioglioma in an 8-year-old girl with intractable complex partial seizures since age 3 years. Interictal and ictal EEG showed epileptiform discharges predominantly over the left temporal lobe (Figure 17-10). The "false lateralization" on EEG may have been due to early spread to the left temporal lobe after onset in an undetected cortical region near the right temporal tumor, because right temporal lobectomy and tumor resection at age 8 years resulted in complete seizure-free outcome and discontinuation of all treatment with antiepileptic medication. (From Wyllie E. A note on temporal lobe epilepsy in preadolescent children with respect to epilepsy surgery. In: Wolf P, ed. *Epileptic seizures and syndromes*. London: John Libbey & Company, 1994:369-74. By permission of the publisher.)

long-term motor deficit. Theoretical benefits of an early operation in young children with Rasmussen's syndrome include forced transfer of neurologic function to the healthier hemisphere when plasticity is greater and protection of the healthier hemisphere from constant bombardment by frequent epileptiform discharges.

TEMPORAL LOBE EPILEPSY

Many children with temporal lobe epilepsy referred for early surgical treatment have low-grade temporal lobe tumors, such as gangliogliomas, dysembryoplastic neuroepithelial tumors, or low-grade astrocytomas or oligodendrogliomas. The detection of a tumor with neuroimaging accelerates the referral process so that the children receive operation at an earlier age. Typically, the only clinical manifestation of the tumor is complex partial seizures. These children usually do not have signs of increased intracranial pressure or focal neurologic deficits, although some have mental retardation.[37]

Computerized tomography (CT) is notoriously poor in detecting low-grade temporal tumors, and MRI is the test of choice. In one series, CT failed to show the lesion in 44% of patients with tumors seen on MRI.[37]

Ictal and interictal EEG findings may be complex (Figure 17-9 and 17-10), but the strategy is resection of the tumor and surrounding epileptogenic cortex. How much surrounding cortex to include in the resection and whether to resect the hippocampus and amygdala are subjects of debate. In any event, it appears that complete tumor resection is a prerequisite for seizure-free outcome.

Some physicians hesitate to refer children for left temporal lobectomy for intractable complex partial seizures, even in the setting of a possible tumor, because of concern about postoperative language and memory deficits. In adults, a new-onset tumor near Wernicke's area can cause significant aphasia, and resection in that area may entail an unacceptable risk for worsened deficit. However, in children with early-onset complex partial seizures, the low-grade temporal lobe tumors are often

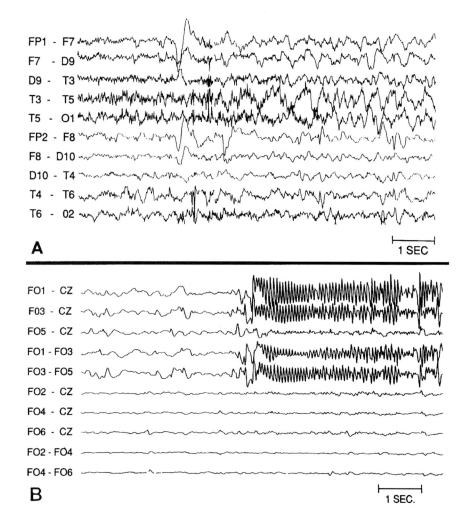

FIGURE 17-10. A. Scalp EEG seizure pattern over the left temporal area, 8 seconds after clinical onset, in the same patient as in Figure 17-9. (The D9 electrode is similar to the T1 or FT9 position.) B. The left temporal seizure pattern was confirmed with foramen ovale electrode recording. (FO1, FO3, FO5: left foramen ovale electrodes, FO1 most distal. FO2, FO4, FO6: right foramen ovale electrodes, FO2 most distal.) (A from Wyllie E. A note on temporal lobe epilepsy in preadolescent children with respect to epilepsy surgery. In: Wolf P, ed. *Epileptic seizures and syndromes*. London: John Libbey & Company, 1994:369-74. By permission of the publisher.)

present since early infancy, allowing left hemisphere language areas to develop in cortical areas not affected by the neoplasm. In a series of patients with epilepsy caused by early left temporal tumors studied at The Cleveland Clinic Foundation,[38] complete resection was usually possible even when the lesion was quite posterior. However, localization of language areas with cortical stimulation was important to guide the resection (Figure 17-11 and 17-12).

Cortical dysplasia may also cause temporal lobe epilepsy, manifesting complex partial seizures in infancy or childhood,[23,28] as discussed above. In the pediatric surgical series of Duchowny and colleagues,[23] cortical dysplasia was the most common pathologic finding.

Hippocampal sclerosis is the most common lesion in adult temporal lobectomy series, but few children with this finding are operated on before adolescence. Although temporal lobe epilepsy due to hippocampal sclerosis may begin in early childhood, patients are often not referred for surgical evaluation until late adolescence or adulthood. Even if complex partial seizures continue despite antiepileptic medication, they may be infrequent or the child's family and physicians may not perceive the

episodes of altered consciousness to be severe enough to warrant an operation. Others believe that in selected cases the developmental and psychosocial impact of daily or weekly complex partial seizures may warrant considering epilepsy surgery before adolescence.

In one series,[37] a small number of children with hippocampal sclerosis had MRI, PET, EEG, and clinical features similar to those typically observed in adolescent or adult patients. The neuroimaging of this disorder is discussed in Chapter 5. However, because so few well-documented cases have been studied in young children, it is possible that other infants and children have hippocampal sclerosis with EEG and clinical features different from those in older patients. Prospective studies will be important to characterize the spectrum of features of this disorder in earliest years.

Pediatric epilepsy surgery series have documented that temporal lobectomy can be as safe and effective for children as for adults, with a 50% to 90% chance for seizure-free outcome.[23,37,39,40] Increased recognition of the possible benefits of epilepsy surgery has gradually resulted in earlier referral of children for surgical consideration.

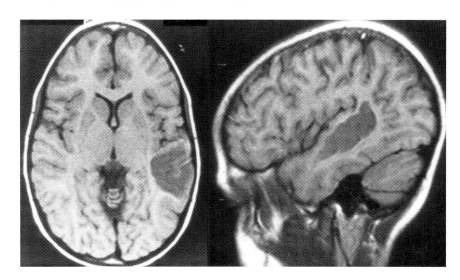

FIGURE 17-11. MRI showing a left posterior temporal dysembryoplastic neuroepithelial tumor in an 8-year-old girl with intractable complex partial seizures since age 4 years. Intracarotid amobarbital testing showed left hemisphere language dominance. (From De Vos et al.[38] By permission of Little, Brown and Company.)

FIGURE 17-12. A. Initial cortical stimulation studies in the same patient as in Figure 17-10. Stimulation revealed frontal and basal temporal language areas but not Wernicke's posterior temporal language area. This led to incomplete tumor resection when the patient was 8 years old, because of concern about potential postoperative language deficit. Seizures decreased in frequency but subsequently occurred at preoperative level. B. Cortical stimulation studies with more posterior electrodes revealed Wernicke's area posterior to the tumor. Complete tumor resection was then performed, resulting in the patient being completely seizure-free and without new language deficit. Because the early tumor probably grew along with the brain during infancy, language developed in an atypical region away from the neoplasm. (A from De Vos et al.[38] By permission of Little, Brown and Company.)

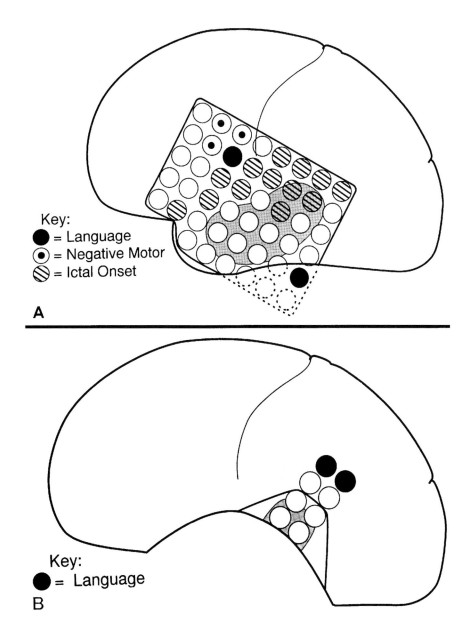

REFERENCES

1. Vigevano F, Bertini E, Boldrini R, et al. Hemimegalencephaly and intractable epilepsy: benefits of hemispherectomy. Epilepsia 1989;30:833–43.

2. Robain O, Floquet C, Heldt N, et al. Hemimegalencephaly: a clinicopathological study of four cases. Neuropathol Appl Neurobiol 1988;14:125–35.

3. Trounce JQ, Rutter N, Mellor DH. Hemimegalencephaly: diagnosis and treatment. Dev Med Child Neurol 1991;33:261–6.

4. Konkol RJ, Maister BH, Wells RG, et al. Hemimegalencephaly: clinical, EEG, neuroimaging, and IMP-SPECT correlation. Pediatr Neurol 1990;6:414–8.

5. King M, Stephenson JB, Ziervogel M, et al. Hemimegalencephaly—a case for hemispherectomy? Neuropediatrics 1985;16:46–55.

6. Kalifa GL, Chiron C, Sellier N, et al. Hemimegalencephaly: MR imaging in five children. Radiology 1987;165:29–33.

7. Barkovich AJ, Chuang SH. Unilateral megalencephaly: correlation of MR imaging and pathologic characteristics. AJNR Am J Neuroradiol 1990;11:523–31.

8. Rasmussen T. Hemispherectomy for seizures revisited. Can J Neurol Sci 1983;10:71–8.

9. Tinuper P, Andermann F, Villemure JG, et al. Functional hemispherectomy for treatment of epilepsy associated with hemiplegia: rationale, indications, results, and comparison with callosotomy. Ann Neurol 1988;24:27–34.

10. Goodman R. Hemispherectomy and its alternatives in the treatment of intractable epilepsy in patients with infantile hemiplegia. Dev Med Child Neurol 1986;28:251–8.

11. Rasmussen T, Villemure JG. Cerebral hemispherectomy for seizures with hemiplegia. Cleve Clin J Med 1989;56 Suppl 1:S62–8.

12. Villemure J-G. Hemispherectomy: techniques and complications. In: Wyllie E, ed. The treatment of epilepsy: principles and practice. Philadelphia: Lea & Febiger, 1993:1116–9.

13. Taylor DC, Falconer MA, Bruton CJ, et al. Focal dysplasia of the cerebral cortex in epilepsy. J Neurol Neurosurg Psychiatry 1971;34:369–87.

14. Hardiman O, Burke T, Phillips J, et al. Microdysgenesis in resected temporal neocortex: incidence and clinical significance in focal epilepsy. Neurology 1988;38:1041–7.

15. Kuzniecky R, Garcia JH, Faught E, et al. Cortical dysplasia in temporal lobe epilepsy: magnetic resonance imaging correlations. Ann Neurol 1991;29:293–8.

16. Palmini A, Andermann F, Olivier A, et al. Focal neuronal migration disorders and intractable partial epilepsy: a study of 30 patients. Ann Neurol 1991;30:741–9.

17. Palmini A, Andermann F, Olivier A, et al. Focal neuronal migration disorders and intractable partial epilepsy: results of surgical treatment. Ann Neurol 1991;30:750–7.

18. Chugani HT, Shields WD, Shewmon DA, et al. Infantile spasms: I. PET identifies focal cortical dysgenesis in cryptogenic cases for surgical treatment. Ann Neurol 1990;27:406–13.

19. Sarnat HB. Cerebral cortical development: normal and pathologic processes. In: Wyllie E, ed. The treatment of epilepsy: principles and practice. Philadelphia: Lea & Febiger, 1993:41–54.

20. Friede RL. Developmental neuropathology. New York: Springer-Verlag, 1989:330–46.

21. Meencke HJ. The density of dystopic neurons in the white matter of the gyrus frontalis inferior in epilepsies. J Neurol 1983;230:171–81.

22. Meencke HJ, Janz D. Neuropathological findings in primary generalized epilepsy: a study of eight cases. Epilepsia 1984;25:8–21.

23. Duchowny M, Levin B, Jayakar P, et al. Temporal lobectomy in early childhood. Epilepsia 1992;33:298–303.

24. Palmini A, Andermann F, Olivier A, et al. Neuronal migration disorders: a contribution of modern neuroimaging to the etiologic diagnosis of epilepsy. Can J Neurol Sci 1991;18 Suppl 4:580–7.

25. Barkovich AJ, Chuang SH, Norman D. MR of neuronal migration anomalies. AJR Am J Roentgenol 1988;150:179–87.

26. Barkovich AJ, Kjos BO. Gray matter heterotopias: MR characteristics and correlation with developmental and neurologic manifestations. Radiology 1992;182:493–9.

27. Barkovich AJ, Jackson DE Jr, Boyer RS. Band heterotopias: a newly recognized neuronal migration anomaly. Radiology 1989;171:455–8.

28. Wyllie E, Baumgartner C, Prayson R, et al. The clinical spectrum of focal cortical dysplasia and epilepsy. J Epilepsy 1994;7:303–12.

29. Kuzniecky R, Andermann F, Guerrini R. The epileptic spectrum in the congenital bilateral perisylvian syndrome. CBPS Multicenter Collaborative Study. Neurology 1994;44:379–85.

30. Alexander GL, Norman RM. The Sturge-Weber syndrome. Bristol, England: John Wright & Sons, 1960.

31. Nellhaus G, Haberland C, Hill BJ. Sturge-Weber disease with bilateral intracranial calcifications at birth and unusual pathologic findings. Acta Neurol Scand 1967;43:314–47.

32. Hoffman HJ, Hendrick EB, Dennis M, et al. Hemispherectomy for Sturge-Weber syndrome. Childs Brain 1979;5:233–48.

33. Arzimanoglou A, Aicardi J. The epilepsy of Sturge-Weber syndrome: clinical features and treatment in 23 patients. Acta Neurol Scand Suppl 1992;140:18–22.

34. Rasmussen T, Olszewski J, Lloyd-Smith D. Focal seizures due to chronic localized encephalitis. Neurology 1958;8:435–45.

35. Rasmussen T, Andermann F. Rasmussen syndrome: symptomatology of the syndrome of chronic encephalitis and seizures: 35-year experience with 51 cases. In: Lüders HO, ed. Epilepsy surgery. New York: Raven Press, 1992:173–82.

36. Andermann F. Chronic encephalitis and epilepsy: Rasmussen's syndrome. Boston: Butterworth-Heinemann, 1991.

37. Wyllie E, Chee M, Granstrom ML, et al. Temporal lobe epilepsy in early childhood. Epilepsia 1993;34:859–68.

38. De Vos KJ, Wyllie E, Geckler C, et al. Language dominance in patients with early childhood tumors near left hemisphere language areas. Neurology 1995;45:349–56.

39. Davidson S, Falconer MA. Outcome of surgery in 40 children with temporal-lobe epilepsy. Lancet 1975;1:1260–3.

40. Whittle IR, Ellis HJ, Simpson DA. The surgical treatment of intractable childhood and adolescent epilepsy. Aust NZ J Surg 1981;51:190–6.

Neuropsychology and Neuroimaging in Epilepsy Surgery

Max R. Trenerry

The reader will observe that there is no expression of opinion as to the very exact part of the brain injury of which produces loss of speech. Whilst I believe that the hinder part of the left third frontal convolution is the part most often damaged, I do not localise speech in any such small part of the brain. To locate the damage which destroys speech and to locate speech are two different things (J.H. Jackson, 1874[1]).

Advances in neuroimaging during the last decade have allowed noninvasive observation of neuroanatomical structures, physiologic characteristics, and even physiologic changes associated with cognitive activity. Neuropsychologic assessment has traditionally provided a quantitative estimation of how well the brain performs different types of tasks. Neuropsychology owes a great debt to the study of the epilepsies and epilepsy surgery.[2] The combination of quantitative neurocognitive data and neuroimaging data in epilepsy surgery has and likely will continue to influence neuropsychologic research and practice in epilepsy surgery settings.

This chapter provides a selective review of functional imaging studies that used techniques to study regional cerebral blood flow and metabolism associated with a particular cognitive task. These investigations have provided fundamental observations. They also have provided hypotheses to be studied with quantitative (for example, volumetric studies or T_2 relaxometry) and functional magnetic resonance imaging (MRI) techniques. This chapter

also reviews the results of studies that have combined neurocognitive data and quantitative MRI data from patients who have had temporal lobectomy and who do not have a structural lesion other than mesial temporal sclerosis (MTS). The chapter also considers the implications of this work for clinical practice and research.

METABOLIC AND BLOOD FLOW IMAGING

Petersen et al.[3,4] studied single-word processing in 17 normal subjects with ^{15}O water positron emission tomorgraphy (PET) during visual and auditory reception, production, and association tasks. They found that metabolic activity increased in expected modality-specific regions during the sensory-receptive word presentation: striate cortex was activated during passive visual word presentation, and auditory cortex was activated bilaterally during passive auditory presentation. Otherwise, output and association tasks produced increased activation in multiple regions. Petersen et al.[3] suggested that the anterior cingulate gyrus has a role in allocating attention to a task. They also found that the left inferior frontal region was activated during a semantic association task. Petersen et al.[3,4] emphasized that although their data did not support serial processing of language, they were consistent with a systemic or multiple-route model of language processing.

Pardo et al.[5] studied regional cerebral blood flow with ^{15}O water PET in eight normal subjects during a Stroop paradigm task. This task requires a subject first to read color names (for example, red, blue, green) printed in black ink or in ink of the same color (for example, "red" printed in red ink). The second component, or interference trial, requires naming the color of the ink used to print the name of a different color (for example, red ink to print the name "blue"). The authors modified the first task so that subjects named the color of ink used to print the same color name. They found metabolic activation of the right anterior cingulate gyrus during the interference trial, as compared with the first trial. Activation was also detected bilaterally in the peristriate cortex, left premotor and postcentral areas, left putamen, supplementary motor area, inferior anterior cingulate cortex, and superior right temporal gyrus. Of interest, no activation was detected in the left anterior frontal cortex, which would be expected, because of the results of Perret.[6] In a follow-up study, Janer and Pardo[7] demonstrated selective attention deficits in a patient after stereotactic anterior cingulotomy. The results of Pardo et al.[5] and Janer and Pardo[7] are consistent with the findings of Petersen et al.,[3] indicating that the anterior cingulate cortex has a prominent role in allocating attentional resources. The results of Pardo et al. are also consistent with those of Petersen et al. in indicating that the multiple cortical sites activated bilaterally did not conform to traditional ideas about lateralization of language function.

Huettner et al.[8] used xenon 133 to study changes in regional cerebral blood flow in three men while they read narrative text. Reading comprehension and the partial pressure of carbon dioxide were monitored in all three men. The authors reported that regional cerebral blood flow increased 12.67% and 14.67% in the left and right hemispheres, respectively, during reading. These results were unexpected and suggested greater hemispheric involvement during the reading of narrative text than expected from the Geschwind model of language. Mazoyer et al.[9] studied regional cerebral blood flow in 16 right-handed French medical students while they were being read stories in French or Tamil. Activation was detected in the left and right superior temporal gyri and temporal poles, and in the left middle temporal, inferior frontal, and superior prefrontal (Brodmann area 8) gyri. Only the left and right superior temporal gyri were activated during the presentation of stories in Tamil. Metabolic activation was relatively greater in the left than in the right hemisphere. Auditory presentation of pseudowords caused activation in the right inferior frontal gyrus. The results of Mazoyer et al.[9] and Huettner et al.[8] also support bilateral hemispheric involvement in language processing. Activation of the right inferior frontal gyrus during pseudoword presentation is of interest because of the hypothesis that the right hemisphere is not "dominant" for visual information as much as for novel information.[10] According to Goldberg[10]:

The right hemisphere is critical for initial orientation in the task and for processing novel information to which none of the representational systems pre-existing in the subject's cognitive repertoire can be successfully applied. The left hemisphere, on the other hand, is critical in any processing which relies upon well-routinized representational systems ensconced in the subject's cognitive repertoire, verbal and nonverbal alike. The left hemisphere's dominance for language is viewed as a special case of this more general principle (p. 474).

Kosslyn et al.[11] used PET to study regional cerebral blood flow in two groups of seven right-handed men who were not taking any medication and who apparently were in good health. Activation of the visual cortex was greater during image generation than during perception of an actual image. The following areas were activated during image generation but not during perception: area 18, left middle temporal, left inferior temporal, and right middle temporal gyri; right superior parietal lobe; right hippocampus; and precuneus area. The following regions were activated during perception but not during imagery: left area 19, right fusiform cortex, right caudate, and right precentral and postcentral gyri. Roland et al.[12] reported on PET studies of changes in regional cerebral blood flow during visual and motor learning and memory. Changes occurred in regional cerebral blood flow during visual learning but not during motor learning in the hippocampus, parahippocampal gyrus, temporal pole, anterior cingulate cortex, and ventral striatum. Increased blood flow was noted in anterior and posterior cingulate cortex and in posterior hippocampus during visual image recall, as compared with learning. The anterior hippocampus, anterior cingulate cortex, temporal pole, and anterior portion of the insula show increased blood flow during visual learning. The difference in anterior versus posterior hippocampal change in blood flow during visual learning and memory may be of interest to neuropsychologists engaged in epilepsy surgery research.

The models of Kosslyn et al. and Roland et al. involved recollection, or memory for, visual information, and in both studies, activation or changes in blood flow occurred in the right hippocampus (Roland et al. indicated bilateral activation of the hippocampus). The findings of Roland et al. suggest that different portions of the hippocampus are involved with different aspects of learning and memory.

Henry et al.[13] used 18-fluoro-2-deoxyglucose PET to study 27 temporal lobectomy patients and found that 25 of them had lateralized regions of abnormal hypometabolism. The lateral and mesial temporal cortices were involved in most patients (78% and 70%, respectively), but 63% of the patients also had hypometabolism in the thalamus. Other extratemporal regions of lateralized hypometabolism were variable. Although the findings in temporal cortex were as expected, Henry et al.[13] suggested that the thalamic hypometabolism may be associated with memory dysfunction or propagation of seizures. Rausch et al.[14] used 18-fluoro-2-deoxyglucose PET to study neuropsychologic measures in 13 patients with intractable complex partial seizures of temporal lobe onset. They found that the relative hypometabolism of the left hemisphere was associated with poorer cognitive test performance. Hypometabolism of the left lateral temporal lobe and thalamus was positively associated with verbal memory performance. That is, decreased metabolism in these regions was also associated with decreased performance on memory testing. However, Rausch et al.[14] did not study changes in metabolism during a specific task.

Parks et al.[15] reviewed research on PET and neuropsychologic test results and noted that several investigators had found *negative* correlations between PET-detected metabolic changes and performance by normal subjects on neuropsychologic tests involving memory and verbal associative fluency. That is, normal subjects who had better neuropsychologic test performances had less metabolic change. That greater ability on cognitive testing is associated with a lower metabolic change from baseline is of particular interest and means that patients with lower cognitive abilities have greater increases in blood flow[8] or metabolism[15] during an activating cognitive task. This suggests that the degree of detectable change in metabolism or blood flow varies among subjects as a function of the baseline ability assessed by a particular activating task. Baseline performance may be an important covariate to use in cerebral activation studies.

Activation patterns may also change with repeated exposure to the same task. The hypothesis developed by Goldberg[10] on hemispheric involvement during exposure to a novel or unfamiliar task suggests that a hemispheric shift in activation from right to left should occur over the course of serial learning trials of an unfamiliar task. On the basis of the results described above, showing lower activation in people who are more facile on a given task, one might expect cerebral activation to decline as learning occurs and as task-specific facility develops over the course of learning trials. The presence or absence of changes in activation and task performance on certain types of cognitive tasks may provide information that is diagnostic of brain dysfunction, at least to the extent that normal variables can be established for any such changes in activation and task performance.

MAGNETIC RESONANCE IMAGING

A major form of operative morbidity after temporal lobectomy, particularly in the language-dominant hemisphere, is a reduction in memory, especially for verbally based information.[16–27] In about 65% of temporal lobectomy patients, mesial temporal sclerosis is the only neuropathologic finding.[28–30] In patients who had mesial temporal sclerosis and left temporal lobectomy, preoperative verbal memory is positively associated with the degree of cell loss in the left hippocampus.[31,32] After left temporal lobectomy in patients with left hemisphere dominance for language, memory change is also associated with the degree of hippocampal cell loss. Patients are at greater risk for impaired verbal memory if they have a relatively normal left hippocampus, as compared with patients who have a high degree of left hippocampal atrophy or cell loss.[22,33,34]

Appropriately conducted and interpreted MRI studies are sensitive to the presence of mesial temporal sclerosis.[35–41] The increased sensitivity to mesial temporal sclerosis has changed dramatically the evaluation of epilepsy surgery candidates. Lencz et al.[40] and Loring et al.[42] have demonstrated that preoperative verbal memory is associated with left hippocampal volume, as determined with MRI, in left temporal lobectomy patients with left hemisphere dominance for language and whose only detectable brain abnormality is mesial temporal sclerosis. Trenerry et al.[43] studied preoperatively and postoperatively the relationships between hippocampal volume as determined with MRI and memory in 36 patients who underwent right temporal lobectomy and 44 who underwent left temporal lobectomy. All these patients had left hemisphere dominance for language and did not have any structural lesion other than mesial temporal sclerosis. Left temporal lobectomy patients who had relative left hippocampal atrophy (as defined by the difference between the volumes of the right and left hippocampi) had improved delayed memory for paragraph-length information after lobectomy. Thus, left temporal lobectomy patients with a left hippocampus that is large relative to the right hippocampus tended to have poorer postoperative verbal memory. After left temporal lobectomy, delayed memory for geometric designs was also positively associated with a relatively small left hippocampus. Right temporal lobectomy patients experienced a decline postoperatively in learning geometric designs *but not in memory*, providing they had a relatively larger right hippocampus.

Trenerry et al.[44] recently investigated sex differences in verbal memory and hippocampal volumes before and after temporal lobectomy. This investigation was prompted by earlier research that demonstrated apparent sex differences in lateralization of verbal and visual perceptual abilities.[45–49] However, others reported conflicting data.[50–52] Geckler and colleagues[53] and McGlone[54] recently have reported that women have better verbal memory outcome than men after left temporal lobectomy.

Trenerry et al.[44] demonstrated that women who underwent left temporal lobectomy had better delayed verbal memory, defined by Logical Memory subtest delayed percent retention on the *Wechsler Memory Scale-Revised*, after left temporal lobectomy. Furthermore, in women in the left temporal lobectomy group, the relationship between delayed verbal memory and the volume of the left and right hippocampi was significant. This relationship was not found in men or in any of the patients in the right temporal lobectomy group. Right temporal lobectomy patients, both men and women, had improved verbal memory after lobectomy. Trenerry et al.[44] posited that their data reflected a sexually dimorphic plasticity of verbal memory that is dependent on the hippocampus. Specifically, Trenerry et al.[44] suggested that the verbal memory abilities measured in women may be more resilient in those with left hippocampal atrophy presumably associated with cerebral insult early in life[55] and, furthermore, because of the prepotency of the left hemisphere for language function, this resilience is not evoked in women who have a similar early insult to the right hemisphere.

Trenerry et al. (Trenerry MR, Jack CR Jr, Cascino GD, et al., unpublished data) studied the same group of patients included in the earlier study to investigate the relationship between visual memory and MRI-determined hippocampal volumes before and after temporal lobectomy. Visual memory was defined by delayed percent retention on the Visual Reproduction subtest of the *Wechsler Memory Scale-Revised*. The associations among preoperative visual memory and postoperative change in visual memory and right hippocampal volume in women in both the left and right temporal lobectomy groups were significant. For women in the right temporal lobectomy group, there was a strong positive relationship between preoperative visual memory and right hippocampal volume and an equally robust but negative relationship between postoperative visual memory change and right hippocampal volume. Thus, a large right hippocampus was associated with better preoperative visual memory, and extirpation of a large right hippocampus was associated with a decline in visual memory postoperatively—but only in women. For women in the left temporal lobectomy group, there was also a positive relationship between preoperative visual memory and right hippocampal volume. In these same women, the volume of the right hippocampus was positively associated with the degree of visual memory change after left temporal lobectomy.

It is unlikely that the extent of hippocampal resection was the cause of the effects described above. Two reports have indicated that the extent of hippocampal resection was not associated with memory change after left temporal lobectomy.[56,57] Also, Hermann et al.[34] demonstrated that the degree of left hippocampal neuronal loss, and not extent of hippocampal resection, was associated with verbal memory change after left temporal lobectomy.

MRI data about hippocampal volume have not been associated with cognitive abilities other than mem-ory in epilepsy surgery patients. Trenerry and Jack[58] found no relationship between MRI-determined hippocampal volume and executive function in temporal lobectomy patients evaluated with the *Wisconsin Card Sorting Test*. Furthermore, the difference between hippocampal volumes was not associated with confrontation naming performance in the same population.[59]

PREOPERATIVE NEUROCOGNITIVE AND MAGNETIC RESONANCE IMAGING VOLUMETRIC DATA: TOWARD A SYNTHESIS

Saykin and colleagues[60,61] studied the relationship between age of "first risk" for central nervous system insult and postoperative memory outcome in temporal lobectomy patients. Reports based on two groups of patients indicated that left temporal lobectomy patients whose first risk was at 5 years of age or younger had a better verbal memory outcome than those whose first risk factor occurred after 5 years of age. The authors included various factors in their definition of first risk: febrile convulsion, discovery of tumor or arteriovenous malformation, head injury, and age of onset of spontaneous seizures. The choice of the age of 5 years as a cutoff was based on the work of Lenneberg[62] on language development in children who had a left hemisphere insult. Krashen[63] elaborated on Lenneberg's research. Curtiss[64] critiqued the research of Lenneberg and Krashen and suggested that the hypothesis proposed by Lenneberg and Krashen may not reflect language *lateralization* as much as it does declining plasticity of brain function over time with regard to language development.

Chelune et al.[65] have proposed the hypothesis of "hippocampal functional adequacy" to guide interpretation of preoperative data with regard to predicting risk to postoperative memory function. Specifically, the data of these authors indicated that left temporal lobectomy patients with higher preoperative verbal memory scores are at greater risk for postoperative memory decline. This seems to be consistent with reports on the relationship between preoperative and postoperative verbal memory and left hippocampal cell loss: (1) better preoperative verbal memory is associated with less cell loss in the left hippocampus, and (2) extirpation of a large hippocampus with little or no cell loss is associated with a greater decline in verbal memory, whereas extirpation of a left hippocampus with marked cell loss is associated with relatively little postoperative change in verbal memory. These findings suggest that patients with better preoperative memory have greater "hippocampal functional adequacy" and, therefore, are at greater risk for impaired memory postoperatively. Hermann et al.[66] have cautioned that the association between higher preoperative memory scores and greater risk for postoperative memory decline is due partly to the statistical artifact of regression to the mean.

Kneebone et al.[67] used Wada's test to show that left lobectomy patients with good recall for material presented after amobarbital was injected into the left internal carotid artery were more likely to have a better verbal memory outcome postoperatively. Thus, patients with greater right hippocampal capacity have better verbal memory outcome. This finding is consistent with the predictive value of preoperative MRI volumetric data: A greater difference between hippocampal volumes in favor of the right hippocampus bodes well for postoperative verbal memory outcome in patients undergoing left temporal lobectomy. Also, Loring et al.[42] demonstrated that MRI hippocampal volume data are well correlated with lateral asymmetries in memory performance on Wada's test. Loring and others have also demonstrated that these same asymmetries detected with Wada's test predict verbal memory outcome after left temporal lobectomy[68] and predict seizure control outcome.[69,70] Although preoperative memory capacity seems to have some prognostic value for postoperative memory outcome, studies that predict postoperative memory outcome (1) from the results of Wada's test or MRI or (2) from the relationship between volumetric data and results of Wada's test suggest that the use of preoperative memory test data alone is insufficient for prediction of postoperative memory. Penfield and Mathieson[71] demonstrated that the status of the right hippocampus is critical for verbal memory outcome after left temporal lobectomy; this is supported by the correlation between hippocampal volume difference and verbal memory outcome.[43] Preoperative verbal memory testing alone evaluates efficiency of the memory system, but currently, it does not separate the functional status of each hippocampus.

Is a patient with a relatively large right hippocampus, a clearly atrophic left hippocampus, and intact verbal memory at risk for reduced verbal memory after left temporal lobectomy? Does the sex of the patient have any prognostic significance with regard to cognitive outcome after left temporal lobectomy? Data from patients described in a previous report[72] were analyzed to address these questions, and results of those analyses are reported elsewhere in more detail.[72] Both preoperative verbal memory and the difference in volume between the left and right hippocampi contribute significantly and independently to the statistical prediction of postoperative delayed verbal memory in men and women. Generally, left temporal lobectomy patients tend to have better postoperative verbal memory (1) the larger the volume of the right hippocampus compared with that of the left hippocampus, and (2) the greater the preoperative delayed verbal memory. Thus, high preoperative delayed verbal memory scores are not necessarily a risk factor for greater verbal memory decline after left temporal lobectomy if there is left hippocampal atrophy, as defined by the difference in volume between the left and right hippocampi. Sex does appear to be a marker for risk of ver-

bal memory decline in left temporal lobectomy patients. On the basis of data from 75 left temporal lobectomy patients, verbal memory change after left temporal lobectomy was defined as "good" if *Wechsler Memory Scale-Revised*[73] Logical Memory percent retention was higher postoperatively than preoperatively.[72] If the percent retention was lower postoperatively than preoperatively, memory outcome was defined as "poor." Verbal memory outcome was good in 30 of 42 women but in only 9 of 33 men. The χ^2 for this 2×2 table (outcome by sex) was 14.4 ($P < 0.0001$), with a phi coefficient of 0.44. This effect appeared to be due largely to a change in the delayed memory portion of the Logical Memory subtest. The preoperative and postoperative Logical Memory immediate recall trial means for men were, respectively, 21.5 (SD = 7.6) and 17.2 (SD = 8.8) (t(32) = -3.2; $P < 0.01$). The preoperative and postoperative Logical Memory immediate recall trial means for women were, respectively, 19.9 (SD = 7.0) and 17.9 (SD = 7.5) (t(41) = -1.98; $P > 0.05$). The preoperative and postoperative Logical Memory delayed recall trial performances for men were, respectively, 13.5 (SD = 7.2) and 9.1 (SD = 8.0) (t(32) = -3.5; $P < 0.01$). The preoperative and postoperative Logical Memory delayed recall trial performances for women were, respectively, 13.3 (SD = 7.6) and 13.5 (SD = 7.4) (t(41) = 0.17; $P > 0.8$). Thus, it appears possible to develop useful information about a patient's postoperative verbal memory by considering preoperative cognitive function, sex, and hippocampal volumes as determined with MRI.

SUMMARY AND COMMENT

Patient sex, preoperative memory function, and MRI characteristics affect the memory ability present after temporal lobectomy. Specifically, the difference between the volumes of the left and right hippocampi (subtracting right from left) is strongly associated with verbal memory after left temporal lobectomy in men and women. However, women tend to have better verbal memory outcome after left temporal lobectomy. The data suggest that the verbal memory abilities supported by the hippocampus in women are more plastic in the face of a developmentally early insult to the left mesial temporal cortex. Conversely, other data suggest that the visual memory abilities supported by the right hippocampus in women may be less robust in comparison with those of men.

Higher preoperative verbal memory scores are not necessarily a risk factor for verbal memory decline after left temporal lobectomy when higher preoperative verbal memory scores occur in the presence of left hippocampal atrophy, as seen on MRI, and a relatively large right hippocampus. Combining quantitative MRI data about hippocampal volumes with neurocognitive test data is clearly useful scientifically and clinically. The addition of data from other studies, such as asymmetries detected with

Wada's test, may increase our ability to determine risk to memory after temporal lobectomy. However, the findings reviewed in this chapter have limited support from studies attempting to replicate them. Other methods of evaluating memory should be compared with those reviewed here, as should other quantitative MRI methods such as T_2 relaxometry.[74] Various methods of memory testing may not be interchangeable, which may also be true of different MRI methodologies that may detect independent pathologic characteristics. The quantitative MRI data and neurocognitive data that have been combined have been obtained from temporal lobectomy patients who had no lesion other than medial temporal sclerosis, and these data may not be generalizable to temporal lobectomy patients with other types of abnormality.

The development of functional MRI may supplant Wada testing and alter the way in which neurocognitive studies are conducted in many patients with disease of the central nervous system, including epilepsy. A challenge to adapting functional MRI to this use will be determining the brain activation variables for certain models or conditions and certain patient characteristics, including sex, age, baseline task performance, and task mastery over trials.

REFERENCES

1. Jackson JH. On the nature of the duality of the brain. Medical Press Circular 1874;i:19, 41, 63. Reprinted in Taylor J, ed. Selected writings of John Hughlings Jackson, Vol 2. New York: Basic Books, 1958:129–30.

2. Novelly RA. The debt of neuropsychology to the epilepsies. Am Psychol 1992;47:1126–9.

3. Petersen SE, Fox PT, Posner MI, et al. Positron emission tomographic studies of the cortical anatomy of single-word processing. Nature 1988;331:585–9.

4. Petersen SE, Fox PT, Posner MI, et al. Positron emission tomographic studies of the processing of single words. J Cognitive Neurosci 1989;1:153–70.

5. Pardo JV, Pardo PJ, Janer KW, et al. The anterior cingulate cortex mediates processing selection in the Stroop attentional conflict paradigm. Proc Natl Acad Sci USA 1990;87:256–9.

6. Perret E. The left frontal lobe of man and the suppression of habitual responses in verbal categorical behaviour. Neuropsychologia 1974;12:323–30.

7. Janer KW, Pardo JV. Deficits in selective attention following bilateral anterior cingulotomy. J Cognitive Neurosci 1991;3:231–41.

8. Huettner MIS, Rosenthal BL, Hynd GW. Regional cerebral blood flow (rCBF) in normal readers: bilateral activation with narrative text. Arch Clin Neuropsychol 1989;4:71–8.

9. Mazoyer BM, Tzourio N, Frak V, et al. The cortical representation of speech. J Cognitive Neurosci 1993; 5:467–79.

10. Goldberg E. Associative agnosias and the functions of the left hemisphere. J Clin Exp Neuropsychol 1990;12:467–84.

11. Kosslyn SM, Alpert NM, Thompson WL, et al. Visual mental imagery activates topographically organized visual cortex: PET investigations. J Cognitive Neurosci 1993;5:263–87.

12. Roland PE, Gulayas B, Seitz RJ. Structures in the human brain participating in visual learning, tactile learning, and motor learning. In: Squire LR, Weinberger NM, Lynch G, et al., eds. Memory: organization and locus of change. New York: Oxford University Press, 1991:95–113.

13. Henry TR, Mazziotta JC, Engel J Jr. Interictal metabolic anatomy of mesial temporal lobe epilepsy. Arch Neurol 1993;50:582–9.

14. Rausch R, Henry TR, Ary CM, et al. Asymmetric interictal glucose hypometabolism and cognitive performance in epileptic patients. Arch Neurol 1994;51:139–44.

15. Parks RW, Crockett DJ, McGeer PL. Systems model of cortical organization: positron emission tomography and neuropsychological test performance. Arch Clin Neuropsychol 1989;4:335–49.

16. Meyer V, Yates AJ. Intellectual changes following temporal lobectomy for psychomotor epilepsy: preliminary communication. J Neurol Neurosurg Psychiatry 1955;18:44–52.

17. Cavazzuti V, Winston K, Baker R, et al. Psychological changes following surgery for tumors in the temporal lobe. J Neurosurg 1980;53:618–26.

18. Delaney RC, Rosen AJ, Mattson RH, et al. Memory function in focal epilepsy: a comparison of nonsurgical, unilateral temporal lobe and frontal lobe samples. Cortex 1980;16:103–17.

19. Novelly RA, Augustine EA, Mattson RH, et al. Selective memory improvement and impairment in temporal lobectomy for epilepsy. Ann Neurol 1984;15:64–7.

20. Ojemann GA, Dodrill CB. Verbal memory deficits after left temporal lobectomy for epilepsy. Mechanism and intraoperative prediction. J Neurosurg 1985;62:101–7.

21. Powell GE, Polkey CE, McMillan T. The new Maudsley series of temporal lobectomy. I: Short-term cognitive effects. Br J Clin Psychol 1985;24:109–24.

22. McMillan TM, Powell GE, Janota I, et al. Relationships between neuropathology and cognitive functioning in temporal lobectomy patients. J Neurol Neurosurg Psychiatry 1987;50:167–76.

23. Hermann BP, Wyler AR. Neuropsychological outcome of anterior temporal lobectomy. J Epilepsy 1988;1:35–45.

24. Ivnik RJ, Sharbrough FW, Laws ER Jr. Effects of anterior temporal lobectomy on cognitive function. J Clin Psychol 1987;43:128–37.

25. Ivnik RJ, Sharbrough FW, Laws ER Jr. Anterior temporal lobectomy for the control of partial complex

seizures: information for counseling patients. Mayo Clin Proc 1988;63;783–93.

26. Katz A, Awad IA, Kong AK, et al. Extent of resection in temporal lobectomy for epilepsy. II. Memory changes and neurologic complications. Epilepsia 1989;30:763–71.

27. Naugle RI, Chelune GJ, Cheek R, et al. Detection of changes in material-specific memory following temporal lobectomy using the Wechsler Memory Scale-Revised. Arch Clin Neuropsychol 1993;8:381–95.

28. Babb TL, Brown WJ. Neuronal, dendritic, and vascular profiles of human temporal lobe epilepsy correlated with cellular physiology *in vivo*. Adv Neurol 1986;44:949–66.

29. Babb TL, Brown WJ. Pathological findings in epilepsy. In: Engel J Jr, ed. Surgical treatment of the epilepsies. New York: Raven Press, 1987:520–4.

30. Mathieson G. Pathology of temporal lobe foci. Adv Neurol 1975;11:163–81.

31. Oxbury J, Oxbury S. Neuropsychology: memory and hippocampal pathology. In: Reynolds EH, Trimble MR, eds. The bridge between neurology and psychiatry. Edinburgh: Churchill Livingstone, 1989:136–50.

32. Sass KJ, Spencer DD, Kim JH, et al. Verbal memory impairment correlates with hippocampal pyramidal cell density. Neurology 1990;40:1694–7.

33. Sass KJ, Westerveld M, Buchanan CP, et al. Degree of hippocampal neuron loss determines severity of verbal memory decrease after left anteromesiotemporal lobectomy. Epilepsia 1994;35:1179–86.

34. Hermann BP, Wyler AR, Somes G, et al. Pathological status of the mesial temporal lobe predicts memory outcome from left anterior temporal lobectomy. Neurosurgery 1992;31:652–6.

35. Berkovic SF, Andermann F, Olivier A, et al. Hippocampal sclerosis in temporal lobe epilepsy demonstrated by magnetic resonance imaging. Ann Neurol 1991;29:175–82.

36. Cascino GD, Jack CR Jr., Parisi JE, et al. Magnetic resonance imaging-based volume studies in temporal lobe epilepsy: pathological correlations. Ann Neurol 1991;30:31–6.

37. Cook MJ, Fish DR, Shorvon SD, et al. Hippocampal volumetric and morphometric studies in frontal and temporal lobe epilepsy. Brain 1992;115:1001–15.

38. Jackson GD, Berkovic SF, Tress BM, et al. Hippocampal sclerosis can be reliably detected by magnetic resonance imaging. Neurology 1990;40:1869–75.

39. Kuzniecky R, de la Sayette V, Ethier R, et al. Magnetic resonance imaging in temporal lobe epilepsy: pathological correlations. Ann Neurol 1987;22:341–7.

40. Lencz T, McCarthy G, Bronen RA, et al. Quantitative magnetic resonance imaging in temporal lobe epilepsy: relationship to neuropathology and neuropsychological function. Ann Neurol 1992;31:629–37.

41. Watson C, Andermann F, Gloor P, et al. Anatomic basis of amygdaloid and hippocampal volume measurement by magnetic resonance imaging. Neurology 1992;42:1743–50.

42. Loring DW, Murro AM, Meador KJ, et al. Wada memory testing and hippocampal volume measurements in the evaluation for temporal lobectomy. Neurology 1993;43:1789–93.

43. Trenerry MR, Jack CR Jr, Ivnik RJ, et al. MRI hippocampal volumes and memory function before and after temporal lobectomy. Neurology 1993;43:1800–5.

44. Trenerry MR, Jack CR Jr, Cascino GD, et al. Gender differences in post-temporal lobectomy verbal memory and relationships between MRI hippocampal volumes and preoperative verbal memory. Epilepsy Res 1995;20:69–76.

45. McGlone J. Sex differences in functional brain asymmetry. Cortex 1978;14:122–8.

46. McGlone J. Sex differences in human brain asymmetry: a critical survey. Behav Brain Sci 1980;3:215–27.

47. Inglis J, Lawson JS. Sex differences in the effects of unilateral brain damage on intelligence. Science 1981;212:693–5.

48. Inglis J, Ruckman M, Lawson JS, et al. Sex differences in the cognitive effects of unilateral brain damage. Cortex 1982;18:257–75.

49. Kimura D. Sex differences in cerebral organization for speech and praxic functions. Can J Psychol 1983;37:19–35.

50. Bornstein RA. Unilateral lesions and the Wechsler Adult Intelligence Scale-Revised: no sex differences. J Consult Clin Psychol 1984;52:604–8.

51. Snow WG, Freedman L, Ford L. Lateralized brain damage, sex differences, and the Wechsler Intelligence Scales: a reexamination of the literature. J Clin Exp Neuropsychol 1986;8:179–89.

52. Snow WG, Weinstock J. Sex differences among non-brain-damaged adults on the Wechsler Adult Intelligence Scales: a review of the literature. J Clin Exp Neuropsychol 1990;12:873–86.

53. Geckler C, Chelune G, Trenerry M, et al. Gender related differences in cognitive status following temporal lobectomy (abstract). Arch Clin Neuropsychol 1993; 8:226–7.

54. McGlone J. Memory complaints before and after temporal lobectomy: do they predict memory performance or lesion laterality? Epilepsia 1994;35:529–39.

55. Trenerry MR, Jack CR Jr, Sharbrough FW, et al. Quantitative MRI hippocampal volumes: association with onset and duration of epilepsy, and febrile convulsions in temporal lobectomy patients. Epilepsy Res 1993;15:247–52.

56. Loring DW, Lee GP, Meador KJ, et al. Hippocampal contribution to verbal recent memory following dominant-hemisphere temporal lobectomy. J Clin Exp Neuropsychol 1991;13:575–86.

57. Wolf RL, Ivnik RJ, Hirschorn KA, et al. Neurocognitive efficiency following left temporal lobectomy: standard versus limited resection. J Neurosurg 1993;79:76–83.

58. Trenerry MR, Jack CR Jr. Wisconsin Card Sorting Test performance before and after temporal lobectomy. J Epilepsy 1994;7:313–7.

59. Trenerry MR, Cascino GD, Jack CR Jr., et al. Boston Naming Test performance after temporal lobectomy is not associated with lateral of cortical resection (abstract). Arch Clin Neuropsychol 1995;10:399.

60. Saykin AJ, Gur RC, Sussman NM, et al. Memory deficits before and after temporal lobectomy: effect of laterality and age of onset. Brain Cogn 1989;9:191–200.

61. Saykin AJ, Robinson LJ, Stafiniak P, et al. Neuropsychological changes after anterior temporal lobectomy: acute effects on memory, language, and music. In: Bennett TL, ed. The neuropsychology of epilepsy. New York: Plenum Press, 1992:263–90.

62. Lenneberg EH. Biological foundations of language. New York: John Wiley & Sons, 1967.

63. Krashen S. Lateralization, language learning, and the critical period: some new evidence. Language Learning 1973;23:263–74.

64. Curtiss S. The development of human cerebral lateralization. UCLA Forum in Medical Sciences no. 26, 1985: 97–116.

65. Chelune GJ, Naugle RI, Lüders H, et al. Prediction of cognitive change as a function of preoperative ability status among temporal lobectomy patients seen at 6-month follow-up. Neurology 1991;41:399–404.

66. Hermann BP, Wyler AR, VanderZwagg R, et al. Predictors of neuropsychological change following anterior temporal lobectomy: role of regression toward the mean. J Epilepsy 1991;4:139–48.

67. Kneebone AC, Chelune GJ, Dinner D, et al. Use of the intracarotid amobarbital procedure to predict material specific memory change following anterotemporal lobectomy (abstract). Epilepsia 1992;33 Suppl 3:87.

68. Loring DW, Meador KJ, Lee GP, et al. Wada memory asymmetries predict verbal memory decline after anterior temporal lobectomy. Neurology 1995; 45:1329–33.

69. Sperling MR, Saykin AJ, Glosser G, et al. Predictors of outcome after anterior temporal lobectomy: the intracarotid amobarbital test. Neurology 1994;44:2325–30.

70. Loring DW, Meador KJ, Lee GP, et al. Wada memory performance predicts seizure outcome following anterior temporal lobectomy. Neurology 1994;44:2322–4.

71. Penfield W, Mathieson G. Memory: autopsy findings and comments on the role of hippocampus in experiential recall. Arch Neurol 1974;31:145–54.

72. Trenerry MR, Westerveld M, Meador KJ. MRI hippocampal volume and neuropsychology in epilepsy surgery. Magn Reson Imaging 1995;13:1125–32.

73. Wechsler D. Wechsler Memory Scale-Revised Manual. San Antonio: Harcourt, Brace & Jovanovich, 1987.

74. Jackson GD, Connelly A, Duncan JS, et al. Detection of hippocampal pathology in intractable partial epilepsy: increased sensitivity with quantitative magnetic resonance T2 relaxometry. Neurology 1993;43:1793–9.

Index